ADOLESCENT PSYCHIATRY

DEVELOPMENTAL AND CLINICAL STUDIES

VOLUME 15

Annals of the American Society for Adolescent Psychiatry

ADOLESCENT PSYCHIATRY

DEVELOPMENTAL AND CLINICAL STUDIES

VOLUME 15

Edited by
SHERMAN C. FEINSTEIN
Editor in Chief

Senior Editors
AARON H. ESMAN
JOHN G. LOONEY
GEORGE H. ORVIN
JOHN L. SCHIMEL
ALLAN Z. SCHWARTZBERG
ARTHUR D. SOROSKY
MAX SUGAR

The University of Chicago Press
Chicago and London

The University of Chicago Press, Chicago 60637
The University of Chicago Press, Ltd., London

© 1988 by The University of Chicago
All rights reserved. Published 1988
Printed in the United States of America

International Standard Book Number: 0-226-24061-4
Library of Congress Catalog Card Number: 70-147017

The paper used in this publication meets the minimum requirements of American National Standard for Information Sciences—Permanence of Paper for Printed Library Materials, ANSI Z39.48-1984. ⊗ ™

CONTENTS

PART IV. PSYCHOTHERAPEUTIC ISSUES IN ADOLESCENT PSYCHIATRY

Special Section

IN MEMORIAM
SOL NICHTERN (1920–1988)

This volume is dedicated to the memory of Sol Nichtern, a Consulting Editor of this journal who was known internationally for his contributions to the field of child and adolescent psychiatry. He was a founding member of the American and International Societies for Adolescent Psychiatry and contributed to their growth and development.

Dr. Nichtern was born in New York City in 1920. His parents were active in bringing many people who were repressed in Eastern Europe to the United States and taking care of them until they were established. He received his medical degree from the University of Health Sciences, Chicago Medical School, and served as a captain in the U.S. Army Medical Corps in World War II. He was among the first medical personnel to enter some of the concentration camps in Germany to provide medical care to those who survived.

He became a pediatrician, and, after many years in private practice, he studied with Lauretta Bender to become a child psychiatrist. I met Dr. Nichtern in 1964 when he became Director of Training in Child and Adolescent Psychiatry at Hillside Hospital in Glen Oaks, New York. It was a great experience to be in training with him. He was an excellent clinician and had a wide range of experience and knowledge, which he shared in a creative and enthusiastic way. He also taught us to be caring physicians and often reminded us that our basic task was to relieve suffering and pain. I met his wife Edith around the same time. She was equally committed to child and adolescent welfare and had been quite active as head of the Child Development Center in New York. When they married in 1968, it was a union of two people rich in providing services to children in need. In 1970, Dr. Nichtern became Director of Psychiatric Services of the Jewish Child Care Association (JCCA). Under his leadership, the JCCA became a highly respected, clinically diversified center for children and adolescents with a variety of emotional problems. I had the pleasure of working with him again in various treatment facilities.

Throughout his career Dr. Nichtern published many important papers and books. Among his books I want to mention *Helping the Retarded Child,* in which he presented a new developmental approach to retardation, with honest, compassionate questions and answers about this field. Dr. Nichtern saw retardation as a developmental variation of the norm. Areas of marginal growth could be traced and methods could be found for modifying differences or turning deficiencies into potentials. It was this compassion and optimism that were so characteristic of Dr. Nichtern. He also started programs with experienced mothers to help disturbed children to be maintained in the regular school program and wrote a book about it. Among his papers he wrote "Has Psychiatry Failed the Acting-Out and Violent Adolescent," "The Missing Adolescent: The Pursuit of the Fantasy Family," and "Gandhi: His Adolescent Conflict of Mind and Body," all published in *Adolescent Psychiatry.* At the time of his death, Dr. Nichtern was working on another book, this time a novel about a young woman with psychological problems.

During the last fifteen years of his life, Dr. Nichtern suffered from Parkinson's disease, which did not adequately respond to medication. Even though in great pain, he creatively sought to understand the disease and find ways to break through the periods of stiffness and discomfort, using his pediatric neurologic experience.

In 1985, he retired from the JCCA because of ill health. He had to close his practice in 1987 but continued contact with many of his patients. In the last months of his life, he became discouraged by his continuous discomfort. On June 6, 1988, Dr. Nichtern and his wife died after a long creative life. They were survived by six children and nine grandchildren.

Dr. Nichtern was respected and honored with life fellowships in most of the professional societies and, as well, received special awards from outside his fields. In the last three years, he still participated as much as possible in the founding of the International Society for Adolescent Psychiatry. I am sure that I speak for all of us in saying that we will miss him not only for his brilliant clinical career but also as a very caring, committed, loyal friend.

ALBERT A. BUYTENDORP

PRESIDENT'S PREFACE

This opportunity to contribute a president's preface is particularly meaningful because it integrates for me two different ways in which I have been involved in the American Society for Adolescent Psychiatry (ASAP). First, there has been the opportunity of helping with the production of *Adolescent Psychiatry.* Over the years I have been on the editorial board and now serve as a senior editor. During this time I have watched the process of manuscripts being circulated for critical review. The final editorial work, of course, has been the responsibility of Sherman C. Feinstein, our editor in chief. I continue to be impressed with and appreciative of his tireless efforts to produce the *Annals,* the official publication of the ASAP.

I also have had the privilege of observing the activities of the ASAP through involvement in the work of constituent societies, committee work, and elected offices. The ASAP is an organization that is in a constant process of refinement and redefinition. However, one thing never changes. The purpose of the organization remains to advance the frontiers of knowledge about the treatment of adolescents. This advancement is achieved through increasing knowledge in three basic areas: normal developmental processes; psychopathological states; and evolving techniques of treatment. The ASAP will continue to advance the frontiers of knowledge about these issues, and *Adolescent Psychiatry* will serve as an instrument to provide our society the widest possible dissemination of this knowledge.

There are important changes both within and without our society. Within the ASAP, we are now in the process of effectively implementing many of the recommendations of our Task Force on Future Directions. For example, we have established a Permanent Program Committee. The establishment of this committee will allow the society more effective programming of the scientific programs of the regional meetings, institutes, and annual meetings. Another major internal change is the centralization of administrative duties in a Washington, D.C., office, under our new executive director, David Lewis. It is clear that, if the organization is to be maximally responsive, such an office location is important. Another major internal issue is a quest for increased membership. The ASAP strives for the membership of psychiatrists devoted to improving the quality of clinical care for adolescents. These psychiatrists come from many backgrounds, many types of practice, and many different types of training experiences. Another major internal change is a more focused attempt to define issues of quality training in adolescent psychiatry. Major efforts are being devoted to consideration of curriculum design both in general psychiatry and in child and adolescent psychiatry fellowship programs.

Many important external changes are taking place. The American Academy of Child Psychiatry has changed its name to the American Academy of Child and Adolescent Psychiatry. In addition to the name change, the academy is actively exploring what it can also do to increase the quality of clinical care for adolescents. Many complicated interface issues are developing between the ASAP and the academy. Your officers, and many key members of the society, are engaging in dialogue with the academy about ways in which this interface can be most productive. A major question remains unanswered. Who treats the adolescents in our nation? The ASAP is participating in a national survey with the American Psychiatric Association to clarify this important issue. The International Society for Adolescent Psychiatry is emerging as a strong organization; the next congress of this organization will be in Geneva during July 1988. The ASAP has been very active in facilitating the organization of the international society. Major organizations such as the Carnegie Corporation and the American Medical Association have begun initiatives in adolescent health issues.

The ASAP is a strong society, poised to be helpful to these organizations, and dedicated to furthering interest in the psychiatric treatment of adolescents.

JOHN G. LOONEY

PART I

ADOLESCENCE: GENERAL CONSIDERATIONS

EDITORS' INTRODUCTION

Recent attention has been focused on the preventive aspects of psychiatry, an examination of the demographics and epidemiology of emotional disorder in children and adolescents. In previous publications, Daniel Offer has presented data from his normal adolescent studies that illustrate the enormity of vulnerability for mental illness in adolescents. The Center for Preventive Psychiatry at the University of California, Los Angeles, confirms these statistics but also shows that many regularly accepted interventions are not effective. The dilemma thus presented demands further study of therapeutic methods as well as insights into the effects of stress and developmental delay. Of general consideration in this part is a series of chapters that enter into examination of some sources of adolescent psychiatric problems and the difficulties thereby engendered by premature approaches that are not based on careful scientific scrutiny.

Among classic examples of the struggles in medicine between bold advances versus a more careful research approach, Susan M. Fisher and Roberta J. Apfel describe the history of the use of diethylstilbestrol (DES) and its effects on the mother-daughter relationship, developing sexuality, and feminine identification. The authors document how DES undermines the bonds of experience between mother and daughter and adversely affects the emotional development of each by remaining as a viable threat to the lives of offspring, male and female. The resulting traumas are described as social and personal, external and internal, public and private, sudden and enduring. The resulting reaction is a posttraumatic emotional disorder manifesting a wide range of symptoms that the authors describe as tragic for the victims as well as the

3

physicians. Norman R. Bernstein discusses Drs. Fisher and Apfel's chapter and focuses on the identity problems young people struggle with as they feel the effect of "medical marketing."

Adrian D. Copeland provides an overview of the effects of childhood sexual trauma on female psychological development, especially trauma resulting from forced sexual involvement with an adult male. The difficulties with data collection concerning sexual trauma are discussed, but it appears that pedophilia constitutes the quantitatively greatest form of illegal sexual involvement of children, followed by exhibitionism, rape, and incest. Cultural considerations seem to vary, and the definition of illegal sexual behavior can change from culture to culture and within cultures. Psychological effects are complex, variable, and multifactorial: sexual activity with significantly older males is usually perceived negatively, the use of force is of major significance in producing trauma, and prior emotional status of the females all contribute to the effects of the sexual involvement. Copeland proposes that, in order to evaluate the effects of sexual traumatization, four parameters be explored: signs and symptoms of psychopathology, the patterns of relationships, self-concept formation, and level of function. He concludes that unanswered questions still inhibit effective preventive efforts.

Rhoda S. Frenkel uses the method of applied analysis to explore development of the ego-ideal—wish fulfillments that are conscious and unconscious resolutions of conflict. Her clinical material, however, is not from her couch but derives from one of the most popular television series, "Star Trek." Frenkel writes that Mr. Spock, the pointed-eared alien (Vulcan) of the starship Enterprise crew, epitomizes developmental adolescence. He represents two worlds (childhood and adulthood) and struggles to deidealize parental figures. Frenkel highlights other adolescent tasks and characteristics: friendships, sexuality, alienation, oedipal issues, and identity formation, among others. The author concludes that the alien tenets of the "Star Trek" series are appealing because they reflect the adolescent process of developing a cohesive sense of self—"having it all together."

1 FEMALE PSYCHOSEXUAL DEVELOPMENT: MOTHERS, DAUGHTERS, AND INNER ORGANS

SUSAN M. FISHER AND ROBERTA J. APFEL

Occasionally an event occurs that, by its impact, reveals previously unseen structural dimensions of complex phenomena. Such was the case with the use of diethylstilbestrol (DES), which was introduced initially to safeguard high-risk pregnancies and then rapidly expanded into vitamin additives or given directly for the perfecting of normal pregnancies. Through the lens of this greatest iatrogenic disaster of our century, using our psychoanalytic understanding, we can fathom some aspects of twentieth-century medicine—its relation to the research establishment, the doctor-patient relationship, the doctor-doctor network of relationships, and some recurrent themes in the history of medicine. This chapter will focus only on what the DES experience can uniquely reveal to us about the mother-daughter relationship and the developing sexuality and feminine identity of young girls.

Though DES has had an extraordinary range of consequences for the female offspring of the women who took it—including a hitherto unknown cancer in a small number of cases, congenital malformations in many others, and severe reproductive problems in a substantial proportion—for many others, numbering in the millions, there are no discernible physiological effects beyond adenosis. Nevertheless, the knowledge in both mothers and daughters that mother took DES sits like a ticking time bomb, as they wait through the physiological maturation of the daughters and watch their sexual and maternal devel-

5

opment to see whether anything happens. For these people—as surely as for those with demonstrable clinical, anatomic, and physiological problems—DES is disastrous even though its effects are only potential. In the real and potential devastation wrought by DES exposure, and in the defensive responses to it, there is an extraordinary opportunity to perceive dimensions and aspects of the female developmental process that might otherwise remain hidden or obscure.

But first let us briefly summarize some history. Diethylstilbestrol, a synthetic estrogen, was synthesized in 1938 in London and Oxford by Charles Dodds, who was later knighted for this achievement, and other academic scientists at the Courtauld Institute, their research sponsored by the British Medical Research Council (Dodds, Goldberg, Lawson, and Robinson 1938). British law required such products to be made available without patent. Diethylstilbestrol was more potent than natural estrogen, it was cheap to produce (from coal tars), and it could be administered pure in oral form. It was tested for numerous sex-related conditions in animals and had many clinical trials. It engendered enormous excitement—in three years 257 papers were written on its possible applications (Noller and Fish 1974). By 1939 it was being used to treat menopausal complaints, to induce menarche, to stimulate genital development, and to suppress lactation in a generation that favored bottle-fed babies for social rather than medical reasons. Its use for conditions ranging from hives to megalomania reflected the fascination with the new science of endocrinology. Like natural estrogen, DES increased cancers in appropriate strains of mice, but this was ignored. During World War II, DES use was extended to agriculture: pellets containing the compound were inserted inside the skin of chickens and lambs to promote their rapid growth. This was later outlawed but remains covertly operant nonetheless. In 1941 the U.S. Food and Drug Administration (FDA), after extensive review of the literature and the positive testimony of fifty out of fifty-four experts, approved the safety of DES. Until 1962 proof of efficacy was not required of a drug. Diethylstilbestrol was expressly licensed to treat vaginitis, gonorrhea, and menopausal complaints as well as to suppress lactation. However, once physicians are permitted to prescribe a drug, they use their judgment on what patients should receive it and for what. From 1941 until 1947, over six years, DES was used in a regime developed at Harvard by George and Olive Smith for pregnant women at high risk with histories of toxemia, diabetes, and repeated spontaneous abortions (Karnaky 1942; Smith and Smith 1946). Only in 1947 did the FDA approve its use for these problem pregnancies. In 1952 DES was declared safe, and its medical usage was made unrestricted.

But if DES was good for high-risk pregnancies, why not use it as a prophylactic drug to prevent spontaneous abortion in routine pregnancies? This switch from treatment to prevention was not a dramatic one, but it was part of an evolving medical and public perception of the role of medicine in modern society. The dizzy success of wonder-drug antibiotics and miracle cures of potentially fatal diseases made medicine shift to technology not only to treat disease but to improve the very quality of life.

The evidence of efficacy was poor. Seven studies from 1948 to 1954 claimed DES was effective for high-risk pregnancies.[1] These studies all lacked blind controls, though the technique had been available since 1948. However, other studies, then and later, showed that almost any treatment has a positive effect on high-risk pregnancies and that DES may have proved of no more value than placebos (Clifford 1964; Jacobson and Reid 1964; King 1953; Mann 1959). Several small studies in the 1950s, well done, controlled, and well placed in the literature, showed DES to be harmful in high-risk pregnancies, but these were ignored and were not used as a basis for larger-scale studies as one would have expected.

Altogether there were seven controlled studies between 1950 and 1955.[2] In 1952 Dieckmann at the University of Chicago, in the largest of these carefully designed controlled studies, showed DES to be ineffective in normal pregnancies (see Dieckmann, Davis, Rynkiewicz, and Pottinger 1953). Later evaluation in England of his data showed DES to be actually harmful (Brackbill and Berendes 1978).

Usage slowed but in spite of this research remained high until 1970, when a rare clear cell adenocarcinoma of the vagina appeared among eight females under twenty years of age.[3] The cancer was not only rare—it had previously been observed only in females over fifty. The link to DES was rapid, and in 1971 DES was banned by the FDA for use in preventing spontaneous abortion. During the years in which it was used routinely in pregnancy, at least 4–6 million mothers and their children had been exposed to DES.

It is worth remembering that there has always been in the history of medicine a conflict between the Promethean tradition leading to public pressure for cure and the Hippocratic tradition that advises

7

physicians to practice a restraint that avoids harm. From ancient times the tension has existed between the desire of the medical profession and the public for bold new advances and the conservative conviction that the art of medicine works best when it helps nature to take its course, a conviction embodied in the writings of Hippocrates: *primum non nocere* (first of all, do no harm). But the contemporary arena in which this ancient struggle is played out has some novel features. Primary among them is the unprecedented rate of medical advance in this century, with attendant leaps in the human stakes involved. Historically, certain ideas become established as proven or reasonable and lead to a medical policy that, one or more generations later, may be abandoned or reversed. Patients are no longer bled, cupped, or purged to remove impurities, as they were well into the nineteenth century. But children, for almost fifty years, routinely had their tonsils removed after tonsillitis, on the false belief that they would otherwise develop rheumatic fever or learning disabilities. Sustained critiques in the literature did nothing to alter this practice until the dramatic connection between tonsillectomy and polio was made in 1941 and 1942. So it was with DES and the cancer connection.[4]

Diethylstilbestrol has left its mark in other ways besides vaginal cancer. It produces in 90 percent of its daughters a benign (with eight exceptions) adenosis (the presence of columnar instead of squamous cell patches in the vaginal lining and on the cervix), cervical and uterine anatomical changes, increases in breast cancer in mothers who took DES and higher risk of squamous cell cervical carcinoma in exposed daughters, probably increased anatomical defects in DES sons' genital and urinary systems, and—the latest—an increase in malignant testicular cancers in DES sons. The rate of reproductive difficulties in DES daughters is 50–60 percent. There is also increasing suggestion of changes in the children in socialization patterns and some related psychiatric problems, possibly related to the fetal brain being bathed in so much female sex hormone.

From the beginning, a central problem with DES has been how to understand what happened. There were no heroes and villains. It engaged a wide range of specialists—biochemists, endocrinologists, pathologists, oncologists, epidemiologists, public health officials, sociologists, legal scholars, and physicians. The DES phenomenon needed to be analyzed and understood as a whole rather than divided into a dozen different specialist perspectives—a central concept was necessary. From interviewing and working with patients, we felt that it was within the framework of the concept of psychological trauma and the terms appropriate to it that the entire DES experience could be understood.

The word "trauma" comes from the Greek word for wound or external assault. Psychologically, trauma is an event or experience that is unexpected and undesired, an event that disrupts, temporarily or permanently, the sense of bodily or psychological integrity, producing a sense of deep personal vulnerability. A trauma is the stroke of the hammer that cracks the previously intact crystal and so reveals the hidden structure—to use Freud's splendid metaphor—and with DES the hidden structure of many aspects of medicine was illuminated.

The whole gamut of experiences associated with trauma has been seen in the aftermath of DES. The insults inflicted by it are social and personal, external and internal, public and private, sudden and enduring. Emotional responses ranging from total denial to mature reintegration can be seen among all those concerned: researchers, physicians, mothers, children, and the community at large.

The DES pill, however, produced trauma in unique ways. Diethylstilbestrol as a medication is related to sexuality and fertility, to the past and the future. It touches on issues at the heart of the mother-child relationship. In all grieving, the childlike parts of us return, and we seek, literally and spiritually, the care of our mothers or of those who represent basic maternal care. But one of the most disturbing features of the DES experience is its isolating nature because the usual sources of help are the very sources of pain. It is the providers of early tender care who have let down the DES daughters and sons—unwittingly. The mothers brought pain to their children; the physicians brought pain to their patients. The ultimate sources of help became the targets of all the feelings involved in mourning—denial, blame, self-accusation, rage, and sadness.

Despite its many complex effects, DES remains most powerfully connected with childbearing, which is both a profoundly private experience and a complex social event involving the extended family and the larger community. Childbirth taps a woman's deepest sense of her own body, intensifies her relationships with her loved ones, and, in addition, awakens fantasied communion with past figures who have been important to her. It involves the continuity of the generations, in her mind and in actuality. The trauma of the DES experience, then, follows from the violation of feelings and relationships that are intensely private and based on the most essential expectations of trust. The obstetrician, trained to deal with the simple, natural problems that can occur in pregnancy, hardly expects or is expected to be the source—however unwittingly—of disasters. The reproductive experience of the mother is obviously not intended to poison the reproductive capacity of her children. As gleaned from the DES exposed, the quality of the experience surrounding DES lies somewhere between a natural disaster and a bad dream in which safe relationships appear uncannily menacing. Diethylstilbestrol, an unnatural substance, touched the most natural process in an area of being that is usually intimate and untouchable. In pregnancy and birth, a woman's expectations of her doctor should be for trust and nurturance; yet childbirth arouses her earliest and most primitive fears. In the healthiest and happiest of persons and families, this combination of external and internal components of the DES trauma reawakened distressing and brutal fantasies and long-buried constellations of conflicts and concerns that had been solved quite satisfactorily in the course of development.

The Mother-Daughter Relationship

The mother-daughter relationship is intimate, powerful, and crucial to the daughter's emergence as a mature woman. It is fraught with possibilities for intense competition and greater hostility than obtains in cross-gender relations. Competition between father and son is more open, a socially accepted step in a boy's progression toward maturity. Women are socialized to subvert their aggressive feelings; thus the negative and hostile dimension of the relation between mother and daughter has fewer explicit outlets. This does not mean that relations between fathers and sons are easier, but it is easier for them to maintain distance between them, which permits a short-run solution to problems of rivalry and tension.

For both daughter and son, the mother is usually the first supportive and nurturing figure. This is not to say that the father cannot do the "mothering" if the mother is absent or otherwise unavailable or that his role as father is not crucial for daughters as well as for sons throughout their development, but the mother has traditionally been the primary object of attachment for both genders during the first year of life.[5] The son switches to his father for gender identification from his initial primary attachment to mother. The daughter switches to her father as love object but retains her gender identification with mother, who remains her model of what it is to be a woman. Her mother is her standard for relating to other people and for handling the whole range of human impulses and appetites. As the child's world expands, mother remains central for the daughter: she can have babies as mother does, and she wants Daddy as mother does. If all goes well in the relationship, if there is affection and tolerance between mother and daughter, the daughter will wait to become a mother—as her mother did—until she is grown up, and she will choose a man who shares her father's virtues.

The daughter will similarly model her experience of her body after her perception of her mother's experience. If mother is comfortable being a woman, comfortable with her sexuality, and happy in her expression of it, her daughter will probably feel comfortable with her own developing sense of her sexuality. If mother is tense and conflicted about being a woman and seductive with her daughter as a means of easing her own sexual tensions and conflicts, the daughter will have problems with femininity.

By eighteen months of age, girls and boys already have a sense of their own genitals. From then on, at every developmental stage there is a new integration of the body image. Studies have shown that, following actual physical injury or a traumatic loss of an important person, small children will experience severe anxiety that will be manifested as fears of bodily defectiveness and mutilation (Roiphe and Galenson 1982).

By adolescence, the genitals begin to be experienced as organs of relationship to other people as well as sources of private pleasure and future childbirth. The anticipated quality of those relationships for a daughter will have a great deal to do with what she senses are her mother's relationships and her mother's comfort and pleasure in sexuality. During the pubertal changes of menstruation, breast development, and altered body configuration, with the abrupt shifts in feelings and self-image they bring, the daughter's anxiety is reduced by her knowledge that mother went through it all and shares her experience. In ideal circumstances, the mother's presence through the course of these changes is a source of confidence and reassurance.[6]

Diethylstilbestrol undermines the bonds of experience between a mother and daughter and adversely affects the development of each. If the relationship between mother and daughter is good, efforts to

11

cope with the inevitable confusion and uncertainty arising from the mother's DES history may be successful, even though painful. But the everyday strains of adolescence on both mother and daughter, with their alternation between rebellion and closeness, their loneliness and separations, are inevitably increased in a DES family. The sense that, unlike her mother, the daughter might not be fertile and able to have children and that mother, however unwittingly, was the principal cause of the daughter's problems intensifies the rivalries, anger, and competitiveness the adolescent girl normally feels. And it confuses her. The mother, who is her natural ally and is needed for support, is also the source of her pain.

The mother's response may include terrible guilt, denial, and even paranoid rage. Such reactions tend to isolate her further from the daughter who needs her. Anything that interferes with a girl's ability to identify with her mother, before or during adolescence, paradoxically inhibits her ultimate ability to separate from mother. Identification is usually a flexible tool. When it works well, it permits the daughter to rebel, to make her own way, to move away from too much intimacy with mother, and to strike out on her own. For some adolescent girls, the fact of DES exposure makes the bond with mother tighter, which inhibits this gradual individuation.[7]

The prepubescent girl organizes a sense of her own femininity and sexuality out of fantasies and sensations, stories and chatter with her friends, and occasional actual explorations. There have been no systematic studies of the effect of knowledge of DES exposure on emerging feminine identity, but other medical conditions that require early and frequent examinations of the genitalia are known to make the pubertal girl unusually self-conscious and confused about those areas, which are supposed to be sources of pleasure but instead yield discomfort and pain. The regular pelvic examination itself sets the adolescent DES girl apart from other girls, who do not have such examinations until much later and have them less frequently. They are repeated reminders that something may not be normal. The experience of younger children and adolescents can be expected to differ from that of adult women, whose sexual identity had been formed before they learned about their DES exposure. For an adult woman, information about her exposure to DES is new and distressing material to be integrated into her already established sense of her womanhood; for a girl, the information becomes part of the very experience of becoming a woman.

The saddest thing about the DES experience for young daughters is that it robs their adolescence of some of its magic. Probably no one has a smooth passage through adolescence. Adolescents mourn for their about-to-be-lost childhood, and most do so with some turmoil. Adolescence is a time when the self becomes strengthened and defined through experimentation with the boundaries of experience, both in reality and in fantasy. It is the sense of limitlessness and omnipotence in the face of reality and separations from home that gives the adolescent years their sense of new horizons. Diethylstilbestrol disrupts the natural developmental process with a too brutal reality too soon. It forces the daughters to consider issues of real death and real damage. The DES adolescent and her mother may have to mourn for the daughter's future loss in adulthood as well. There may be a premature closure on identity formation. Too many serious decisions must be made in response to DES at a time when youth and play should still contain a sense of infinite possibility:

A twelve-year-old DES daughter nearing puberty anticipated her first examination with great dread. One day an elastic band on her ballet slipper broke, and, with uncharacteristic fury and tears, the girl yelled at her mother for "not letting me be a ballet dancer." As she sobbed, she told of the fantasy she had developed on the way to dance class. She would be such a beautiful ballerina in Class II that she would be rapidly accelerated to Class V and asked to solo in the *Nutcracker*. Being a prima ballerina had become an especially powerful compensatory daydream since she had learned about DES and had been anticipating a visit to the gynecologist. The broken elastic snapped her back to reality, where she was a good, but novice, ballet student. "I need to be a ballerina if I can't be a mommy."

For some daughters fears related to DES expand into preoccupying fears of cancer or a relentless focusing on bodily deficiencies and paralyzing fantasies about what is going on inside them. Such women will require additional expert help to put their concerns in perspective:

An attractive, poised, well-to-do college student came for treatment because of anxieties about her schoolwork. The academic concerns quickly turned out to mask depression, drug use, trouble

13

having orgasms, poor self-esteem, and fears about social and personal intimacy. Her sophisticated physical presentation disguised massive confusion about her body's functions, disgust at the appearance of her genitals, and poor self-care—alcohol and cocaine use, poor nutrition, and excessive use of douches and perfumed genital sprays.

All these concerns were the subject of her psychotherapy. When she consciously acknowledged, perhaps in response to the treatment, that she was a DES daughter, all her self-hate and self-revulsion crystallized around her identity as a DES-flawed individual. Her fantasies and fears of genital damage, which were being discovered, explored, and understood in the therapy as deriving from guilt and shame over her ambivalent identification with her mother and her eroticized, guilt-ridden relationship to her father, now became anatomic reality to her, on the basis of this one fact of personal history.

Painstaking work was done concerning the actualities of her DES history, the condition of her genitals, the difference between the harm her mother had actually caused and the harm she fantasized, whether she was adequate to attract a man of her own, and whether she could separate from the parents she considered responsible for her condition. Eventually, all the development she required was achieved in therapy—but always through the lens of DES.

Other DES daughters have experienced life-threatening illness and responded with courageous resourcefulness:

> A young woman of eighteen, a physician's daughter attending a liberal arts college, developed vaginal cancer. She had radical surgery to remove her ovaries, uterus, and vagina and subsequent plastic surgery to create an artificial vagina. She was able to use warm, close friendships, her family and physicians, and her own unconflicted intellect to support herself emotionally through this crisis. She became interested in a career in medicine for herself during her own recuperation. At age twenty-five, she decided to go to medical school.

These two cases present an interesting contrast. In the first, the mere revelation of DES exposure despite minimal physical pathology could have stalemated the emotional development of this ordinarily neurotic woman had she not been in psychotherapy. The second woman was not a therapy patient, nor did she need psychotherapy for any underlying difficulties. She was able to transcend the massive disappointments she suffered and use her crisis in the service of her new career.

These cases are unusual because they represent so graphically the two poles of relatively severe maladaption and extraordinary courage, resilience, and sublimation. More often the response in a healthy woman is mixed. Very often the DES daughter will not experience anger at her mother for taking the drug. She will fully appreciate that her mother's intentions were absolutely the best, and a good relationship between them will help them through the period of uncertainty about DES changes and questions of future fertility.

In other daughters, anger toward the mother about DES will unite with an underlying and barely controlled rage against her that has characterized the daughter's feelings from earliest childhood. This anger will appear as extreme pathology:

A talented seventeen-year-old musician entered a music conservatory. Her history revealed her to be an anxious, dependent young woman who had a difficult time separating from a difficult and restricting mother. When she learned during her first pelvic exam at the college health service of her probable DES exposure, she became unable to practice, attend classes, or think of anything besides her defective body. She went home and saw her mother's obstetrician-gynecologist, who confirmed the diagnosis of adenosis. She dropped out of school and, with her mother's support, made the rounds of numerous gynecologists in her vicinity until she found one whom she convinced to do a prophylactic hysterectomy at age twenty-one.

Her concerns about her genitals had achieved delusional proportions, and she continued to have symptoms in her vagina. This led to frequent gynecological visits for biopsies, laser-beam treatments, and cautery.

At this point she was referred for psychiatric consultation. She proclaimed that her mother, by taking DES, had poisoned her body and that she would stop at nothing to remove all consequences of the poisoning. Immediate psychiatric hospitalization occurred.

Even without DES this woman probably would have become deeply upset, even psychotic, on leaving home and would have been forced to return to the mother she hated and needed. Perhaps she would ultimately have required hospitalization in any case. Though her delusion formed around the seed of DES exposure, it could have achieved such magnitude only in a fragile personality.

A studious, religious, middle-class fourteen-year-old required medical hospitalization for her self-induced starvation. She had rapidly lost thirty pounds, become amenorrheic, and lost all her female body contours.

She was initially polite but cool to the consulting psychiatrist. Eventually she revealed that her obsessions about food centered around long-term struggles with her mother. These struggles had escalated in the past few years around her dating and emerging sexuality. She learned about her DES exposure when her mother, aware of her own exposure to DES, insisted that the girl have a gynecological exam. The daughter thought the mother was intruding on her and looking for evidence of petting and masturbation.

When the gynecologist confirmed adenosis and explained its origins to this young girl, she became quietly enraged at her mother and determined that she would get revenge by starving herself. Prolonged psychiatric treatment was useful in allowing this girl to develop comfortable acceptance of her sexuality and achieve age-appropriate distance from her mother.

This case illustrates how learning of DES exposure can traumatically unleash massive bodily anxieties in psychologically vulnerable individuals who might otherwise have managed at least marginal adjustment had there been no physical correlate of their worst fantasies.

Sexuality and Identification

Women's capacity to create life gives rise to fantasies about their fecundity and power. Every culture has myths of the *magna mater* and female seasonal symbols of fertility.[8] In the twentieth century, however, mothers have been singled out for their power to harm. They have, at various times, been deemed totally responsible for childhood schizophrenia and accused of causing all developmental problems of infancy, either through rejection or through overindulgence. The pendulum has swung back in recent years, but the milieu into which DES was introduced was one in which mothers were particularly aware of their power to do damage to their children. Child-care manuals during the post–World War II baby boom were concerned with the psychological and physical vulnerability of children. Historian Nancy Weiss (1977) has written an interesting comparison of these manuals with the turn of the century "infant care" manuals produced by the U.S. Children's Bureau. All these were filled with practical advice, but the tone of the earlier government pamphlets was more matter of fact and solicitous of the mother.

The sense of potential destructiveness is, of course, implicit in every relationship of caring: if I can help, then I can withdraw my help and thus hurt. What I can give I can take away. Certainly, all mothers are conscious of the helplessness of their infants and their power over them. No normal mother wants to do harm in reality, and for the mother who learns that out of love and a desire to give birth she may have caused harm there is terrible pain.

Fears about sexuality are tied in with the particular emotional charge the DES experience has for everyone involved, whether she is the innocent victim or the unwitting vehicle or perpetrator of what she feels to be destructive forces. The fact that the genitals are the target of the DES hormone has provoked some unusual responses that point to deeper aspects of the DES trauma, concerning DES sons as well as daughters.

The initial reports of DES-associated damage focused on female offspring (Herbst, Ulfelder, and Poskanzer 1971). It was five years before any follow-up study of DES-related effects on exposed males was reported (Bibbo, Al-Naqeeb, Baccarini, Gill, Newton, Sleeper, Sonek, and Wied 1975), and clinical follow-up of DES sons is still less thorough and more controversial than that of daughters.[9] One wonders why workers in this field did not consider male genital damage sooner and whether the seeming absence of concern had to do with the difficulty both researchers and victims had in acknowledging potential genital damage in males.

Our culture is more familiar with castration fear in males than in females. We believe that the DES experience has shed some light on female concerns. The concept of "castration anxiety" is technically based on Freudian oedipal theory, which focuses on fears in the boy aged four to six about penile castration by the father as punishment for the boy's sexual wishes toward the mother (Freud 1923, 1924, 1925, 1931). Castration anxiety is often generalized to refer to all anxiety about the loss of body intactness in males and females of any age. Since in the male body genitals are exposed, the castration fears of males tend to focus concretely on the loss of the penis.

Both men and women, however, tend to underestimate the impact of genital damage on women, as if—as Freud thought—they see women as already castrated. This leads to an inflation of the impact genital damage would have on males and a corresponding minimizing of the potential impact of such damage on women (Horney 1933). The frequency with which unnecessary hysterectomies have been performed on premenopausal women—as documented by the National Institutes of Health—relates to this point.[10] It seems to us that, in spite of our increasingly sophisticated understanding of female sexual development, our culture retains the view that intact male genitals are more to be prized and can be devastated more easily than female genitals and that the penis is valued for its symbolic significance even more than for its anatomic function. Both men and women participate in developing and maintaining this value system. As a result, both men and women tend to exhibit greater anxiety in the face of potential danger to the penis because it is both more valued and more visible; thus there is also a greater tendency toward denial.

Women's relative ability to face and adjust to genital harm may reflect the fact that women are more accustomed to attending to bodily changes. Each month they anticipate and experience menses and with it the expectation of menopause. All through life women have, in addition, at least some subliminal awareness of childbirth, with its temporary changes in contour and physiology. Males, by contrast, lack such experiences and are socialized from earliest childhood to idealize bodily integrity.

Recent psychoanalytic work throws a different light on the developmental value of the genitals. In people with anomalous sexual organs, the most valued organ is the one they are supposed to have, not necessarily the penis. Females born without a vagina yearn for a vagina and value that above all.[11]

Female castration anxiety then is not generally recognized. We refer here not to women's anxiety about having somehow been castrated or to the anxiety that males and females share about the general loss of body intactness but to specific apprehensions about losing the female genitalia. When asked by an interviewer about fears that they had never expressed spontaneously, and when talking with trusted therapists, many young women exposed to DES said that their primary fear was of losing their vaginas (Belsky 1978). It was found that the fear of organ loss was even more prominent than the potential loss of fertility. Everyone is most afraid of losing what he or she already has.

It may be that the male physicians' tendency grossly to underestimate the trauma that even the idea of losing a female organ has for women is a means of mastering their own castration anxieties. This may well be related to the period in the early 1970s when partial vaginectomy, the removal of the inner third of the vagina, was briefly recommended as the treatment for DES daughters at risk for vaginal adenocarcinoma (Sherman, Goldrath, Berlin, Vakhariya, Banooni, Michaels, Goodman, and Brown 1974). Fortunately, these "prophylactic" vaginectomies were performed on only a relatively few DES daughters who showed early adenosis. But other treatments used on DES daughters—cautery, laser, excision, "weeding," conization, all shown to be unnecessary and replaced by clinical observation and waiting—may connect with a need to deny castration fears.

Such treatments also relate, however, to an attribution throughout history of illness to the unseen and unknown and with attempts to solve a problem by eliminating such mysterious influences. Special power and mystery have been ascribed since ancient times to the organs of reproduction, particularly female organs, hidden from view and for a long time poorly understood.[12]

Remember that the ovaries were seen as the basis of neurosis for a time in the nineteenth century and that their removal was a recommended treatment for mental illness. Even in the early twentieth century, castration of males and removal of the ovaries were experimental treatments for psychosis. Charcot and his colleagues used ovarian compresses for the treatment of hysteria until the mid-nineteenth century, and clitoridectomy was practiced as late as the 1920s in the United States as a treatment for compulsive masturbation and for orgasmic dysfunction. Astonishingly, in 1981 DES was prescribed to control masturbation in mentally retarded boys.[13]

Diethylstilbestrol was developed and became popular because of the universal human wish to control the mysteries of our own sexuality and mortality. It was one treatment that seemed within the control of the individual doctor-patient pair; yet it simultaneously connected the doc-

19

tor to the frontiers of endocrinological research. No one imagined just how powerful the drug was or how extensively it would be used. It was prescribed to make nature better, especially to assist in the scientific conquest of aging and mortality, to create control of reproduction and sexuality. Mortality and sexuality are two central areas of human concern. The fantasies and expectations around DES touched the core of both. It was a unique wonder drug in that it promised to prevent mishap, not merely to cure illness. It may have been among the first modern medical substances that seemed likely to improve on nature and to prevent natural defects and unwanted outcomes from occurring in the first place. It became a means by which life itself could be mastered. It could help create life and then maintain youth and inhibit aging. It promised to be an elixir of youth, the goal of an eternal human search.

Conclusions

The story of DES, for all its modernity, bears as well many of the marks of classical tragedy. Everyone acted in good faith, with the best of intentions, and within the established norms of medical procedures of the day. Thus the consequences seem unavoidable. What we can learn from the story is not who to blame or what technical procedure we can employ to avoid the errors of our predecessors but that we are subject to the same stresses and temptations as the actors in the DES tragedy. The story is a sad one, but it need not be futile if we can learn from it. In the words of Aeschylus, "From suffering comes wisdom," not only about what it means to be human but, in this case, about what it means to be female.

NOTES

Portions of this chapter have been adapted from R. J. Apfel and S. M. Fisher, *To Do No Harm: DES and the Dilemmas of Modern Medicine* (New Haven, Conn.: Yale University Press, 1984).

1. The seven papers were Davis and Fugo (1950), Gitman and Koplowitz (1950), Pena (1954), Plate (1954), Ross (1953), Smith and Smith (1954), and White, Koshy, and Duckers (1953). The last group studied diabetes.

2. The seven controlled trials were Crowder, Bills, and Broadbent (1950), Dieckmann, Davis, Rynkiewicz, and Pottinger (1953), Ferguson

(1953), Randall, Beatz, Hall, and Birtch (1955), Reid (1955), Robinson and Shettles (1952), and Swyer and Law (1954).

3. In that year three reports of cases in young females appeared in the scientific literature: Droegemuller, Makowski, and Taylor (1970), Herbst, Green, and Ulfelder (1970), and Herbst and Scully (1970).

4. From 1939 through the early 1950s numerous articles appeared in the medical literature linking tonsillectomy and poliomyelitis, especially of the bulbar type (see, e.g., Aycock 1942; Krill and Toomey 1941; and Pederson 1947). Francis, Krill, Toomey, and Mack (1942) highlighted this dangerous association in their report of the experience of the "K" family of Akron, Ohio. Of the six children in the family, five were tonsillectomized on August 22. By September 7 all five had bulbar poliomyelitis; three of the children later died of this disease. The one child who was not operated on showed no sign of illness, although the polio virus was recovered from his stool.

5. Thoughtful commentaries on the primary maternal relationship can be found in Bibring, Dwyer, Huntington, and Valenstein (1961), Chodorow (1978), Cohler and Grunebaum (1981), Ehrensaft (1980), Friday (1977), Friedl (1975), Hammer (1975), and Newton (1973).

6. Comprehensive discussions of female adolescent development can be found in Kirkpatrick (1980), Nadelson and Notman (1982), Notman and Nadelson (1978), and Sugar (1979).

7. Exposure to DES, like other physical problems, can disrupt optimal growth and development. There is a growing body of literature in adolescent psychiatry on the problems of serious illness and its effects on adolescence (see Schowalter 1977, 1983a, 1983b).

8. Universal fantasies about the power of women are discussed in Lederer (1968) and Lerner (1974). For presentations of mythic forms and symbolism, see Neumann (1963) and Weigert (1970).

9. Fewer studies have been conducted of DES male offspring than of female, there are fewer investigators, and there have been less cooperation and follow-up involving males. For reports of work on DES sons, see Bibbo, Gill, Azizi, Blough, Fang, Rosenfeld, Schumacher, Sleeper, Sonek, and Wied (1977), Conley, Sant, Ucci, and Mitcheson (1983), Cosgrove, Benton, and Henderson (1977), Driscoll and Taylor (1980), Gill, Schumacher, and Bibbo (1976), Gill, Schumacher, Bibbo, Strauss, and Schoenberg (1979), Henderson, Benton, Cosgrove, Baptista, Aldrich, Townsend, Hart, and Mack (1976), Hoefnagel (1976), and Mills and Bongiovanni (1978).

10. Hysterectomy statistics have been compiled by the Centers for Disease Control and are summarized in a report on premenopausal U.S. women aged fifteen to forty-four (U.S. Department of Health and Human Services 1981).

11. There are individuals who are genetically male but appear to be anatomically female at birth; they are reared as females and have their femininity affirmed by appropriate parental attitudes and behavior. When such people reach adolescence and are discovered to have ambiguous genitals and to lack a normal vagina and uterus, they wish for a vagina and a uterus, not for the male organs that may also be present in rudimentary form. With the exception of rare cases of hermaphroditism, involving a sexual hormone enzyme defect in genetic males that allows for prenatal androgen priming of the developing brain tissue but causes anatomic female genitals, the people studied want the organs that go with their assigned gender. This assumes normal parenting and does not apply to transsexuals who are clearly physiologically male or female but nevertheless desire to have the organs of the opposite anatomic gender (see Money and Ehrhardt 1972a, 1972b; Money, Hampson, and Hampson 1957; and Stoller 1979).

12. Veith (1965) traces the history of hysteria from ancient Egypt to Charcot and twentieth-century psychoanalysis. Simon (1978) relates the wandering uterus concept to interpersonal relations in ancient Greece.

13. Bassuk (1983) discusses ovarian surgery as a widespread treatment of insanity in the late nineteenth century. References from that time document the conviction that castration was a valuable treatment for mental illness (see Barnes [1890], Clark [1888], and Wells, Hegar, and Battey [1886] and also Tyrone [1952], a review of late nineteenth-century gynecologic practice). Although Freud (1911) discussed Schreber's paranoia about castration as if it were completely delusional, the use of sadistic restraining devices in Schreber's childhood has been documented by psychoanalyst William Niederland (1974). Schreber's doctor, Flechsig, had promoted castration as a treatment for insanity. Spitz (1952) describes clitoridectomy as a treatment for masturbation. A journal was published on the subject from 1892 until 1923. The *Washington Post* carried an article about the current use of DES to inhibit masturbation in the mentally retarded ("University of Maryland Doctor Gives DES to Retarded Youths" 1981). Celia Bertin, in her

1982 biography of Marie Bonaparte, describes a procedure for operating on the external female genitals to enable orgasmic pleasure. Genital-mutilative surgery is still practiced on women throughout the world for complex reasons beyond this discussion (see Thiam 1983). Nonpathological conditions in women continue to be made into medical problems (see Love, Gelman, and Silen 1982).

REFERENCES

Aycock, W. L. 1942. Tonsillectomy and poliomyelitis. *Medicine* 21:65–94.

Barnes, R. 1890. On the correlations of sexual functions and mental disorders of women. *British Journal of Gynecology* 6:390–430.

Bassuk, E. L. 1983. "Normal" ovariotomy, 1872–1893: sadism or humanitarian health care. Paper presented to the Bunting Institute, Radcliffe College, Cambridge, Massachusetts, March 8.

Belsky, D. E. 1978. DES daughters: adaptation to bodily uncertainty. Unpublished manuscript. Northampton, Mass.: Smith College, School of Social Work.

Bertin, C. 1982. *Marie Bonaparte: A Life*. New York: Harcourt Brace Jovanovich.

Bibbo, M.; Al-Naqeeb, M.; Baccarini, I.; Gill, W.; Newton, M.; Sleeper, K. M.; Sonek, M.; and Wied, G. L. 1975. Follow-up study of male and female offspring of DES-treated mothers: a preliminary report. *Journal of Reproductive Medicine* 15:29–32.

Bibbo, M.; Gill, W. B.; Azizi, F.; Blough, R.; Fang, V. S.; Rosenfeld, R. L.; Schumacher, G. F. B.; Sleeper, K.; Sonek, M. G.; and Wied, G. L. 1977. Follow-up study of male and female offspring of DES-exposed mothers. *Journal of Obstetrics and Gynecology* 49:1–8.

Bibring, G.; Dwyer, T.; Huntington, D.; and Valenstein, A. F. 1961. A study of the earliest mother-child relationship. *Psychoanalytic Study of the Child* 16:9–72.

Brackbill, Y., and Berendes, H. W. 1978. Dangers of diethylstilbestrol: review of a 1953 paper. *Lancet* 2:520.

Chodorow, N. 1978. *The Reproduction of Mothering*. Berkeley and Los Angeles: University of California Press.

Clark, A. C. 1888. Relations of the sexual and reproductive functions to insanity. *American Journal of Insanity* 45:292–297.

Clifford, S. H. 1964. High risk pregnancy: prevention of prematurity, the *sine qua non* for reduction of mental retardation and other neurologic disorders. *New England Journal of Medicine* 271:243–249.

Cohler, B. J., and Grunebaum, H. U. 1981. *Mothers, Grandmothers and Daughters*. New York: Wiley.

Conley, G. R.; Sant, G. R.; Ucci, A. A.; and Mitcheson, H. D. 1983. Seminoma and epididymal cysts in a young man with known diethylstilbestrol exposure in utero. *Journal of the American Medical Association* 249:1325–1326.

Cosgrove, M. D.; Benton, B.; and Henderson, B. E. 1977. Male genitourinary abnormalities and maternal diethylstilbestrol. *Journal of Urology* 117:220–222.

Crowder, R. E.; Bills, E. S.; and Broadbent, J. S. 1950. The management of threatened abortion: a study of 100 cases. *American Journal of Obstetrics and Gynecology* 60:896–899.

Davis, M. E., and Fugo, N. W. 1950. Steroids in the treatment of early pregnancy complications. *Journal of the American Medical Association* 142:778–785.

Dieckmann, W. J.; Davis, M. E.; Rynkiewicz, L. M.; and Pottinger, R. E. 1953. Does the administration of diethylstilbestrol during pregnancy have therapeutic value? *American Journal of Obstetrics and Gynecology* 66:1062–1081.

Dodds, E. C.; Goldberg, L.; Lawson, W.; and Robinson, R. 1938. Oestrogenic activity of certain synthetic compounds [letter to editor]. *Nature* 141:247–248.

Driscoll, S. G., and Taylor, S. H. 1980. Effects of prenatal maternal estrogen on the male urogenital system. *Journal of Obstetrics and Gynecology* 56:47–50.

Droegemuller, W.; Makowski, E. L.; and Taylor, E. S. 1970. Vaginal masonephric adenocarcinoma in two prepubertal children. *American Journal of Diseases of Children* 119:168–170.

Ehrensaft, D. 1980. When women and men mother. *Socialist Review* 10:37–74.

Ferguson, J. H. 1953. Effects of stilbestrol on pregnancy compared to the effect of a placebo. *American Journal of Obstetrics and Gynecology* 65:592–601.

Francis, T., Jr.; Krill, C. E.; Toomey, J. A.; and Mack, W. N. 1942. Tonsillectomy in five members of a family. *Journal of the American Medical Association* 119:1392–1396.

Freud, S. 1911. Psychoanalytic notes on an autobiographical account of a case of paranoia (dementia paranoides). *Standard Edition* 12:3–82. London: Hogarth, 1958.

Freud, S. 1923. The ego and the id. *Standard Edition* 19:28–39. London: Hogarth, 1961.

Freud, S. 1924. The dissolution of the Oedipus complex. *Standard Edition* 19:171–179. London: Hogarth, 1961.

Freud, S. 1925. Some physical consequences of the anatomical distinction between the sexes. *Standard Edition* 19:248–258. London: Hogarth, 1961.

Freud, S. 1931. Female sexuality. *Standard Edition* 21:225–243. London: Hogarth, 1961.

Friday, N. 1977. *My Mother Myself: The Daughter's Search for Identity*. New York: Dell.

Friedl, E. 1975. *Women and Men: An Anthropologist's View*. New York: Holt, Rinehart & Winston.

Gill, W. B.; Schumacher, G. F. B.; and Bibbo, M. 1976. Structural and functional abnormalities in the sex organs of male offspring of mothers treated with diethylstilbestrol (DES). *Journal of Reproductive Medicine* 16:147–153.

Gill, W. B.; Schumacher, G. F. B.; Bibbo, M.; Strauss, F. H.; and Schoenberg, H. W. 1979. Association of diethylstilbestrol exposure in utero with cryptorchidism, testicular hypoplasia and semen abnormalities. *Journal of Urology* 122:36–39.

Gitman, L., and Koplowitz, A. 1950. Use of diethylstilbestrol in complications of pregnancy. *New York State Journal of Medicine* 50:2823–2824.

Hammer, S. 1975. *Daughters and Mothers, Mothers and Daughters*. New York: Quadrangle.

Henderson, B. E.; Benton, B.; Cosgrove, M.; Baptista, M. A.; Aldrich, J.; Townsend, D.; Hart, W.; and Mack, T. 1976. Urogenital tract abnormalities in sons of women treated with diethylstilbestrol. *Pediatrics* 58:505–507.

Herbst, A. L.; Green, T. H., Jr.; and Ulfelder, H. 1970. Primary carcinoma of the vagina. *American Journal of Obstetrics and Gynecology* 106:210–218.

Herbst, A. L., and Scully, R. E. 1970. Adenocarcinoma of the vagina in adolescence: a report of 7 cases including 6 clear-cell carcinoma (so-called mesonephromas). *Cancer* 25:745–757.

Herbst, A. L.; Ulfelder, H.; and Poskanzer, D. C. 1971. Adenocarcinoma of the vagina: association of maternal stilbestrol therapy with tumor appearance in young women. *New England Journal of Medicine* 284:878–881.

Hoefnagel, R. 1976. Prenatal diethylstilbestrol exposure and male hypogonadism. *Lancet* 17:152–153.

Horney, K. 1933. The denial of the vagina: a contribution to the problem of the genital anxieties specific to women. *International Journal of Psycho-Analysis* 14:55–70.

Jacobson, H. N., and Reid, D. E. 1964. High risk pregnancy: a pattern of comprehensive maternal and child care. *New England Journal of Medicine* 271:302–307.

Karnaky, K. J. 1942. The use of stilbestrol for the treatment of threatened and habitual abortion and premature labor: a preliminary report. *Southern Medical Journal* 35:838–847.

King, A. G. 1953. Threatened and repeated abortion: present status of therapy. *Journal of Obstetrics and Gynecology* 1:104–114.

Kirkpatrick, M. 1980. *Women's Sexual Development: Exploration of Inner Space*. New York: Plenum.

Krill, C. E., and Toomey, J. A. 1941. Multiple cases of tonsillectomy and poliomyelitis. *Journal of the American Medical Association* 117:1013–1017.

Lederer, W. 1968. *The Fear of Women*. New York: Harvest.

Lerner, H. E. 1974. Early origins of envy and devaluation of women. *Bulletin of the Menninger Clinic* 38:538–553.

Love, S. M.; Gelman, R. S.; and Silen, W. 1982. Fibrocystic disease of the breast—a non-disease? *New England Journal of Medicine* 307:1010–1014.

Mann, E. C. 1959. Habitual abortion: a report in 2 parts of 160 patients. *American Journal of Obstetrics and Gynecology* 77:706–718.

Mills, J. L., and Bongiovanni, A. M. 1978. Effect of prenatal estrogen exposure on male genitalia. *Pediatrics* 62(suppl.): 1160–1164.

Money, J., and Ehrhardt, A. A. 1972a. Gender dimorphic behavior and fetal sex hormones. *Recent Progress in Hormonal Research* 28:735–763.

Money, J., and Ehrhardt, A. A. 1972b. *Man and Woman: Boy and Girl*. Baltimore: Johns Hopkins University Press.

Money, J.; Hampson, J. G.; and Hampson, J. L. 1957. Imprinting and the establishment of gender role. *Archives of Neurology and Psychiatry* 77:333–336.

Nadelson, C. C., and Notman, M. T. 1982. *The Woman Patient*. Vol. 2, *Concepts of Femininity and the Life Cycle*. New York: Plenum.

Neumann, E. 1963. *The Great Mother: An Analysis of the Archetype*. New York: Pantheon.

Newton, M. 1973. Editorial about ACOG Technical Bulletin on DES, encouraging casefinding. *ACOG Newsletter* 17(5): 2.

Niederland, W. G. 1974. *The Schreber Case*. New York: Quadrangle.

Noller, D. L., and Fish, C. R. 1974. Diethylstilbestrol usage: an interesting past, important present, and questionable future. *Medical Clinics of North America* 58:793–810.

Notman, M. T., and Nadelson, C. C. 1978. *The Woman Patient*. Vol.1, *Sexual and Reproductive Aspects of Women's Health Care*. New York: Plenum.

Pederson, P. M. 1947. A statistical study of poliomyelitis in relationship to tonsillectomy. *Annals of Otolaryngology, Rhinology, and Laryngology* 56:1281–1293.

Pena, E. F. 1954. Prevention of abortion. *American Journal of Surgery* 87:95–96.

Plate, W. P. 1954. Diethylstilbestrol therapy in habitual abortion. *Proceedings of the International Congress of Obstetrics and Gynecology* (Geneva) 751–757.

Randall, C. L.; Beatz, R. W.; Hall, D. W.; and Birtch, P. K. 1955. Pregnancies observed in the likely-to-abort patient with or without hormone therapy before or after conception. *American Journal of Obstetrics and Gynecology* 69:643–656.

Reid, D. D. 1955. Use of hormones in the management of pregnancy in diabetes. *Lancet* 2:833–836.

Robinson, D., and Shettles, L. B. 1952. The use of diethylstilbestrol in threatened abortion. *American Journal of Obstetrics and Gynecology* 63:1330–1333.

Roiphe, H., and Galenson, E. l982. *Infantile Origins of Sexual Identity*. New York: International Universities Press.

Ross, J. W. 1953. Further report on the use of diethylstilbestrol in the treatment of threatened abortion. *Journal of the National Medical Association* 45:223 ff.

Schowalter, J. E. 1977. The adolescent with cancer. In E. M. Pattison, ed. *The Experience of Dying*. Englewood Cliffs, N.J.: Prentice-Hall.

Schowalter, J. E. 1983a. Mood disturbance in physical illness in adolescence. In H. Golombek and B. D. Garfinkel, eds. *The Adolescent and Mood Disturbance*. New York: International Universities Press.

Schowalter, J. E. 1983b. The psyche and soma of physical illness in adolescence. *Psychosomatics* 24:453–461.

Sherman, A. I.; Goldrath, M.; Berlin, A.; Vakhariya, V.; Banooni, F.; Michaels, W.; Goodman, P.; and Brown, J. 1974. Cervical-vaginal adenosis after in-utero exposure to synthetic estrogens. *Journal of Obstetrics and Gynecology* 44:531–545.

Simon, B. 1978. *Mind and Madness in Ancient Greece: The Classical Roots of Modern Psychiatry*. Ithaca, N.Y.: Cornell University Press.

Smith, G. V., and Smith, O. W. 1946. Increased excretion of pregnanediol in pregnancy from diethylstilbestrol with special reference to the prevention of late pregnancy accidents. *American Journal of Obstetrics and Gynecology* 51:411–415.

Smith, G. V., and Smith, O. W. 1954. Prophylactic hormone therapy: relation to complication of pregnancy. *Journal of Obstetrics and Gynecology* 4:129–141.

Spitz, R. A. 1952. Authority and masturbation. *Psychoanalytic Quarterly* 21:490–527.

Stoller, R. J. 1979. A contribution to the study of gender identity. *International Journal of Psycho-Analysis* 60:433–441.

Sugar, M., ed. 1979. *Female Adolescent Development*. New York: Brunner/Mazel.

Swyer, G. I. M., and Law, R. G. 1954. An evaluation of the prophylactic antenatal use of stilbestrol: preliminary report. *Journal of Endocrinology* 10:6–7.

Thiam, A. 1983. Women's fight for the abolition of sexual mutilation. *International Journal of Social Science* 35:747–756.

Tyrone, C. 1952. Certain aspects of gynecologic practice in the late nineteenth century. *American Journal of Surgery* 84:95–106.

University of Maryland doctor gives DES to retarded youths. 1981. *Washington Post* (November 15).

U.S. Department of Health and Human Services. Centers for Disease Control. *Morbidity and Mortality Weekly* (April 24, 1981).

Veith, I. 1965. *Hysteria: The History of a Disease*. Chicago: University of Chicago Press.

Weigert, E. 1970. The cult and mythology of the Magna Mater from the standpoint of psychoanalysis. In *The Courage to Love: Selected Papers of Edith Weigert*. New Haven, Conn.: Yale University Press.

Weiss, N. P. 1977. Mother, the invention of necessity: Dr. Benjamin Spock's *Baby and Health Care*. *American Quarterly* 29:519–546.

Wells, T. S.; Hegar, A.; and Battey, R. 1886. Castration in mental and nervous diseases: a symposium. *American Journal of Medical Science* 92:455–490.

White, P.; Koshy, P.; and Duckers, J. 1953. The management of pregnancy complicating diabetes and of children of diabetic mothers. *Medical Clinics of North America* 37:1481–1496.

2 DISCUSSION OF FISHER AND APFEL'S "FEMALE PSYCHOSEXUAL DEVELOPMENT: MOTHERS, DAUGHTERS, AND INNER ORGANS"

NORMAN R. BERNSTEIN

Fisher and Apfel's chapter represents the confluence of several different views of a major medical problem involving millions of women. It provides a social history of personal tragedy. It is also an elegant and sensitive study of the dynamics of skewed mother/child relationships in adolescent girls with present or threatened damage to their genitalia, and it locates this whole discussion in the context of classical Greek tragedy. It is both scholarly and moving in the best tradition of scientific humanism while it illuminates many developmental issues.

In adolescent practice, we all see girls who are concerned about their self-concepts and body images, the patients who say, "I am the same fat girl with psoriasis that I was at ten," or the young woman executive who reports, "My weight is normal but I'm still an anorexic inside." We know how the personal mythology about our bodies lives on in later life. Enuretics often grow up to have sexual concerns and feel damaged self-confidence. Chronically ill children commonly grow up socially behind their peers. But few of these situations combine the interior concerns about one's body with the real threat of cancer and malformation of the genitals. A visible physical defect such as a harelip thrusts someone into a different social role. She feels acutely the horror, scorn, and rejection that society often shows her. Adolescents with cryptic or nonvisible defects follow a different developmental course:

they have emotions of personal mortification and damage to self-esteem, a situation that is sometimes harder to deal with because it is masked and diffusely located.

Some patients with major and serious handicaps seem to evade their roles as handicapped children, often by moving to a lower level of functioning and accepting it, remaining in the role of the "good kid" patient or child. Others take the more complex road of fighting to create an adolescent identity that engages the sense of damage and threat—for example, the "Damocles Syndrome," as some have characterized the situation of patients who live under the threat of cancer. This is the grimmer background—the "ticking bomb"—that Fisher (1984) notes as the climate in which her adolescent patients mature. They show increased anxiety and difficulty functioning because they feel they have deficient inner organs. Common results of chronic disorders in childhood are delayed maturation and ego constriction. Fisher's patients do not show this, but they demonstrate how it is harder for children at risk to find validation and a sense of worth. Added anxiety defines a phase of adolescent development for the DES (diethylstilbestrol) experience with its real threat of genital abnormality and cancer.

As Fisher and Apfel have so beautifully described, these females have also lost the normal, expectable, secure matrix of their relationship with their mothers; the fulcrum for hammering out identity problems with mother is tinged with guilt and alarm. These young women try to build their self-concepts in the midst of threat: all aspects of the self system—health, attractiveness, and physical competence—are at risk. Their social selves are shaky; even the transient shifts in self-esteem, which adolescents show so readily, are shadowed by a threat of serious illness. The inner geography of the body image is marked by fantasies of damage and a skewed sense of selfhood. The internal world of private experiences about body parts and the feeling that the private self is a comfortable place to lodge have become tinged with destructive imagery.

Studies of chronically ill and handicapped children show not that the uses of adversity are sweet but rather that chronic illness engenders bitterness, guilt, feelings of rejection, and a lingering self-doubt. This self-doubt can be masked, as Fisher and Apfel's case shows, where a college student's "sophisticated physical presentation disguised massive confusion about her body's functions . . . her identity as a DES-flawed individual" (p. 000). We need to give these children opportunities to bring out what they feel on this endopsychic level of functioning if we are best

31

to give them help. For some distancing from the problem can be achieved, even if it is within the body system. "It is not that I am handicapped— I have a handicap," rather than, "It has me."

Today, in a different world of medical marketing, we are seeing hundreds of thousands of young women striving to remove body-image defects through plastic surgery. Over a million cosmetic procedures are done each year in this country, and, with the advent of lipectomy, the rapid suctioning out of fatty tissue, young women are attempting to sculpt and contour their bodies to rid themselves of adolescent concerns that they could not remove, such as saddle bags, chubby knees, and rounded bellies. Camouflaged by the technology and quick-fix mentality, the inner unresolved concerns about the teenage body image go quietly onward. For cosmetic patients, the reaction is one of "fixing themselves up"; there is no threat of terrible disease, no sense of the vulnerability Weisman (1972) described in studies on reactions to cancer.

Weisman paired many of the feelings to assess how cancer patients were coping: hopeful or hopeless, perturbed or composed, despondent or responsive, helpless or autonomous, exhausted or energetic, isolated or secure, denying/avoidant or aware, and truculent or appreciative. These antinomies can also be seen in DES adolescents and young women.

Burch (1985) has described "identity foreclosure," a developmental impairment in adolescents who "appear mature but function well below this level." Goffman (1963) spoke of "spoiled identity" as the result of a stigmatizing role. That is what these adolescents and young women risk.

Fisher and Apfel (1984) have pursued studies that cross over from individual psychology to family structure and the anatomy of scientific progress while examining the bodily threats to developing sexuality in adolescent females. They report the best and worst of medicine and some of the catastrophies and triumphs of these young women and their mothers.

REFERENCES

Burch, C. 1985. Identity foreclosure in early adolescence. *Adolescent Psychiatry* 12:145–161.

Fisher, S., and Apfel, R. 1984. *To Do No Harm*. New Haven, Conn.: Yale University Press.

Goffman, E. 1963. *Stigma: Notes on the Management of Spoiled Identity*. Englewood Cliffs, N.J.: Prentice-Hall.

Weisman, A. 1972. *On Dying and Denying: A Psychiatric Study of Terminality*. New York: Behavioral Publications.

3   THE EFFECT OF CHILDHOOD SEXUAL
     TRAUMA ON FEMALE PSYCHOLOGICAL
     DEVELOPMENT: AN OVERVIEW

ADRIAN D. COPELAND

Psychological trauma is generally defined as an emotional shock that makes a lasting impression on the unconscious part of the mind and exerts a negative influence on psychological development. Sigmund Freud (1893), responsible to a large degree for the enunciation of the concept of psychic trauma, stresses the importance of the individual's sense of helplessness as a key element in the psychological damage that occurs. Psychological traumatization of young girls can occur through family strife, maternal deprivation (Bowlby 1952), parental separation and divorce, neglect, and physical abuse. Forced sexual involvement with an adult male is another important means of traumatization and is the subject of this chapter.

Objective data collection about sexual trauma has been difficult in a society that, until recently, has frowned on discussion of the subject. While it is true that Freud postulated childhood seduction as a cause of neurosis nearly 100 years ago, it was not until 1953 that pedophilia and incest were again brought to the public's attention (Kinsey 1953). The post–World War II advent of the women's movement brought further attention to the subject of sexual abuse with its concern for the rape victim. These same feminist groups, in conjunction with pediatricians and social workers, extended the focus beyond rape to a whole new area, that of child sexual abuse. Pertinent data were gathered from crisis centers (Herman 1981), from general surveys of women (Finkelhor 1979; Russell 1986), and from college campuses (Rooth 1973). As a consequence, evidence of widespread adult-child sexual involvement and traumatization became clear and compelling. Estimates of the extent of sexual traumatization of children vary and are fraught with a number of methodological and philosophical problems. One such problem is low reportage of sex crimes, owing to a strong cultural taboo concerning sexual issues and even stronger needs to suppress feelings of guilt, shame, and fear. This is not only on the part of the victim but on the part of the perpetrator as well, as I have noted in an evaluation of more than 200 convicted sexual offenders (Copeland and Pedigo 1988).

Absence of an adequate, multidisciplinary nosology and classification system, common to both law and psychiatry, is another problem that thwarts data collection and communication between the two fields, and it impedes necessary cross-disciplinary research. For instance, DSM-III, the psychiatric classification system, has no specific term for incest, and one would have to infer that a child diagnosed as having an adjustment disorder of childhood has been thus exposed. Nor is there a precise diagnostic term for the incestuous father, with pedophilia or atypical psychosexual disorder the diagnostic terms most closely approximating this behavior. Legal terminology is often ambiguous as well. For example, the term "sodomy" refers to both homosexual and heterosexual anal intercourse. The psychiatric term "exhibitionism" may be referred to legally in a number of ways—indecent exposure, open lewdness, and corrupting the morals of a minor.

Lack of a comprehensive research design is another complicating factor that results in confusing and sometimes contradictory research findings. For instance, with regard to incest, the incidence has been variously reported as 1.9 cases per million (Gleuck 1956; Weinberg 1976), 5,000 cases per year (DeFrancis 1971), 100,000 cases per year (National Center for Child Abuse and Neglect 1981), and sixteen cases per hundred (Russell 1986). These variations may be attributable to methodological differences, including those of statistical analysis to derive projections for incidence and prevalence (Mayer 1983), and to differences in the types of populations studied (Kempe and Kempe 1984).

Reporter bias constitutes yet another barrier to objective understanding of the problem owing to the intense feelings evoked by the subject of sexual abuse. Overidentification with the victim may lead to possible overreporting, as seen in some of the rape statistics that include unsubstantiated reports and attempted rapes (Herman 1981). Overidentification with the offender has traditionally resulted in underreportage of incestuous fathers and sexually abusive members of professional groups such as physicians, psychologists, lawyers, and clergymen.

With all the imperfections in data collection taken into consideration, it appears that pedophilia constitutes the quantitatively greatest form of illegal sexual involvement of children. Russell (1984) reports an incidence of eighty-five per 100,000 cases of sexual abuse of underage females annually, and Herman (1981) estimates that between one-fifth and one-third of underage females have sexual contact with adult males. The Pennsylvania *Child Abuse Report* (1985) shows that roughly half of all substantiated child abuse cases reported were of a sexual nature and that pedophilia constituted 71 percent of all sexual crimes.

Exhibitionism is the next most frequent form of illegal sexual behavior, constituting almost one-third of all sexual abuse cases and producing the greatest number of jailings for misdemeanors, with a recidivism rate of 11 percent (Rossman 1980; Snaith 1983; Smith 1978). Cox and Daitzman (1980) point out that about 27 percent of the exhibitionist group is also pedophilic. It might be added that, in general, the preferred target for the exhibitionist, whether leading to pedophilia or not, is the pubertal and prepubertal girl.

Rape has been characterized as one of the fastest growing crimes of violence in the United States, with a reported incidence of 56,000 in 1975 (U.S. Department of Justice 1975) and 72,000 in 1983 (Prescott 1985), with the actual incidence possibly four to ten times higher (Delin 1978). Roughly one-third of these victims are eighteen years old or younger (Hicks, Halpern, and Crenshaw 1978). The incidence of nonadult female rapes in Pennsylvania in 1985 was 322, or 6 percent of all sexual crimes against children (*Child Abuse Report* 1985).

With regards to incest, variations in reportage have already been noted, with incidence estimates ranging from as low as one per million (Weinberg 1976) to 16 percent (Russell 1986).

Cultural Considerations

Societal standards often influence the individual's perception of whether an experience is traumatic. Culturally approved behaviors and experiences are usually perceived more positively and are ego syntonic.

Those behaviors and experiences perceived as socially unacceptable are seen as more ego dystonic and often psychologically traumatic. For instance, the perception of one's imminent violent death usually evokes fear and dread, but not among World War II Japanese kamikaze pilots, ready to die for their emperor and fortified by social sanction. In Bolivia, a country that embraces and institutionalizes the use of the coca leaf, there is far less psychobiological breakdown than in the United States, where its use runs counter to societal mores and standards of health. In 1985, there were almost 40,000 cocaine-caused hospital admissions in this country and 563 cocaine-induced fatalities (*U.S. Journal of Drug and Alcohol Dependence* 1986). By extension, cultural attitudes also influence the individual's perceptions about his or her sexual behaviors and experiences. A sexual behavior defined as illegal and viewed as abusive in one country may be considered neither illegal nor abusive in another.

Abel, Becker, and Skinner (1980) point out that violent sex is indigenous among the Siriono and Chorati people, and Rada (1978) reports that certain Kenyan tribes practice ceremonial rape and that among the Zatopecs, where there is much incest and adultery, there is no word for rape. Pursuing the issue of cultural relativism and sexual abuse, Mrazak and Kempe (1981, p. 86) note that "researchers have cited clitoridectomy in areas as diverse as Australia, Brazil, Malaya, Pakistan, El Salvador, Egypt, Nigeria and the Soviet Union. Quite obviously child sexual abuse takes on an entirely different meaning in such cultures. Any evaluation of whether such practices should be redefined as sexual abuse must be done by the people of those particular countries." Thus, sexual behaviors that appear abusive to us may not be viewed as harmful in other cultures, and whether these behaviors and practices are necessarily traumatic is difficult to determine. A better understanding of the effect of a sexual event on an individual requires an understanding of the cultural context from which that individual springs.

Mores, even within one society, change with time, as noted in the sexual revolution witnessed in the United States in the last quarter of a century and in the antisexual reaction to the AIDS problem just now occurring. Sometimes, these changes occur more slowly. Traditional codes of Western sexual behavior, derived from Judeo-Christian religious doctrine, were initially extreme and harsh. Today, these are less so.

37

In the Old Testament, incest was punishable by death by stoning, and early Christianity forbade marriage even among distant relatives. It was not until the era of the Protestant Reformation and the Catholic Counterreformation that the definition of incest became more liberalized (Maisch 1972). The late nineteenth century was again an era of sexual suppression and Victorian moralism. Freud's initial hypothesis of pedophilia and incest as causes of psychopathology in adult women evoked considerable negative reaction, especially among the laity, and it was not until almost a century later that sexual attitudes had relaxed sufficiently to permit open discussion of the subject of childhood seduction. Paradoxically, it might be noted that, at the same time that Victorian mores were suppressive and the era prudish, the age of sexual consent in the United States in 1886 was ten to twelve years (Schultz 1980). Yesterday's age of consent became today's statutory rape and sexual abuse.

It seems apparent, then, that illegal sexual behavior may vary from culture to culture and within one culture at different times. It is extremely difficult to judge whether sexual practices, illegal in one culture and believed to be traumatic, are traumatic in another culture in which such practices are legal. More research is necessary to understand the effect of cultural and subcultural mores on sexual experience and the process of traumatization, especially in a pluralistic society such as ours.

Psychological Effect

The response on the part of girls to sexual activity with adult males in American society is complex, variable, and determined by a number of factors (Landis 1956). Finkelhor (1979) contends that, in general, sexual experience with adults is usually perceived negatively, with the age spread between adult and child being an important issue. The use of force is also a factor of major significance in producing sexual trauma (Rose 1986; Schultz 1975). Abel et al. (1980) note that, unfortunately, child molesters often use violence during the commission of sex acts with children; they cite a 5–10 percent incidence of physical injury in cases of incest and pedophilia. In the Pennsylvania *Child Abuse Report* (1985), sexually related physical injuries were noted to have increased by 28 percent over the prior year.

Another key factor influencing traumatization is the girl's mental condition and the quality of her life circumstances prior to the sexual involvement. For instance, Schultz (1980) found that 79 percent of child sex victims suffered from prior emotional neglect and that 11 percent experienced prior physical abuse. Maisch (1972) reported that a number of incestuously involved girls in his study had symptoms of behavioral disturbances and depression before the sexual involvement began.

Age spread, the use of force, and prior psychological maladjustment are three factors cited that appear to influence a child's response to early sexual exposure. Since children are plastic, they may react in different manners, with psychological trauma not always resultant (Herman, Russell, and Trucki 1986; Schultz 1975). Renshaw (1987, p. 263) notes that "at times the child experiences quite natural sexual arousal and orgasmic responses from the sexual contact," and Bender and Blau (1937) also suggest that some children may derive emotional satisfaction from such sexual experience.

Browning and Boatman (1977), Gomez-Schwartz, Horowitz, and Sanzier (1985), Herman and Schatzow (1984), Klein (1932), and Miller, Moeller, and Kaufman (1978) disagree. Herman and Schatzow see major psychological trauma produced not only in childhood but also later on in adult life. A pattern of repeated victimization is also noted (Burgess and Holmstrom 1974).

The following case illustrates the relation between early childhood neglect and sexual abuse and a pattern of later victimization. A twenty-five-year-old separated mother of two small children, in her fifth month of pregnancy, came to the Joseph J. Peters Institute for treatment of her chief complaints of anxiety, insomnia, and a repetitive dream of being raped by a man, with only the top of his head and his hands appearing. In addition, she had flashbacks of being punched in the face. These symptoms developed six weeks before, when she had been raped by an employee of her husband. The man was a convicted rapist who had been recently released from prison and hired by her husband as a construction work helper. His hiring was a source of much acrimony as the patient told her husband of her fears concerning this man. This dispute was one of many, as there was basic disagreement in the marriage, and she had been considering leaving. The offender gained admission to her house on a weekend when her husband was away. The offender not only raped her but beat her about the face and head as well. This memory was the basis of her flashbacks and night terrors. Shortly after the man was arrested, she and her husband separated.

From a developmental standpoint, her parents separated when she was three years old, and her mother gave her to her own mother and stepfather to raise. The patient remained with her maternal grandmother and step-grandfather until she was eleven, when she rejoined her mother. From the ages of seven to eleven, she was sexually abused by her step-grandfather during her grandmother's frequent absences. He would frequently force his way into her bed, mount her, and make "crushing movements that hurt." She was perpetually frightened but afraid to tell anyone. She revealed the abuse to her mother only when she rejoined her, but nothing was done. From a symptomatic standpoint, she suffered from enuresis until she was fourteen and was a chronic nail biter. In her later adolescent and early adult years, she suffered from frequent bouts of depression when the men she was involved with would leave her. She often entertained suicidal thoughts on the weekends that her husband would disappear. The pattern of abandonment, abuse, chronic mental illness, and victimization was complete.

Burgess and Holmstrom (1974) find that psychological damage may be produced in three ways: ethically, in terms of installing false standards regarding what constitutes usual sexual behavior between adults and children; emotionally, in terms of instilling fear, shame, and guilt; and physically, in terms of anatomic harm. In cases of rape, Rada (1978) points out that sense of being overpowered and made a helpless victim generates fear that can become generalized and paralyzing.

Common Symptoms and Signs of Sexual Trauma

As noted, assessing the effect on a nonadult female of sexual involvement with an adult male must include evaluation of her prior psychological status as well as the prevailing sociosexual mores under which she lives. Once these basic issues are clarified, her current psychological condition may be evaluated according to four parameters: (1) symptoms and signs of psychopathology, (2) the pattern of relationships, (3) self-concept, and (4) level of function.

SYMPTOMS AND SIGNS OF PSYCHOPATHOLOGY

Indicators of sexual traumatization may be physical or psychological/behavioral, and many of these are equivocal and nonspecific (American Medical Association 1985). With regard to physical findings, A. Finkel (1986, personal communication) has developed a more precise method

40

of examination of sex trauma victims. With the use of colposcopy, he is able to collect more significant data than simply the presence or absence of perineal bruises, an intact hymen, semen, pregnancy, or venereal disease, information collected in the routine physical examination for sexual abuse.

Schultz (1980) categorizes psychological/behavioral symptoms according to age, and, as already noted, many of these are nonspecific. Their presence, however, should alert the clinician to investigate further the possibility of sexual abuse. In infants, he cites changes in eating and sleeping patterns. Toddlers may present insomnia, enuresis, symptoms of anxiety and phobia, stomachaches, and precocious sex play. The latency child may present obsessive-compulsive behavior, increased masturbatory activity, separation anxiety, and disturbed sleeping and eating patterns. The adolescent can show a variety of symptoms, including pavor nocturnus (Maisch 1972), emotional instability (Carman, Renker, and Mills 1984), and a pattern of repeated victimization (Swanson and Biaggio 1985) and masochistic behavior (Smith 1978). In addition, there may be delinquent behavior in the form of running away, substance abuse, and sexual promiscuity, with the development of subsequent venereal disease and/or pregnancy (Schultz 1980; Smith 1978).

Specifically with regard to incest, Maisch (1972) notes that depression with suicidal behavior was notable in 20 percent of his studied population. He also reported a pregnancy rate of 20 percent. In cases of rape, posttraumatic stress disorders with flashbacks were often reported (Burgess 1979; Herman and Schatzow 1984; Rose 1986). Conversion symptoms, depersonalization, dissociation, and fugue were also reported, along with a whole range of anxiety reactions and depression (Renshaw 1987). With regard to exhibitionism, both Cox and Daitzman (1980) and Landis (1956) independently agree that the long-term negative effects on girls are usually minimal.

PATTERN OF RELATIONSHIPS

Young females who have been sexually traumatized often withdraw and manifest a general mistrust (Burgess 1979; Butler 1978; Carman et al. 1984). In cases of incest, withdrawal from siblings is also noted (Butler 1978), as are problems of intimacy in adult life (Herman and Schatzow 1984). The pattern of delinquent behavior and sexual acting out has already been noted.

SELF-CONCEPT

Girls who have been sexually traumatized often suffer from a negative image of themselves as well as a lowered self-esteem (Herman et al. 1986; Smith 1978). In cases of rape, victims may lose a sense of autonomy and wholeness (Rose 1986).

LEVEL OF FUNCTION

In younger girls, activity levels change and may increase or decrease after a sexual assault (Smith 1978). Academically, there may be a decrease in attention span, refusal to attend school (Burgess 1979), and school failure (Schultz 1980). Sexual dysfunction may develop in postpubertal females (Herman et al. 1986).

Conclusions

Sexual involvement of nonadult females with adult males is generally traumatic. Although well-substantiated epidemiologic data is lacking, the problem may be growing. Collection of data is hampered by a number of methodological and philosophical problems, including faulty reportage, clinical bias, absence of an adequate classification system, and absence of a coordinated, interdisciplinary research design. Sexual traumatization of nonadult females by adult males is associated with the presence of preexisting psychopathology, the use of force, and age spread. Subcultural mores and family standards must also be considered in assessing the effect of sexual involvement. After establishing the presexual psychological status, four parameters are proposed to assess sexual traumatization: symptom pattern, relationship pattern, level of function, and self-concept. Indications are that not all underage females are traumatized by sexual involvement, and more research needs to be done to clarify this issue so that preventive efforts can be undertaken.

REFERENCES

Abel, G.; Becker, J.; and Skinner, L. 1980. Aggressive behavior and sex. *Psychiatric Clinics of North America* 3:133–150.

American Medical Association. 1985. *Diagnostic and Treatment Guidelines concerning Child Abuse and Neglect.* Chicago: American Medical Association.

Bender, L., and Blau, A. 1937. The reaction of children to sexual relations with adults. *American Journal of Orthopsychiatry* 7:500–581.

Bowlby, J. 1952. *Maternal Care and Mental Health.* Geneva: World Health Organization.

Browning, D., and Boatman, B. 1977. Incest: children at risk. *American Journal of Psychiatry* 134:69–72.

Burgess, A. 1979. *Sexual Assault of Children and Adolescents.* Lexington, Mass.: Lexington.

Burgess, A., and Holmstrom, L. 1974. Rape trauma syndrome. *American Journal of Psychiatry* 131:981–986.

Butler, S. 1978. *Conspiracy of Silence.* San Francisco: Neo Glide.

Carman, E.; Renker, P.; and Mills, T. 1984. Victims of violence and psychiatric illness. *American Journal of Psychiatry* 141:378–383.

Child Abuse Report. 1985. Harrisburg, Pa.: Commonwealth of Pennsylvania.

Copeland, A., and Pedigo, J. 1988. Pedophiles and incestuous fathers: new perspectives. Typescript. Philadelphia: Jefferson Medical College.

Cox, D., and Daitzman, R. 1980. *Exhibitionism: Description, Assessment and Treatment.* New York: Gartland.

DeFrancis, V. 1971. Protecting the child victim of sex crimes committed by adults. *Federal Probation* 35:15–20.

Delin, B. 1978. *The Sex Offender.* Boston: Beacon.

Finkelhor, D. 1979. *Sexually Victimized Children.* New York: Free Press.

Freud, S. 1893. Studies on hysteria. *Standard Edition* 2:133–134. London: Hogarth, 1955.

Gleuck, B. 1956. *Final Report.* Research Project for the Study and Treatment of Persons Convicted of Crimes Involving Sexual Aberrations. Minneapolis: University of Minnesota.

Gomez-Schwartz, B.; Horowitz, J.; and Sanzier, M. 1985. Severity of emotional distress among sexually abused pre-school, school-age and adolescent children. *Hospital and Community Psychiatry* 36:503–508.

Herman, J. 1981. *Father-Daughter Incest.* Cambridge, Mass.: Harvard University Press.

Herman, J.; Russell, D.; and Trucki, K. 1986. Long-term effects of incestuous abuse in childhood. *American Journal of Psychiatry* 143:1243–1296.

Herman, J., and Schatzow, E. 1984. Time limited group therapy for women with a history of incest. *International Journal of Group Psychotherapy* 34:605–616.

Hicks, D.; Halpern, S.; and Crenshaw, T. 1978. *Rape: Helping the Victim.* Oradell, N.J.: Economic Press.

Kempe, R., and Kempe, C. 1984. *The Common Secret: Sexual Abuse of Children and Adolescents.* New York: Freeman.

Kinsey, A. 1953. *Sexual Behavior in the Human Female.* Philadelphia: Saunders.

Klein, M. 1932. *The Psychoanalysis of Children.* London: Hogarth.

Landis, J. 1956. Experiences of five hundred children with adult sexual deviation. *Psychiatric Quarterly* 30(suppl.): 91–109.

Maisch, H. 1972. *Incest.* New York: Stein & Day.

Mayer, A. 1983. *A Treatment Manual with Victims, Spouses and Offenders.* Holmes Beach, Fla.: Learning Publications.

Miller, J.; Moeller, D.; and Kaufman, A. 1978. Recidivism among sex assault victims. *American Journal of Psychiatry* 135:1103–1104.

Mrazak, P., and Kempe, C. 1981. *Sexually Abused Children and Their Families.* New York: Pergamon.

National Center for Child Abuse and Neglect. 1981. *National Study of Incidence and Severity of Child Abuse.* Washington, D.C.: National Center for Child Abuse and Neglect.

Prescott, W. 1985. The violent sex offender. Paper presented at National Conference on Managing the Sex Offender in Correctional Systems, St. Elizabeth's Hospital, Washington, D.C., November 7.

Rada, R. 1978. *Clinical Aspects of the Rapist.* New York: Grune & Stratton.

Renshaw, D. 1987. Evaluating suspected cases of child sexual abuse. *Psychiatric Annals* 17:262–270.

Rooth, G. 1973. Exhibitionism, sexual violence and pedophilia. *British Journal of Psychiatry* 122:705–710.

Rose, D. 1986. Worse than death: psychodynamics of rape victims and the need for psychotherapy. *American Journal of Psychiatry* 143:817–824.

Rossman, P. 1980. The pederasts. In L. Schultz, ed. *The Sexual Victimology of Youth*. Springfield, Ill.: Thomas.

Russell, D. 1984. *Sexual Exploitation*. Beverly Hills, Calif.: Sage.

Russell, D. 1986. *The Silent Trauma: Incest in the Lives of Girls and Women*. New York: Basic.

Schultz, L. 1975. *Rape Victimology*. Springfield, Ill.: Thomas.

Schultz, L. 1980. *The Sexual Victimology of Youth*. Springfield, Ill.: Thomas.

Smith, S. 1978. *The Maltreatment of Children*. Baltimore: University Park Press.

Snaith, P. 1983. Exhibitionism: a clinical conundrum. *British Journal of Psychiatry* 143:231–235.

Swanson, L., and Biaggio, M. 1985. Therapeutic perspectives on father-daughter incest. *American Journal of Psychiatry* 142:667–673.

U.S. Department of Justice. Federal Bureau of Investigation. 1975. *Uniform Crime Reports for the United States*. Washington, D.C.: U.S. Government Printing Office.

U.S. Journal of Drug and Alcohol Dependence (Pampano Beach, Fla.) (August 1986).

Weinberg, S. 1976. *Incest*. New York: Citadel.

4   LATE ADOLESCENCE:
SPOCK AND THE EGO-IDEAL

RHODA S. FRENKEL

Twenty-four centuries ago, when Sophocles wrote *Oedipus Rex,* he had not heard of Freud or the Oedipus complex. The esteem and endurance of this masterpiece demonstrate not only Sophocles' greatness as a playwright but also the universality of the truths he dramatized. Similarly, in our century, through the media of television and film, I believe Gene Roddenberry has created a representation of a universal truth in "Star Trek" as a whole and in the character of Spock in particular. This chapter explores some thoughts about Spock and the ego-ideal.

Using the method of applied analysis enables me to present a richness of detail from public sources that is not possible, for reasons of confidentiality, with case presentations. Significantly, my observations originated from my clinical work in general, but especially from my work with adolescent boys. Although devotion to "Star Trek" spans nationalities, generations, and gender, initially it was targeted for viewing by youths. Because it was created, written, acted, and produced primarily by men, it evolved from a masculine perspective. While this chapter emphasizes adolescent male development, the ego-ideal is relevant to both sexes and to youths of all ages.

For years, many of my patients, as well as some friends and family members, unsuccessfully tried to share with me their enthusiasm for this unique television and film series. Their dedication baffled me. Recent concurrent experiences in my clinical work and personal life stirred me to watch some reruns of the original television series.

RHODA S. FRENKEL

The "Star Trek" Phenomenon

After a nineteen-year voyage, the *USS* (United Space Ship) *Enterprise*, an intergalactic spacecraft and a starship of the United Federation of Planets, picked me up as a passenger and in May 1985 introduced me to the world of "Star Trek." It is no accident that its science-security mission in the twenty-third century—to seek out new life and new civilizations in outer space, beyond our known galaxy—continues to influence millions of viewers. By cleverly disguising its commentary on the often-primitive nature of the behavior and beliefs of twentieth-century civilization, it provides us with a format to explore another great frontier, that of our inner space. Before looking inward, let us examine some information about this living legend.

The range of the *Enterprise* and her crew is extraordinary. Two decades after its first telecast on September 8, 1966, "Star Trek" stubbornly insists on living and has spawned an ever expanding universe. All around the planet Earth, probably at any hour, accounting for time differences, millions of our species stop and avidly watch daily syndicated reruns of the original television series. In addition, there are reruns of an animated series being shown on cable television, four movies, local and national conventions and miniconventions, magazines, fanclubs, fanclub magazines, several series of pocketbooks, games, cards, and even calendars, to mention just some of the "Star Trek" universe. In addition, 10,000 fans have created 30,000 literary and artistic works that have appeared in amateur publications called fanzines (Bacon-Smith 1986). In 1985, the videocassettes of the movie *Star Trek III: The Search for Spock* ranked first in sales and the seventy-nine original television episodes third. What is so compelling about this show? It seems to be more than great escape.

In examining the components of any pervasive fantasy (Bettelheim 1976; Freud 1908), we find wish fulfillments that are conscious and unconscious resolutions to conflicts. It is not difficult to understand the appeal, even at times the need, to escape from painful life experiences. More germane to my topic, the ego-ideal, is how some fantasies (i.e., defensive mental operations) can be transformed into behavior—real actions that make alterations in the individual and the environment. Many children dream of flying. Some extend their arms and pretend to have wings. For them, the illusion is sufficient. With age, a few may become interested in gliders. Two glider enthusiasts dreamed of a motor-driven airplane. Others may have had similar dreams, but, in 1903, the Wright brothers tested theirs in Kitty Hawk. Their dream became reality, and our world changed. We can make some wishes come true. This spirit suffuses "Star Trek" and partially explains why, while "Star Trek" unquestionably provides excellent entertainment, its effect on many viewers is more profound.

In 1968, when the National Broadcasting Company (NBC) wanted to cancel the show at the end of its second season, almost a million fans petitioned the network to reverse their decision (Gerrold 1973). The entire graduating class of Princeton wrote in protest; Massachusetts Institute of Technology students picketed the station; and NBC reversed itself and renewed "Star Trek" for another season. This is but one example of the power the illusion of "Star Trek" has to affect the actual behavior of individuals and groups and thus change reality. It is important to remember that this show is an illusion. Compare it to any documentary on the National Aeronautics and Space Administration (NASA) and to the television coverage of the *Challenger* disaster. Yet, like in a dream, behind its manifest content, are latent truths, sufficiently potent to change people's lives (Lichtenberg, Marshak, and Winston 1975). A real life Captain Kirk (Captain Pierre D. Kirk) described how he organized his military unit, using the format of the *Enterprise*'s personae and dialogue, to bluff his company's way through a Viet Cong ambush (Blish 1972). "Star Trek" fans got the first space shuttle to be renamed the *Enterprise*. In the halls of the Smithsonian Institute, paying tribute to man's efforts to go where no man has gone before, next to Lindbergh's *Spirit of St. Louis,* is the *USS Enterprise.*

Integral to the "Star Trek" lore is the enduring appeal of the show's most popular character, the pointed-eared alien Mr. Spock. The unprecedented response to Mr. Spock is a phenomenon that this chapter can only partially explain. As the only alien among the starship's crew, his half-Vulcan, half-human inheritance produced a constant internal war that contributed to Spock's emergence as the show's most interesting and beloved character. Though not the star of the show, from the very beginning Spock's presence was considered essential to the ideas that Gene Roddenberry, the show's creator, wanted to convey. Though kept in the background initially, the positive reaction to Mr. Spock's character had an incredible effect on the show, on his fans, and on the life of Leonard Nimoy, the actor whose portrayal made Spock seem real. One fan legally changed his name to Spock. Spock is more than a popular cult–comic book hero (Widzer 1977). He commands respect and attention, perhaps as a metaphor for something important about ourselves. Over the years, several patients tried to impress me with their great admiration for Mr. Spock and how each, in his own way, went to great lengths to emulate him. Our discussions would end with their frustration at my inability to understand why they preferred Mr. Spock to the dashing hero, Captain Kirk. I thought it was defensive (and, to some degree, it was), but I missed the "point."

Following one such session, during a period in my life when memories from my own adolescence were resurfacing, I began to watch an occasional late-night rerun of "Star Trek." Other times, after a few minutes' viewing, I had discounted the show as somewhat trivial overacted melodrama. Before long, that opinion was revised. This was a high-quality production, with breadth of concept and, at times, exceptional writing and acting. It was fun, funny, yet often moving. It raised intelligent, philosophical questions about the choices and directions our civilization could make. In difficult times, it portrayed effective ways for individuals to cope; it was a source of hope. What happened to my initial enmity to the show? (This is a problem for a psychoanalyst, so I had to analyze it.) Reflecting and reading about the show, I learned my response was not unique. Lichtenberg, Marshak, and Winston (1975, p. 9) write, "It's something like discovering gold. . . . There you are in the midst of whatever personal demons or small annoyances that haunt your own life and the rather large problems that haunt your planet, and then—suddenly there is 'Star Trek.' " They continue describing how, after discovering that you love it, you become aware that so do an astonishing variety of other people of every age and ilk, dockworkers and doctors, children and businessmen, stagehands and NASA scientists and missionaries. Unknowingly summarizing the feelings of many fans, Nimoy (1975, p. 3) wrote, "The show has certainly given me a sense of self worth and particularly the relationship with the character Mr. Spock has given me a constant guideline for a dignified approach to life as a human being." Recognizing a universal appeal in "Star Trek" and Mr. Spock, I began to explore its genesis and meaning in my patients, myself, and others. It began in the character and dream of one man.

Gene Roddenberry

Gene Roddenberry is the acknowledged father of "Star Trek," its creator-producer. In 1960, long before we landed a man on the moon, he began to develop a new concept for a television series. Writing about his initial efforts (Lichtenberg, Marshak, and Winston 1975, p. ix), Roddenberry says, "If television can bend minds and capture imaginations while in its present, rather primitive stage of development, what of tomorrow? It seems to be necessary that we begin to use today's telecommunications marvels to draw all of humanity together in a free exchange of ideas, art and knowledge . . . or its great mind-bending potential will be used by a powerful few to own and manipulate the rest of us. The making of 'Star Trek' was very much our effort to make the right choice now for myself and the remarkable cast, production staff and crew, who somehow came together during those bruising, exhausting, completely lovely years, it was an effort to prove that people are willing to think beyond the petty beliefs which have for so long kept humanity divided. We used to joke that we suspected that there was intelligent life out there, and we aimed to use our show to signal some of our thoughts to them, but never in our wildest imaginings did we expect the volume and intensity of the replies we received."

Roddenberry knew life; he knew his medium; he knew television was a tough and often brutal industry. Although realistic, he was also idealistic. The creation, writing, and producing of "Star Trek" was an act of love. In psychoanalytic terms, we might say that, in large measure, it was the external embodiment of Roddenberry's internal mature ego-ideal.

The Mature Ego-Ideal

The mature ego-ideal is a beacon, a North Star for the soul. While the early ego-ideal provides an inner source of ease and contentment for the child and younger adolescent, it is normally more self-centered and egoistic. By contrast, the mature ego-ideal transcends self-interests and physical comforts. Freed from early attachments, it provides inner strength and direction for our endeavors to attain less selfish goals and higher values. Generally, the ego-ideal is defined as "the image of the self to which the individual aspires both consciously and unconsciously and against which he measures himself" (Moore and Fine 1968, p. 43). According to Blos (1974), the mature ego-ideal emerges late in adolescence and thereafter remains the primary influence on adult behavior. Originating in primary narcissism, it progresses through the secondary narcissism of childhood and adolescence. Blos believes its final emergence in young adulthood, where it continues to evolve, is the highest level of psychic development. Paradoxically, the goals of the mature ego-ideal are never fully attainable. Nevertheless, they provide the courage and integrity that compel, guide, and inspire our greatest achievements in our relationships and work.

Historically and ontologically, the ego-ideal has its origins in the concept of the superego. As its name indicates, the superego arises as a precipitate from the ego, after the ego has achieved a fair degree of maturation, in order to facilitate, protect, and guide the ego's further growth. Similarly, when the mature ego-ideal emerges from the superego with some ego attributes, it functions with relative independence, facilitating greater autonomy and growth of the individual. The superego encompasses mental representations of moral attitudes, conscience, and the sense of guilt. "Superego functions may be divided into two categories: 1) the protective and rewarding functions, which set up ideals and values that are grouped under the term ego-ideal; 2) the critical and punishing functions which evoke the sense of guilt and the pangs of conscience" (Moore and Fine 1968, p. 90).

First let us deal with the punitive function of the superego. In structural theory, the id, ego, and superego constitute the three systems of the psychic apparatus. In the preoedipal years, the child complies with the moral demands and prohibitions of parents, or parental surrogates, out of fear of physical punishment or loss of love. As Freud (1923) first pointed out, it is only with the dissolution of the Oedipus complex that the parental demands and moral standards become an internal affair; the superego is the heir of the Oedipus complex. In order to relinquish, repress, or otherwise repudiate the incestuous and parricidal wishes (oedipal strivings), the child transforms these drives into an identification with the object of those drives—the parents. What is primarily introjected and identified with are the prohibitions and demands (the authority) of the parent of the same sex as well as that parent's idealized image. These reflect that parent's superego and cultural heritage. Acquiescing to superego demands, the ego develops defenses against the forces of the instinctual drives (id derivatives), insisting that their expression be restrained or forgotten. By submitting to the parental demands through the threat of guilt from the superego, the child renounces direct instinctual gratification and, thus, is able to maintain an affectionate, desexualized relationship with his parents.

To the extent the young child identifies with and acts like the loving and beloved parent, he establishes a source for an inner sense of well-being. According to Sandler (1960, p. 151), "The esteem in which the omnipotent and admired object [parent] is held is duplicated in the self and gives rise to self-esteem." Thus, with the idealized parental image in the ego-ideal, the child can recapture, albeit transiently, a sense of closeness and oneness that recalls the earliest days of life, of primary narcissism. As we know, relative resolution of the oedipal complex first occurs around six years, when the child is still very dependent on parents and others in the environment. Therefore, the child's identifications are enhanced and expanded by the pride, approval, and love from real objects in his environment, which increase his sense of worth and well-being. It is important to note that the change to relative independence from these early objects usually occurs in late adolescence.

The establishment of both components of the superego releases energy for aim-inhibited pursuits. Thus, in the ensuing latency years, secondary process thinking (i.e., logical thought processes) increasingly dominates cognition, and there is enormous development in social, nonsexual physical, intellectual, and cultural skills (Bornstein 1951). The stellar achievement of superego formation, however impressive, represents only a partial and temporary resolution of the oedipal complex. With the onslaught of the hormonal and bodily changes of puberty, there is a resurgence of all the oedipal issues. The new biologic capacity brings about a massive psychic disorganization. Reorganization occurs only with a more definitive resolution of oedipal drives and fantasies, which is the essential task of adolescence.

While latency dealt primarily with the resolution of the positive oedipal constellation, with puberty both positive and negative oedipal issues come to the fore. We are more familiar with the positive strivings whereby the child's incestuous longings are directed toward the parent of the opposite sex and the jealous murderous wishes toward the parent of the same sex. The negative Oedipus complex is always present, though usually less intense. Here, the child wishes for the exclusive loving and sexual union with the parent of the same sex and the death or disappearance of the parent of the opposite sex. Bisexuality is less conflictual in latency and early adolescence. However, resolution of the negative strivings becomes critical in late adolescence.

Blos (1974) believes that the ego-ideal as it emerges at the end of adolescence is heir to the negative Oedipus complex and that this is a more crucial and difficult problem in treating adolescent boys. My clinical experience to some extent confirms his findings with boys. More than cultural determinants seem to be involved. One of the girl's major developmental tasks is to change her object from mother to father. By contrast, for the boy, the essential task is to change his identity. Among my patients, adolescent girls complain more frequently about their problems establishing and maintaining a fulfilling heterosexual object relationship. Adolescent boys most often seem involved in a Herculean struggle to establish a separate masculine identity.

The biologic changes of puberty require the adolescent boy to renounce his libidinal attachment to his mother more forcefully. However, with biologic capability, identification with the father is dangerous on two accounts: it puts father and son back in competition for the mother and/or arouses an upsurge of homosexual libido in the adolescent by reestablishing a close relationship with his father. If this negative oedipal position is not resolved, the adolescent remains rivalrous with his mother, a feeling often expressed as contempt, and adapts a passive feminine attitude with respect to his father and men, which threatens his masculine identity. Nonincestuous heterosexual object choice is blocked, and appropriate phallic assertiveness in meeting his own aspirations (realistic efforts in job and career choices) is inhibited.

More than it is in latency, the task in adolescence is one of internalization. According to Loewald (1973, pp. 82–83), "Internalization involves a giving up of both the libidinal-aggressive as well as the identification elements in object relations. . . . Identification tends to erase a difference: subject becomes object and object becomes subject. Identification is a way-station to internalization, but in internalization, if carried to completion, a redifferentiation has taken place by which both subject and object have been reconstituted, each on a new level of organization. . . . Internalization as a completed process implies an emancipation from the object . . . the individual is enriched by the relationship . . . but not burdened by identification and fantasy relations with the object." Renouncing father in this sense allows the adolescent boy to establish his separate masculine identity.

In my opinion, the internalization of both maternal and paternal ideals is critical in freeing the adolescent from both infantile objects. This coalescence of both parental value systems, augmented by some ego attributes, establishes the mature ego-ideal. Any separation from infantile objects, even in latency, involves a sense of loss, some mourning, and a search for new objects. With adolescence, when internalizations replace early identifications, the search for new objects becomes more intense. Peers, teachers, and other environmental figures, both real and fictional, as they actually are, as they were in the past, or as they are idealized, become objects for new identifications and internalizations. They help in the separation and mourning and also become incorporated as part of the mature ego-ideal. It is important to note that multiple sources interact and coalesce to form the mature ego-ideal.

This discussion concerns mental operations in which we create internal images, illusions, out of our need both to defend and to grow. The early ego-ideal is clearly defensive, reparative. Yet, as Hartmann (1958) described, mental structures during the course of development can change functions. The mature ego-ideal emerges with relative autonomy, promoting growth and adaptation to reality. Hartmann wrote, "It is general knowledge that fantasy . . . can be fruitful even in scientific thought supposedly the undisputed domain of rational thought. (Although apocryphal, recall Fisher's dream of the benzene ring.) . . . the relationship to reality is learned by way of detours (recall the real function of play in children, the initial normal regression in adolescence, not to mention the psychoanalytic process). . . . Fantasy may fulfill a synthetic function by provisionally connecting our needs and goals with possible ways of realizing them" (p. 18). Keeping in mind the potential for powerful illusions to be transformed into positive progressive actions, let us return to "Star Trek" and Mr. Spock.

Mr. Spock

The evolution of Mr. Spock's character bears striking similarities to the mature ego-ideal. They are both complex composites in which the multiple factors fuse. Both emerge initially from an interaction of maternal and paternal components and mature over time, gaining depth by assimilating new elements. Although this is true for "Star Trek" as a whole, it is particularly germane to Mr. Spock. In what follows, it is difficult to distinguish each element or even to include them all. As stated earlier, this show seems to be an external representation of Roddenberry's mature ego-ideal. As stated, this ideal would encompass both maternal and paternal values as well as other influences from his life. Nevertheless, he is the father. Initially, he selected the key actors, writers, production staff, and crew carefully, inseminating them with his concepts for the show. In surmounting the innumerable obstacles in the six-year effort to get "Star Trek" on the air and keep it there for three years (Whitfield and Roddenberry 1968), for many of the participants it was an act of love.

This was true for Leonard Nimoy, the actor who portrays Spock. Acknowledging his physical and spiritual involvement in Spock's birth, Nimoy (1975, p. 17) wrote, "I was present. . . . I suffered the labor pains, but I don't think I am the mother. . . . I don't know exactly when it happened. I recall vividly when the seed of this life was planted. I can still see the face of Gene Roddenberry, the man who did the planting." Frustrated at not knowing exactly when this birth took place, in contrast to other characters, he decided that perhaps Spock had many births. Like the mature ego-ideal, various aspects of the character were born at different times. Nimoy's own character, acting style, and contributions to the scripts enhanced the shape of both Spock and the show. Talented writers like Dorothy Fontana, Theodore Sturgeon, and Gene Coon (also coproducer) added depth and history to Spock's character. Others, especially William Shatner as Captain Kirk and DeForest Kelley as Dr. McCoy, modified and highlighted Spock's uniqueness. Thus, like the mature ego-ideal, Spock was born from the sublimated union of a father and son in which all three maintained separate identities and autonomy. Furthermore, Spock's evolution resulted from the merged contributions of a variety of people. The following data expand and support this hypothesis.

From the beginning, Roddenberry wanted Nimoy to play the slightly satanic appearing alien as a "regular" character in the series. Mr. Spock was the only character to survive the first pilot, "The Cage." This beautiful show was rejected as too good, too cerebral.[1] The networks wanted an action-adventure series and wanted many of the original character types and relationships changed, especially the alien. Roddenberry writes (Whitfield and Roddenberry 1968, p. 125), "They were nervous about Spock as a character. They were afraid his satanic appearance would repulse people. They were sure no one would ever identify with a person from another world. My own idea on that was that in a very real sense we are all aliens on our strange planet. We spend most of our lives reaching out and trying to communicate. If during our whole lifetime we could reach out and really communicate with just two people, we are indeed very fortunate; and this is exactly what Spock is trying to do."

Roddenberry fought for Spock, wondering why no one else believed in him. He refused to do a second pilot without Spock, explaining that a space show had to have at least one such person on board as a constant reminder that you are out in space, in a world of the future. He did not reveal that an alien was essential as a primary cover for his social commentary. Only through an alien (the alien's perspective and how he was perceived) could Roddenberry risk his statements about the fallibility of our current human customs and institutions. The network agreed, but only if the alien were kept in the background and subdued by merging his personality with the quiet, controlled first officer. This fortuitous combination became the hallmark of the Vulcan species— total mental control over all bodily functions and feelings. Ironically, Spock's inherent conflict opened dramatic potential that forced him to the forefront, where he remains.

Who are Vulcans? What do we know about Spock? Terrans seem insatiably curious (that should tell us something) about everything that is Vulcan. Contrast that to our interest in the backgrounds of Captain Kirk or Dr. McCoy. Much that emerged in the "Star Trek" series, books, and movies details in depth information about Spock, his parents, the Vulcan planet, language, and culture, and so on. Vulcans apparently have something to teach us. They have superior mental and physical characteristics as a result of inheritance and the long evolution of their species on a planet with a heavy gravity and hot climate. Stoic and formal, they place great value on duty to family and Vulcan traditions. Complete adherence to logic is the primary motivating factor in Vulcan mores. To ensure pure logic, Vulcans practice both total concentration and complete suppression of emotion. From birth, a Vulcan child is taught that any display of emotion is highly improper and offensive. Many centuries ago, at the beginning of their species, the Vulcans were more violent than humans. Concluding that emotion was dangerous, they set about to repress it and replace it with logic. They point out that emotion has killed more people on Earth than any other cause. After centuries of practice and custom, they are almost incapable of feeling emotion. Logic became breath, a sensation as exhilarating (they would say energizing) as any emotion. They believe the Vulcan way to be superior to that of men of Earth, as they have had ten centuries of peace.

Critical to the Vulcan philosophy is the tenet of nonviolence. Given a rational reason, a Vulcan can kill very efficiently in self-defense, but only after excluding all other means of defense. Physical violence of a lesser degree is permitted if logical. Thus, the Vulcan neck pinch causes instant unconsciousness.[2] Additionally, the Vulcan diet is restricted to the simplest of vegetable life forms. Nevertheless, once every seven years the Vulcan pays a price for this repression. At this time, the Pon Farr, the Vulcan male is overcome with the mating urge, much like a rutting season. Their behavior becomes savage; however, it is sanctioned and to some degree limited by Vulcan law, ritual, and tradition.

As science officer, Mr. Spock is in charge of all scientific departments aboard the *Enterprise*. As executive officer, he is second in command. Stationed at the library-computer, his intellect and skill, extraordinary even for a Vulcan, enable him to extract and interpret complex information rapidly. The product of an interplanetary marriage between his mother, Amanda, a teacher and scientist from Earth, and his father, Sarek, a physicist and ambassador from Vulcan, he inherited characteristics from both parents. Considering himself Vulcan, his dominant Vulcan inheritance is seen in his physical appearance. As a half human, Spock constantly struggles with himself to repress his feelings. Deeply ashamed of his emotions, he denies them with "logical" rationalizations. As a Vulcan, he has the capacity to "mind-meld." Inducing a trance-like state to lower mental barriers, he can meld his mind with the thoughts and feelings of another intelligence through the physical contact of his fingers. This is difficult for Mr. Spock as it reveals to him and others the exquisite range of his human emotions and his capacity for total empathy. With his distinguished Vulcan heritage, Sarek expected Spock to enter the Vulcan Science Academy. Spock realized his mixed heritage would never be accepted on Vulcan. Thus, he entered the Space Academy, gaining acceptance and fame on the basis of his talents and abilities. This was a logical decision, but Sarek disagreed as it ran counter to Sarek's sense of duty to the family and Vulcan tradition. For eighteen years, father and son did not speak. Can Vulcan logic be flawed?

Parallel Development of Spock and the Ego-Ideal

The growth and development of Spock and the mature ego-ideal have many parallels. At first glance, Spock appears as a faintly devilish creature who evokes conscious or unconscious associations to the fires of hell, the volcanic eruptions of sexuality, and aggression. Next, we note that, even for a Star Fleet officer, his grooming is impeccable. In a full, low-pitched voice, he speaks with authority and at times an annoying preciseness. His movements are laconic but decisive and without extraneous gestures. These images fuse into an impression of violent forces under strict control (Vulcan history) but also of the history of the id, ego, and superego. His physical, emotional, and intellectual control, combined with high functional capacity, imply that this is not latency, whereas his function in the script, his conflicts, and his behavior point to adolescence. Who, more than the adolescent, feels a part of two worlds, child and adult, yet belongs to neither? Who, more than the adolescent, feels compelled to criticize the discrepancies in the adult world? Unlike latency, Spock's behavior reflects the extremes that are the hallmarks of adolescence—the urgent and virulent reemergence of oedipal drives and attendant demands for control and mastery. Emergency measures are needed, and the ego responds with defenses of regression and reaction formations to all earlier phases. For example, in reaction to oral drives, Mr. Spock needs little sleep and can go for long periods without food or water. His rigid vegetarian diet and revulsion to meat control his oral aggression (cannibalistic fantasies). Derivatives of this drive are seen occasionally in Spock's biting sarcasm. Reaction to anal drives can be seen in his fastidiousness. The basic Vulcan tenets of nonviolence and suppression of all emotion from birth reflect reaction to all three phases—oral, anal, and phallic. His asceticism is profound, reflecting the strength of the drives it opposes. Even Vulcan hairstyle resembles a Franciscan monk. However, his insatiable curiosity and the Pon Farr clearly indicate that the conflict is predominantly oedipal. Biologic potency indicates at least puberty. During the Pon Farr, Vulcans are sanctioned to kill rivals for a mate, and they die if their mating is not consummated. In Spock, we see both the punishing and the loving aspects of the superego. Failure to follow Vulcan prohibitions brings acute shame and guilt. Identification with his father's interest in science and adherence to Vulcan values gives him a sense of worth and pride.

As described earlier, the mature ego-ideal emerges in late adolescence, following the resolution of negative oedipal strivings. Jacobson (1964, p. 187) noted, "The final stages in the development of the ego-ideal demonstrate beautifully the hierarchical recognition and final integration of different—earlier and later—value concepts, arising from both systems (ego and superego), into a new, coherent structure and functional unit." When the maturing ego-ideal engages the services of the ego, it achieves some autonomy and weakens the punitive power of the superego. We see this occur in Spock, particularly in his relationship with Kirk. It is also built into the evolution of the series format.

Consider this formulation: prior to entering the Star Fleet Academy, Spock is faced with an adolescent crisis. Spock's father is authoritative, stern, and demanding. Unintentionally, Spock's mother, Amanda, is seductive. She loves both sides of Spock, but wishes he could acknowledge his human half—her. Is she not sometimes lonely? Could Spock not share with her some things that Sarek cannot? Could this be why Sarek demanded, and Spock complied, that Spock behave more Vulcan than Vulcans? Spock is probably smarter than his father. Following in his footsteps, Spock might surpass Sarek, symbolically eliminating him as a rival for his mother's love. Although he has renounced his human heritage, his mother, Vulcans never completely accept him. Maybe they do not believe him; neither do we. In his valiant efforts to out-Vulcan Vulcans, he gains Sarek's admiration. If he stopped his development here, Spock would be an admirable, but irritating, obsessional. The potential for a more intimate relationship with his father would evoke homosexual strivings and a wish to be in a passive, feminine position with respect to Sarek. It seems a "logical imperative" that Spock leave Vulcan to study at the Space Academy, thereby renouncing his aggressive-libidinal attachment to both parents. It is at this phase that we first see him.

As the series progresses, he gradually internalizes the values of both parents, human and Vulcan, by modifying his identification with his father. This occurs, in part, because violence is often necessary in the space service as part of the duty to protect the United Federation of Planets, which includes both Earth and Vulcan. Spock's close relationship to his captains, first Captain Pike, then Kirk, facilitates this action. Both can command him, but they are more his peers, more flexible and less threatening than his father. Under their orders, Spock can be more aggressive and even command the ship. However, they also respect Spock, taking his advice and modifying their actions. Kirk and Spock are complementary, as different as salt and pepper (Nimoy 1975). This is also true of Nimoy and Shatner, the actor who portrays Kirk. Similar friendships often occur as a normal part of adolescent development. We observe them when a brainy kid becomes best friends with a "jock," who is usually also a sexual athlete. Both learn from

59

the other. Kirk's heterosexuality is legion, which allows Spock more freedom to feel and act pleasurably heterosexual, if only occasionally and under unusual circumstances. This is in marked contrast to when Spock reverts to the Vulcan mode at the time of Pon Farr, as in the episode "Amok Time," when his sexuality strips away his veneer of civilization and brings a madness that almost destroys him and his captain. Because the Spock-Kirk relationship is desexualized, Spock can be effective and masculine and gradually allow himself to express his maternal/human half. Through the years, he becomes more understanding, patient, and caring. His relationship with Kirk deepens as they become something more than brothers or close friends, willing to sacrifice all they have or are for each other. Spock and especially Kirk have love affairs, but neither marries. Aside from the fact that this would probably ruin the plot, it implies some incompletion in their development, their autonomy.

Spock's loyalty to Kirk is above and beyond duty or friendship.[3] They are bound together, like two parts of a whole, in their mutual devotion (sublimated love) to each other and to their mother ship, the *Enterprise,* and her crew. The three central characters, Kirk, Spock, and McCoy, are all flawed. Were they perfect, they would be as unbelievable as the early comic book heroes whose strengths were acquired magically. We care for them because their search for new worlds and new life forms is as much in their inner space as in outer space. We watch them struggle, strive, and grow. The mature ego-ideal is, by definition, a continuing endeavor. Outstanding as Spock's disciplined intellect, strength, and skills are, combined with his unselfishness, loyalty, and courage, he is not a superman but superhuman, a metaphor for a heroic mature ego-ideal.

Added to these formulations, the following data are significant. In the first pilot, the executive officer, second in command, was a slim dark woman of indeterminate age, named Number One. More efficient and knowledgeable of the ship's equipment and personnel than the captain, she had an expressionless, cool manner with the strength and respect to become acting commander. However, Number One also was romantically attached to the captain. The manifest reason for NBC's eliminating her was that no female could have command responsibilities. A better reason was her romance with the captain, which limited his involvement with other women. But the Captain needed an executive officer. Desexualizing the role for Mr. Spock, he acquired her qualities, but not her gender, adding depth and interest to his character.

Roddenberry stated (Lichtenberg, Marshak, and Winston 1975, p. 144), "Kirk and Spock were sort of dream images of myself. Two sides of me . . . of my own fantasies. . . . At the beginning . . . 'Star Trek' was my baby. . . . Everyone on it was some expression of some dream very personal to me." He carefully selected all major members of the cast and production crew, choosing Majel Barrett to act Number One. In the series, she was recast as Nurse Chappell, whose unrequited love for Mr. Spock emphasized his alien nature. It is not surprising that, at the end of the third season, Majel Barrett symbolically married both Mr. Spock and her captain in her marriage to the real character of Gene Roddenberry.

Much of Spock's magnetism is Leonard Nimoy. Learning more about Nimoy helps expand some of the negative oedipal issues. A consummate actor, he has an exceptional sensitivity to nuances of character. Prior to portraying Spock, Nimoy valued expressing emotions in his work. Through Spock, he learned the value of restraint. Like Spock, he is intense, articulate, dignified, demanding of himself, and constantly seeking challenge and growth in his life. It seems likely that Roddenberry was attracted to Nimoy's personal integrity as much as his professional skills. Nimoy respected Roddenberry but had to be seduced by Roddenberry's ideas and idealism. This sublimated union produced Spock. Nimoy's capacity to bring to the forefront elements of himself that define Spock and voluntarily suspend his own reality as Nimoy gave Spock life. Ruefully, Nimoy (1975, p. 19) once commented, "Oh, how he lives." At the end of the series, he made a virtual three-year crusade to dissociate himself from Spock and reestablish Leonard Nimoy as an individual and an actor. In addition to publishing two books of poetry and photography, he received critical acclaim for his acting in a variety of roles. Despite professional recognition and personal satisfaction, Mr. Spock followed him everywhere, even while performing different characters. His voyage away from Spock parallels Spock's sojourn on Vulcan to erase his human half. Neither attempt succeeded. In the first "Star Trek" movie, returning to the *Enterprise* after a three-year absence, Spock says Kirk can never know the price it cost him to return to the *Enterprise*. Spock might be speaking for Nimoy as well.

Nevertheless, Nimoy (1975) knew he wanted this birth and worked harder physically for Spock than for other roles. However, he noted that somewhere he lost control and felt possessed by this alien life. Six years after completing the role, Nimoy wrote how the character of Spock changed his life and, in a sense, gave him a career. "It also

61

affected me very deeply and personally, socially, psychologically and emotionally. To this day I sense Vulcan speech patterns, Vulcan social attitudes, and even Vulcan patterns of logic and emotional suppression in my behavior. . . . It became a constant and ongoing influence in my thinking and lifestyle" (pp. 22–23). Perhaps Spock seems so real because he became a real part of Nimoy, in terms of being an important aspect of Nimoy's mature ego-ideal. Powerful ideas, illusions, apparently can change reality.

Conclusions

We know the Vulcan tenet of total emotional suppression is fallacious. Although Vulcan is a hypothetical planet, we know it exists because we know Vulcans. They are us. "Being cool," unemotional, is our misconception of "having it all together." Total suppression or denial of emotions leads to catatonic states; to psychosis, not health; to loss of reality, not intellectual achievement. Spock's internal and external struggles are ours. We meet prejudice everyday, our own and others'. His alienation from those around him, from himself, is us. He is Everyman. His ability gradually to resolve his conflicts gives us hope. If he can, maybe we can. At least we can try. His triumph could be ours. Facing problems, whatever the difficulties or pain, he strives for solutions and actions helpful to himself and others. Neither wild savage nor cold computer, he has assimilated and accommodated to the best of both his parents' worlds, Vulcan and Earth, male and female, ego and id.

Paradoxically, in our culture, which values conformity, an alien became a hero. We all have "pointed ears" we try to hide. Spock lives with his and does so with dignity. Accepting what cannot be changed, he devotes his energies to what can. Outer space can be less terrifying if we conquer our inner space, our own inner fears of raging monsters. With reason (logic combined with compassion), we can understand, tame, even come to love, what scares us most. Despite the tragedies, chaos, and despair that the media records or we experience, this series, this character, encourages us not to retreat or give up but to reenter or continue in our everyday lives. Nimoy says (Lichtenberg, Marshak, and Winston 1975, p. 74) that people view Spock as a person they would want to spend time with as he could know and understand them in a way no one else could. "He would know what I mean when I tell

him how I feel. He would have insight that nobody else seems to have.
. . . He would acknowledge . . . verify my existence in a way that few
other people would." This sounds like an ideal psychiatrist, a metaphor
for our own mature ego-ideal.[4]

NOTES

Based on the author's talk to the North Texas Branch of the American
Society for Adolescent Psychiatry, Dallas, March 12, 1986.

1. "The Cage" was later incorporated into the two-part "The Me-
nagerie," among the best and most popular episodes of the television
series.

2. Nimoy invented the neck pinch, objecting to a script requiring
Spock to assault an adversary from behind, anathema to Vulcan mores.

3. He denies any "affection," maintaining that his interest is logical
as Kirk is an unusually good commander and the odds are against
getting a better replacement.

4. Another excellent summary is provided by Kirk's words at the
end of the second movie. Believing Spock dead, at his space burial,
Kirk said (McIntyre 1982, p. 215), "Of my friend, I can only say that
of all the souls that I have encountered, his was the most human."

REFERENCES

Bacon-Smith, C. 1986. Spock among women. *New York Times Book Review* (November 16, 1986), p. 1.

Bettelheim, B. 1976. *The Uses of Enchantment.* New York: Knopf.

Blish, J. 1972. *"Star Trek" 6.* New York: Bantam.

Blos, P. 1974. The genealogy of the ego ideal. *Psychoanalytic Study of the Child* 29:43–88.

Bornstein, B. 1951. On Latency. *Psychoanalytic Study of the Child* 6:279–285.

Freud, S. 1908. Creative writers and daydreaming. *Standard Edition* 9:141–154. London: Hogarth, 1971.

Freud, S. 1923. The ego and the id. *Standard Edition* 19:3–66. London: Hogarth, 1961.

Gerrold, D. 1973. *The World of "Star Trek."* New York: Ballantine.

Hartmann, H. 1958. *Ego Psychology and the Problem of Adaptation.* New York: International Universities Press.

Jacobson, E. 1964. *The Self and the Object World*. New York: International Universities Press.

Lichtenberg, J.; Marshak, S.; and Winston, J. 1975. *"Star Trek" Lives*. New York: Bantam.

Loewald, H. 1973. On Internalization. In *Papers on Psychoanalysis*. New Haven, Conn.: Yale University Press, 1980.

McIntyre, V. 1982. *"Star Trek": The Wrath of Khan*. New York: Pocket.

Moore, B., and Fine, B. 1968. *A Glossary of Psychoanalytic Terms and Concepts*. New York: American Psychoanalytic Association.

Nimoy, L. 1975. *I Am Not Spock*. Millbrae, Calif.: Celestial.

Sandler, J. 1960. On the concept superego. *Psychoanalytic Study of the Child* 15:128–162.

Whitfield, S., and Roddenberry, G. 1968. *The Making of "Star Trek."* New York: Ballantine.

Widzer, M. 1977. The comic book superhero: a study of the family romance fantasy. *Psychoanalytic Study of the Child* 22:565–603.

PART II

CREATIVITY AND ADOLESCENCE

CREATIVITY AND ADOLESCENCE:
INTRODUCTION TO SPECIAL SECTION

HARVEY A. HOROWITZ

We shall know a little more by dint of rigor and imagination, the two great contraries of mental process, either of which by itself is lethal. Rigor alone is paralytic death, but imagination alone is insanity. [Bateson 1979]

Rigor and Imagination: Creativity and the Great Contraries

The story is told of Jean Piaget that, when a colleague spoke of an interest in studying creativity, the Swiss psychologist skeptically replied, "Tout y touche" (Everything bears on it). Indeed, the idea of the unmanageable, even unknowable, nature of creativity deterred serious inquiry for many years. Nevertheless, Piaget's colleague, Howard Gruber, went on to do his psychological study of scientific creativity, *Darwin on Man,* which contributed to and reflects the emergence of creativity as a legitimate domain of scientific inquiry and discourse (Gruber 1981). More important, today creativity and the related subjects mind, metaphor, and symbol are a focus for the combined interests of dynamic psychiatrists, cognitive and developmental psychologists, artists, poets, and philosophers. It is in this interdisciplinary spirit that the American Society for Adolescent Psychiatry held a conference on the theme of creativity in Philadelphia in September 1986.

Meetings and symposia on creativity are generally greeted with excitement in many quarters of the intellectual community. Reflecting on this response, one is struck by the intensity with which the topic brings forth an acute awareness of change, a sense of something happening. This sense may in part have to do with the historical shift in the root metaphor of science in the twentieth century, a shift from the mechanistic and reductionistic metaphor of the machine to the constructivist metaphor of the symbol. Related, and perhaps even more compelling, are more fundamental discussions of creativity and mind that focus attention on what Bateson called the "great contraries" and lead to the experience and exploration of the tensions immanent in a world of opposites, of polarities. Four of Bateson's "great contraries" are central to any discussion of creativity.

SUBJECT OBJECT

The subject-object contrary distinguishes and articulates the tension present in the relationship of the subjective experience of ourselves, the knower, and our descriptions of that experience, the construction of an objective self and world, the known. The subjective experience, and the meaningful whole made of it, provides us with our knowledge, our personal epistemology, for we have no direct access to our environment, what Kant called the *Ding an Sich*. We have only our symbols, metaphors, and languages with which to refer and to express that universal experience. Those who bring a unique sensibility and awareness of the unity of the subject-object duality in human experience, and express it in a particular medium, are the creative, the artists and poets among us.

A more specific form of the subject-object dualism is seen in the integration of cognition and motivation in the lived life of the creative individual, where affects, motives, and wishes arise in the subjective experience, providing the contents, the "what," of creative products. Simultaneously, cognition, the ordering and organizing of experience, the skill and technique that provides the "how," gives outline and structure to creative activity.

Nowhere in the life cycle is this subject-object dynamic more intense and apparent than in the universal experience of adolescence and in the unique developmental transitions of the gifted adolescent. Here motivations and goals are reintegrated with newly acquired cognitive abilities and emerging talents into an identity. It is in the flowering of

68

adolescence that the gifted child develops into a working, creative adult.

NATURE NURTURE

The nature-nurture contrary distinguishes and articulates the tension immanent in the relationship of the biological individual and the environment. This dynamic dialectic process has long been rigidly reified into two poles, with thinking and research in the field of creativity reflecting a more broadly held scientific and cultural model. In this view one pole reflects the assertion that creativity is biological endowment, intelligence, or trait, while the opposite pole reflects the assertion that creativity is a stimulating and reinforcing environment at work on a tabula rasa.

Recently, this static general model has been challenged, and a more dynamic view has been put forth by Csikszentmihalyi and Robinson (1986), Feldman (1980), and Gardner (1986). Grounding their work in the constructivist developmental model of Piaget, these investigators hold that talent cannot be observed except against a backdrop of well-specified cultural expectations. In this view, creativity is a relation between culturally defined opportunities for action and personal skills or capacities to act. Four vectors describe and express this relation over time: (1) the psychosocial, which examines change in the organization of motives across the life span of the individual, as in Erikson's epigenetic schema; (2) the cognitive, which examines the transitions between the stages, marking the discontinuous reorganizations in the way the individual thinks, as in the genetic epistomology of Piaget; (3) the domain, which examines culturally structured bodies of knowledge, as in mathematics, music, or poetry, each of which has its own principal structures, operations, and patterns of opportunity; (4) the social field, defined as the social organization within which the individual and the domain exist and interact, the surrounding, supportive, and changing sociohistoric context.

This "evolving systems approach" (Gruber 1981) maintains that creativity and the creative process, the genius of a Freud or an Einstein, can be understood only as a unity, a systemic integration of a specific biopsychological potential interacting with a ripe domain at a particular moment in a unique sociohistorical context. In this vision of creativity as a necessary unity, we begin to see a synthesis of the givenness of biology-nature and the unpredictability of experience-nurture.

UNCONSCIOUS CONSCIOUS

Though Pascal taught us that "the heart has reasons the reason knows not of," our Cartesian epistemology split the mental world into an irrational unconscious and a rational conscious. Freud called this division the primary and secondary processes, with unconscious primary process, including the intuitive and the figurative modes of knowing, and the conscious secondary process, including the analytic and linear modes of knowing. Langer (1942), in *Philosophy in a New Key,* makes a similar distinction between two forms of symbolism. The discursive form, analogous to the secondary process, consisting of words and mathematical symbols, is abstract and logical. The presentational form, analogous to primary process, presents organized, complex, and meaningful information in metaphor, as in a dream, painting, or ritual.

Whereas it was once held, particularly in Western science, that these two ways of knowing were separate, distinct, and as unrelated as a theorem and a dream, reflection on the creative process in art, poetry, science, and psychotherapy, as in the work of Arieti (1976) and Bateson (1972), produces a different view.

Bateson writes that the unconscious is what is most deeply learned and most profoundly known, both in the root metaphors, myths, and rituals of a culture and in the structured constellation of beliefs, skills, and values of an individual. The unconscious embraces the implicit meanings and metaphors from which our explicit meanings and metaphors are built. This "knowing" is always personal and subjective, a knowing learned in contexts of relation, abstraction, and analogy found in the experience of things and persons. In contrast, conscious secondary process is knowing of an objective, real world wherein we talk with the grammatical logic of language about things and persons as if they existed independently of the observer and the conversation.

The creative process, in this view, is the integration of the unconscious ways of knowing in image and context with conscious ways of knowing in language and logic, or what Arieti (1976) calls "the magic synthesis."

70

RIGOR AND IMAGINATION

The last contrary, referred to by Bateson in the epigraph as rigor and imagination, embraces the preceding three and draws us to the realization that the human creative process is a minor version of the great stochastic processes of life. As with evolution, human creative activity has two fundamental characteristics. It is a dynamic system dependent on a stable organization or structure (rigor) interacting with a source of the random (imagination) and thus giving rise, unpredictably, to the new. While the process produces change, it conserves its own organization and is, therefore, self-organizing and self-regenerating.

This process of autonomously generating change while regenerating structure seems analogous to the central and universal mission of the developmental unity we call the self, that is, to construct meaning out of the ambiguous flux of the world. The creative person, unlike universal man, strives for and risks more, bringing a unique meaning—making activity and sensibility to the diverse possibilities provided by both conscious and unconscious experience and the inner and outer environments. The visionary makes a poem or a painting in the acutely experienced moment, while the rest of us pass by, blindly.

The idea suggested here is that the pairs of opposites, of which rigor and imagination, order and chaos, are the most basic, put tension into the world, a tension that sharpens our sensitivity and roughens our awareness of ourselves and, perhaps more important, of our interrelatedness and interdependency. This awareness is the core of empathy and our aesthetic, empathic, and creative activities, be they painting or dreaming, science or psychotherapy.

Perhaps Piaget was correct that everything bears on creativity, and we might add that creativity bears on everything. Certainly, in reading the chapters to follow there will be unfamiliar ideas and unexpected images, bringing forth the tension immanent in the relation of order and chaos. It is hoped that, on reading these essays, the reader will, with rigor and imagination, construct new metaphors.

Creativity, Constructivism, and Experience

Constructivism is that branch of philosophy and science that holds that there is no objective reality independent of an observer and no objects independent of the observer's experiences and descriptions of objects, be they experiences of persons or landscapes. Constructivism does not deny an environment but posits that we cannot know one directly, and so we devote the totality of our mental faculties, our cognition, to the construction of a world of models and metaphors.

Freud founded his psychoanalysis on the constructivist premise of psychic reality and the dynamic, symbolic unconscious. Piaget based his developmental psychology on the transformations in the child's construction of reality. Surely, creative individuals, poets, painters, and therapists, whose lives are focused on the construction of meaning through the use of symbol, are reality and world makers.

The question then arises as to how such worlds are made, how such realities are constructed. This is the subject of Heinz von Foerster's classic lecture "On Constructing a Reality," originally delivered in 1973. In this chapter one of the founders of cybernetics and modern constructivism explores the steps of this process from first premises, that is, from the realization that the environment as we perceive it is our invention, to the neurophysiological mechanisms of these perceptions and cognitions, and, finally, to the ethical and aesthetic imperatives drawn from these constructs.

Howard Gardner and Constance Wolf, in their chapter, focus on a synthetic-scientific approach to the psychology of creativity. Adopting a systems and dialectic model, they describe five perspectives that must be integrated into a process view of creativity. First are (1) subpersonal-biological and (2) personal-cognitive, in which is described Gardner's theory of multiple intelligences. Here the authors cite Freud's unique blend of talents in logical-mathematical, interpersonal, and linguistic domains and Picasso's talents in visual-spatial and kinesthetic domains. Then follow (3) personal-emotional, having to do with personality, affect, and motive; (4) impersonal-domain, bodies of knowledge as in music or mathematics; and (5) multipersonal-field, a sociological concept consisting of people in roles, institutions, and other social entities. The creative individual, from this systems-interactive view, is marked not by synchrony across and within levels but by asynchrony; not by a perfect match but by a mismatch. It is through asynchronies that the possibility arises of new creations.

The poet C. K. Williams, in his chapter "Poetry and Consciousness," focuses on the complex relation of emotion, consciousness, and language and specifically on the imprecision and reflective uncertainty of language in describing experience and emotion. He puts forth the view that the construction of images from the interior world onto the "screen of consciousness," and the extension of this image making to narrative and fantasy, is the major activity of the poet's mind. Moreover, this constant flow of image, narrative, and language is arbitrary and non-determined. It is the arbitrary, unpredictable character of mental phenomena, which is the foundation of imagination.

With the indeterminateness and simultaneity of mental events as first premise, emotions are held by Williams to be complex, ambiguous, and perhaps unknowable. He maintains that, if one is to know one's soul, there is need for "education"; the most useful method for that education, Williams contends, is the poem. He concludes the essay by describing and giving an example of how the poem speaks of emotion and consciousness to the soul of man.

Painter and teacher Frank Galuszka, in his chapter "Art and Inspiration," asserts that artwork is an accumulation of decisions, solutions to problems formulated according to code or intuition. In order to make decisions, each artist carries a mental catalog of alternative possibilities. No catalog is comprehensive but rather provides economy, constraint, and tension. Galuszka describes the operation of the catalog as a rapid, dynamic process, involving a continuous flow of imagery "streaking through the mind," a "parade of imagery" moving to colution and leading to visualization, the projection of the internal image the artist wants to see on the canvas.

Galuszka's visualization, the projection of the internal image, is not a linear, logical process but rather a process of synthesis and symbolization that brings together intuitive openness and critical faculties in inspiration. Inspirations are proposals arising out of "floating configurations of catalog possibilities past the problem." These proposals are "keys to locks," which never fit the actual artwork, but lead, through empathy, to mysterious solutions. Galuszka concludes with the assertion that works of art are not ideas but models, samples of mind proclaiming the presence of human consciousness, which can be appreciated but never exhausted.

The Psychology and Psychopathology of Art

In the "Puzzle of Art," psychologist Ellen Winner notes that relatively little attention has been paid to the study of the arts by psychology despite the fact that artistic activity has, from earliest times, accompanied the evolution of human culture. This neglect has, in part, been due to the perception that the arts are mysterious and not open to empirical study. As a consequence, even a satisfactory definition of art remains a modern problem for those interested in the studies of the psychology of art. Winner presents a new definition of art that may have pragmatic usefulness to psychology. Grounded in the work of Nelson Goodman, she defines artwork as aesthetic symbol with three features: relative syntactic repleteness, metaphorical exemplification, and nontransparency. With the definition of artwork as aesthetic symbol, Winner goes on to describe a psychology of art that examines the artistic process from the point of view of the two essential questions. What motivates the artist to create? What cognitive processes are involved in the creating of art? It is these questions that now seem amenable to empirical study.

The relation of art and psychopathology, a complex and controversial matter that has fascinated since Plato, is approached in Aaron H. Esman's chapter, from the standpoint of "outsider" art. Outsider art is work produced by persons frequently psychotic, at the least eccentric, who operate outside the norms of art and the art world and who are untrained and seemingly unaware of the coda. Surveying this outsider art in the twentieth century, particularly that work collected and studied by Hans Prinzhorn, a German art historian and psychiatrist, Esman addresses the essential theoretical questions, Does psychopathology generate or unharness creativity? Does psychopathology preclude creative achievement? In those disturbed individuals who do produce artwork, does the work contribute to the reintegration of the personality and the organization of experience? Esman concludes in agreement with Prinzhorn, Dubuffet, and Kris that at the core of the creative process is the urge for order, symbolization, formalization, and communication. This is true of artists as well as outsiders and is the message of outsider art. The related question, What is art then? seems to have more to do, in Esman's view, with the sociohistoric context and the perceptions of the audience.

Creativity and Psychotherapy

Psychotherapy as an artful human activity that has much in common with other forms of creative work is a view held by many psychotherapists and is the focus of the chapters by Russell E. Phillips and E. James Anthony.

Phillips explores the analogy between the tasks of the jazz improvisor and the creative psychotherapist, where improvisation means the simultaneous creation and execution of ideas. Though psychotherapists use their preferred theories and methods as guidelines, the actual conduct of a given session is highly individualized and thus is improvisational. Phillips defines four psychological characteristics of the improvisor, jazz musician or psychotherapist, that must be integrated with fundamental technical mastery: access to the past; the ability to focus attention intensely on the present; comfort in relaxing control and experimenting; and recognition of the significance of accident. The author presents clinical examples of his own use of improvisation and personal metaphor in the psychotherapy of a hospitalized adolescent.

Through a series of clinical vignettes depicting encounters with gifted adolescent patients, Anthony eloquently demonstrates the unfolding of the creative process in psychoanalytic psychotherapy. The gifted adolescent, intelligent and witty beyond her years, curious, spontaneous, flexible, and filled with the urge to explore, brings a great deal to psychotherapy. When gifted patient and gifted therapist share the same space, the therapist is "grasped" by a process in which imagination and play are primary. Acknowledging his debt to Winnicott, Anthony asserts that the capacity to play is an expression of the therapist's creativity and a source of creativity to the patient, particularly vital to the creative process of psychotherapy with gifted adolescents. Anthony looks beyond the creative forces within the patient and within the therapist to the contribution of the context, the psychotherapeutic situation, which he calls a "stage" for the externalization of internal representations. Believing that the most creative aspect of psychodynamic psychotherapy may be the way in which the past grows out of the present, Anthony draws the analogy between the artistic act and the therapeutic situation, each involving the articulation of the forbidden, unattainable, and the repressed, each fundamentally a making-meaning enterprise.

REFERENCES

Arieti, S. 1976. *Creativity: The Magic Synthesis*. New York: Basic.
Bateson, G. 1972. Style, grace, and information in primitive art. In G. Bateson. *The Steps to an Ecology of Mind*. New York: Chandler.

Bateson, G. 1979. *Mind and Nature*. New York: Dutton.

Csikszentmihalyi, M., and Robinson, R. E. 1986. Culture, time, and the development of talent. In R. J. Sternberg and J. E. Davidson, eds. *Conceptions of Giftedness*. New York: Cambridge University Press.

Feldman, D. H. 1980. *Beyond Universals in Cognitive Development*. Norwood, N.J.: Ablex.

Gardner, H. 1986. Freud in three frames: a cognitive-scientific approach to creativity. *Daedalus* 115(3): 105–134.

Gruber, H. E. 1979. The evolving systems approach to creativity. In S. Modgil and C. Modgil, eds. *Toward a Theory of Psychological Development*. Windsor: NFER.

Gruber, H. E. 1981. *Darwin on Man: A Psychological Study of Scientific Creativity*. 2d ed. Chicago: University of Chicago Press.

Langer, S. K. 1942. *Philosophy in a New Key*. Cambridge, Mass.: Harvard University Press.

5 ON CONSTRUCTING A REALITY

HEINZ VON FOERSTER

Draw a distinction! [Brown 1972, p. 3]

The Postulate

I am sure you remember the plain citizen Jourdain in Molière's *Le bourgeois gentilhomme* who, nouveau riche, travels in the sophisticated circles of the French aristocracy and who is eager to learn. On one occasion his new friends speak about poetry and prose, and Jourdain discovers to his amazement and great delight that whenever he speaks, he speaks prose. He is overwhelmed by this discovery: "I am speaking Prose! I have always spoken Prose! I have spoken Prose throughout my whole life!"

A similar discovery has been made not so long ago, but it was neither of poetry nor of prose—it was the environment that was discovered. I remember when, perhaps ten or fifteen years ago, some of my American friends came running to me with the delight and amazement of having just made a great discovery: "I am living in an Environment! I have always lived in an Environment! I have lived in an Environment throughout my whole life!"

However, neither M. Jourdain nor my friends have as yet made another discovery, and that is when M. Jourdain speaks, may it be prose or poetry, it is he who invents it, and, likewise, when we perceive our environment, it is we who invent it.

Every discovery has a painful and a joyful side: painful, while struggling with a new insight; joyful, when this insight is gained. I see the sole purpose of my presentation to minimize the pain and maximize the joy for those who have not yet made this discovery; and for those who have made it, to let them know they are not alone. Again, the discovery we all have to make for ourselves is the following postulate.

The environment as we perceive it is our invention. The burden is now upon me to support this outrageous claim. I shall proceed by first inviting you to participate in an experiment; then I shall report a clinical case and the results of two other experiments. After this I will give an interpretation, and thereafter a highly compressed version of the neurophysiological basis of these experiments and my postulate of before. Finally, I shall attempt to suggest the significance of all that to aesthetical and ethical considerations.

Experiments

The blind spot. Hold book with right hand, close left eye, and fixate star of figure 1 with right eye. Move book slowly back and forth along line of vision until at an appropriate distance (from about 12 to 14 inches) round black spot disappears. With star well focused, spot should remain invisible even if book is slowly moved parallel to itself in any direction.

This localized blindness is a direct consequence of the absence of photo receptors (rods or cones) at that point of the retina, the "disk," where all fibers leading from the eye's light-sensitive surface converge to form the optic nerve. Clearly, when the black spot is projected onto the disk, it cannot be seen. Note that this localized blindness is not perceived as a dark blotch in our visual field (seeing a dark blotch would imply "seeing"), but this blindness is not perceived at all, that is, neither as something present, nor as something absent: whatever is perceived is perceived "blotchless."

Scotoma. Well-localized occipital lesions in the brain (e.g., injuries from high-velocity projectiles) heal relatively fast without the patient's awareness of any perceptible loss in his vision. However, after several weeks motor dysfunction in the patient becomes apparent, for example,

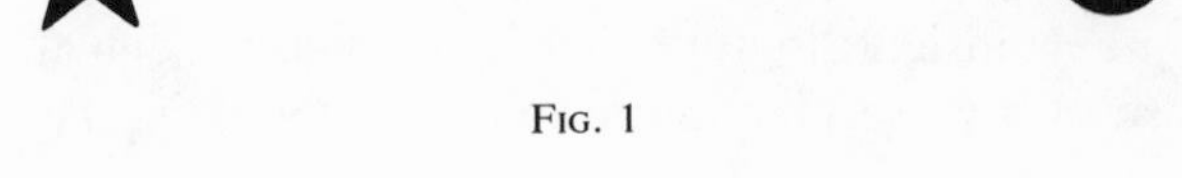

Fig. 1

loss of control of arm or leg movements of one side or the other. Clinical tests, however, show that there is nothing wrong with the motor system, but that in some cases there is substantial loss (fig. 2) of a large portion of the visual field (*scotoma*) (Teuber 1961). A successful therapy consists of blindfolding the patient over a period of one to two months until he regains control over his motor system by shifting his "attention" from (nonexistent) visual clues regarding his posture to (fully operative) channels that give direct postural clues from (proprioceptive) sensors embedded in muscles and joints. Note again absence of perception of "absence of perception," and also the emergence of perception through sensorimotor interaction. This prompts two metaphors: perceiving is doing; and if I don't see I am blind, I am blind, but if I see I am blind, I see.

Alternates. A single word is spoken once into a tape recorder and the tape smoothly spliced (without click) into a loop. The word is repetitively played back with high rather than low volume. After one or two minutes of listening (from fifty to 150 repetitions), the word clearly perceived so far abruptly changes into another meaningful and clearly perceived word: an "alternate." After ten to thirty repetitions of this first alternate, a sudden switch to a second alternate is perceived, and so on (Naeser and Lilly 1971). The following is a small selection of the 758 alternates reported from a population of about 200 subjects who were exposed to a repetitive playback of the single word "cogitate": "agitate," "annotate," "arbitrate," "artistry," "back and forth," "brevity," "ça d'était," "candidate," "can't you see," "can't you stay," "Cape Cod you say," "card estate," "cardiotape," "car district," "catch a tape," "cavitate," "cha cha che," "cogitate," "computate," "conjugate," "conscious state," "counter tape," "count to ten," "count to three," "count yer tape," "cut the steak," "entity," "fantasy," "God to take," "God you say," "got a date," "got your

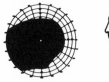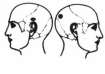

F<small>IG</small>. 2

79

pay," "got your tape," "gratitude," "gravity," "guard the tit," "gurgitate," "had to take," "kinds of tape," "majesty," "marmalade."

Comprehension.[1]   Into the various stations of the auditory pathways in a cat's brain microelectrodes are implanted that allow a recording (electroencephalogram) from the nerve cells first to receive auditory stimuli (cochlea nucleus, CN) up to the auditory cortex (Worden 1959). The cat so prepared is admitted into a cage that contains a food box whose lid can be opened by pressing a lever. However, the lever-lid connection is operative only when a short single tone (here C_6, which is about 1,000 hertz) is repetitively presented. The cat has to learn that C_6"means" food. Figures 3–6 show the pattern of nervous activity at eight ascending auditory stations and at four consecutive stages of this learning process. The cat's behavior associated with the recorded neural activity is for "random search" in figure 3, "inspection of lever" in figure 4, "lever pressed at once" in figure 5, and "walking straight toward lever (full comprehension)" in figure 6. Note that no tone is perceived as long as this tone is uninterpretable (figs. 3–4, pure noise), but the whole system swings into action with the appearance of the first "beep" (figs. 5–6, noise becomes signal), when sensation becomes comprehensible, when *our* perception of "beep, beep, beep" is in the *cat's* perception "food, food, food."

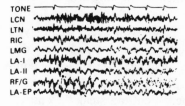

Fig. 3.—Session 3, trial 1

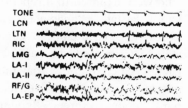

Fig. 4.—Session 3, trial 13

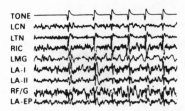

Fig. 5.—Session 4, trial 20

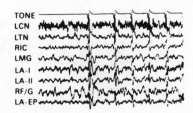

Fig. 6.—Session 6, trial 9

Interpretation

In these experiments I have cited instances in which we see or hear what is not "there," or in which we do not see or hear what is "there" unless coordination of sensation and movement allows us to "grasp" what appears to be there. Let me strengthen this observation by citing now the "principle of undifferentiated encoding":

> The response of a nerve cell does *not* encode the physical nature of the agents that caused its response. Encoded is only "how much" at this point on my body, but not "what."

Take, for instance, a light-sensitive receptor cell in the retina, a "rod" that absorbs the electromagnetic radiation originating from a distant source. This absorption causes a change in the electrochemical potential in the rod, which will ultimately give rise to a periodic electric discharge of some cells higher up in the postretinal networks (see fig. 15 below), with a period that is commensurate with the intensity of the radiation absorbed, but without a clue that it was electromagnetic radiation that caused the rod to discharge. The same is true for any other sensory receptor, may it be the taste buds, the touch receptors, and all the other receptors that are associated with the sensations of smell, heat and cold, sound, and so on: they are all "blind" as to the quality of their stimulation, responsive only as to their quantity.

Although surprising, this should not come as a surprise, for indeed "out there" there is no light and no color, there are only electromagnetic waves; "out there" there is no sound and no music, there are only periodic variations of the air pressure; "out there" there is no heat and no cold, there are only moving molecules with more or less mean kinetic energy, and so on. Finally, for sure, "out there" there is no pain.

Since the physical nature of the stimulus—its *quality*—is not encoded into nervous activity, the fundamental question arises as to how does our brain conjure up the tremendous variety of this colorful world as we experience it any moment while awake, and sometimes in dreams while asleep. This is the "problem of cognition," the search for an understanding of the cognitive processes.

The way in which a question is asked determines the way in which an answer may be found. Thus it is upon me to paraphrase the "problem of cognition'' in such a way that the conceptual tools that are today at our disposal may become fully effective. To this end let me paraphrase (→) "cognition" in the following way:

cognition → computing a reality.

With this I anticipate a storm of objections. First, I appear to replace one unknown term "cognition," with three other terms, two of which, "computing" and "reality," are even more opaque than the definiendum, and with the only definite word used here being the indefinite article "a." Moreover, the use of the indefinite article implies the ridiculous notion of other realities besides *the* only and one reality, our cherished environment; and finally I seem to suggest by "computing" that everything, from my wristwatch to the galaxies, is merely computed, and is not "there." Outrageous!

Let me take up these objections one by one. First, let me remove the semantic sting that the term "computing" may cause in a group of women and men who are more inclined toward the humanities than to the sciences. Harmlessly enough, computing (from *com-putare*) literally means to reflect, to contemplate (*putare*) things in concert (*com*), without any explicit reference to numerical quantities. Indeed, I shall use this term in this most general sense to indicate any operation (not necessarily numerical) that transforms, modifies, rearranges, orders, and so on, observed physical entities ("objects") or their representations ("symbols"). For instance, the simple permutation of the three letters *a, b, c,* in which the last letter now goes first—*c, a, b*—I shall call a computation; similarly the operation that obliterates the commas between the letters—"cab"—and likewise the semantic transformation that changes "cab" into "taxi," and so on.

I shall now turn to the defense of my use of the indefinite article in the noun phrase "a reality." I could, of course, shield myself behind the logical argument that solving for the general case, implied by the "a," I would also have solved any specific case denoted by the use of "the." However, my motivation lies much deeper. In fact, there is a deep hiatus that separates the "the" school of thought from the "a" school of thought in which, respectively, the distinct concepts of "confirmation" and "correlation" are taken as explanatory paradigms for perceptions. The "the" school: my sensation of touch is *confirmation* for my visual sensation that here is a table. The "a" school: my sensation of touch in *correlation* with my visual sensation generates an experience that I may describe by "here is a table."

I am rejecting the "the" position on epistemological grounds, for in this way the whole problem of cognition is safely put away in one's own cognitive blind spot: even its absence can no longer be seen.

Finally one may rightly argue that cognitive processes do not compute wristwatches or galaxies, but compute at best *descriptions* of such entities. Thus I am yielding to this objection and replace my former paraphrase by

cognition → computing descriptions of a reality.

Neurophysiologists, however, will tell us (Maturana 1970b) that a description computed on one level of neural activity, say, a projected image on the retina, will be operated on again on higher levels, and so on, whereby some motor activity may be taken by an observer as a "terminal description," for instance, the utterance, "Here is a table." Consequently, I have to modify this paraphrase again to read

cognition → computing descriptions of ⌐

where the arrow turning back suggests this infinite recursion of descriptions of descriptions, et cetera. This formulation has the advantage that one unknown, namely, "reality," is successfully eliminated. Reality appears only implicit as the operation of recursive descriptions. Moreover, we may take advantage of the notion that computing descriptions is nothing else but computations. Hence

cognition → computations of ⌐

In summary, I propose to interpret cognitive processes as never-ending recursive processes of computation, and I hope that in the following tour de force of neurophysiology I can make this interpretation transparent.

Neurophysiology

Evolution. In order that the principle of recursive computation be fully appreciated as being the underlying principle of all cognitive processes—even of life itself, as one of the most advanced thinkers in biology assures me (Maturana 1970a)—it may be instructive to go back for a moment to the most elementary—or as evolutionists would say, to the very "early"—manifestations of this principle. These are the "independent effectors," or independent sensorimotor units, found in protozoa and metazoa distributed over the surface of these animals (fig. 7). The triangular portion of this unit, protruding with its tip from the surface, is the sensory part: the onion-shaped portion, the contractile motor part. A change in the chemical concentration of an agent in the immediate vicinity of the sensing tip, and "perceptible" by it, causes an instantaneous contraction of this unit. The resulting displacement of this or any other unit by change of shape of the animal or its location may, in turn, produce perceptible changes in the agent's concentration in the vicinity of these units, which, in turn, will cause their instantaneous contraction, and so on. Thus we have the recursion

⌐→change of sensation → change of shape ⌐

Separation of the sites of sensation and action appears to have been the next evolutionary step (fig. 8). The sensory and motor organs are now connected by thin filaments, the "axons" (in essence degenerated muscle fibers having lost their contractility), which transmit the sensor's perturbations to its effector, thus giving rise to the concept of a "signal": see something here, act accordingly there.

The crucial step, however, in the evolution of the complex organization of the mammalian central nervous system (CNS) appears to be the appearance of an "internuncial neuron," a cell sandwiched between the sensory and the motor unit (fig. 9). It is, in essence, a sensory cell, but specialized so as to respond only to a universal "agent," namely,

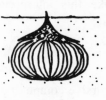

FIG. 7

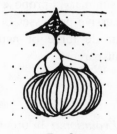

FIG. 8

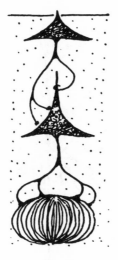

Fig. 9

the electrical activity of the afferent axons terminating in its vicinity. Since its present activity may affect its subsequent responsivity, it introduces the element of computation in the animal kingdom and gives these organisms the astounding latitude of nontrivial behaviors. Having once developed the genetic code for assembling an internuncial neuron, to add the genetic command "repeat" is a small burden indeed. Hence, I believe, it is now easy to comprehend the rapid proliferation of these neurons along additional vertical layers with growing horizontal connections to form those complex interconnected structures we call "brains."

The neuron. The neuron, of which we have more than 10 billion in our brain, is a highly specialized single cell with three anatomically distinct features (fig. 10): (1) the branchlike ramifications stretching up and to the side, the "dendrites"; (2) the bulb in the center housing the cell's nucleus, the "cell body"; and (3) the "axon," the smooth fiber stretching downward. Its various bifurcations terminate on dendrites of another (but sometimes—recursively—on the same) neuron. The same membrane that envelops the cell body forms also the tubular sheath for dendrites and axon, and causes the inside of the cell to be electrically charged against the outside with about one-tenth of a volt. If in the dendritic region this charge is sufficiently perturbed, the neuron

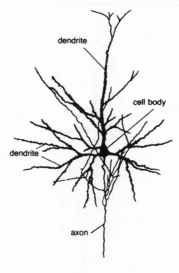

dendrite

cell body

dendrite

axon

Fig. 10

"fires" and sends this perturbation along its axon to its termination, the synapses.

Transmission.   Since these perturbations are electrical, they can be picked up by "microprobes," amplified and recorded. Figure 11 shows three examples of periodic discharges from a touch receptor under continuous stimulation, the low frequency corresponding to a weak stimulus, the high frequency to a strong stimulus. The magnitude of the discharge is clearly everywhere the same, the pulse frequency representing the stimulus intensity, but the intensity only.

Synapse.   Figure 12 sketches a synaptic junction. The afferent axon (Ax), along which the pulses travel, terminates in an end bulb (EB), which is separated from the spine (sp) of a dendrite (D) of the target neuron by a minute gap (sy), the "synaptic gap." (Note the many spines that cause the rugged appearance of the dendrites in fig. 10.) The chemical composition of the "transmitter substances" filling the synaptic gap is crucial in determining the effect an arriving pulse may have on the ultimate response of the neuron: under certain circumstances it may produce an "inhibitory effect" (cancellation of another simultaneously arriving pulse), in others a "facilitory effect" (augmenting another pulse to fire the neuron). Consequently, the synaptic gap can be seen as the "microenvironment" of a sensitive tip, the spine, and

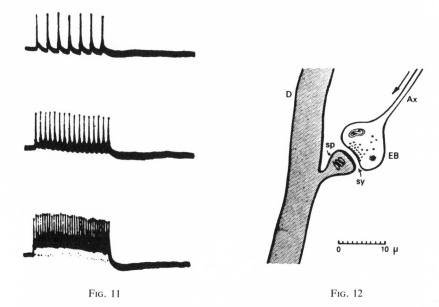

FIG. 11   FIG. 12

with this interpretation in mind we may compare the sensitivity of the CNS to changes of the *internal* environment (the sum total of all micro-environments) to those of the *external* environment (all sensory receptors). Since there are only 100 million sensory receptors, and about 10,000 billion synapses in our nervous system, we are 100,000 times more receptive to changes in our internal than in our external environment.

The cortex. In order that one may get at least some perspective on the organization of the entire machinery that computes all perceptual, intellectual, and emotional experiences, I have attached figure 13 (Sholl 1956), which shows a magnified section of about two square millimeters of a cat's cortex by a staining method that stains only cell body and dendrites, and of those only 1 percent of all neurons present. Although you have to imagine the many connections among these neurons provided by the (invisible) axons, and a density of packing that is 100 times that shown, the computational power of even this very small part of a brain may be sensed.

Descartes. This perspective is a far cry from that held, say, 300 years ago (Descartes 1664, p.142):

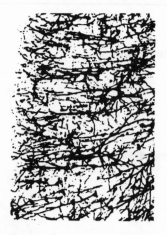

Fig. 13

If the fire *a* is near the foot *b* [fig.14], the particles of this fire, which as you know move with great rapidity, have the power to move the area of the skin of this foot that they touch; and in this way drawing the little thread, *c,* that you see to be attached at base of toes and on the nerve, at the same instant they open the

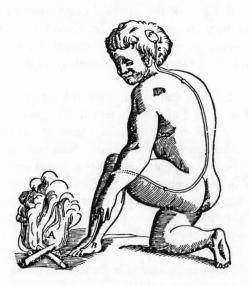

Fig. 14

entrance of the pore, *d, e,* at which this little thread terminates, just as by pulling one end of a cord, at the same time one causes the bell to sound that hangs at the other end. Now the entrance of the pore or little conduit, *d, e,* being thus opened, the animal spirits of the cavity *f,* enter within and are carried by it, partly into the muscles that serve to withdraw this foot from the fire, partly into those that serve to turn the eyes and the head to look at it, and partly into those that serve to advance the hands and to bend the whole body to protect it.

Note, however, that some behaviorists of today still cling to the same view (Skinner 1971), with one difference only, namely, that in the meantime Descartes's "animal spirit" has gone into oblivion.

Computation.   The retina of vertebrates, with its associated nervous tissue, is a typical case of neural computation. Figure 15 is a schematic representation of a mammalian retina and its postretinal network. The layer labeled 1 represents the array of rods and cones, the layer 2 the bodies and nuclei of these cells. Layer 3 identifies the general region

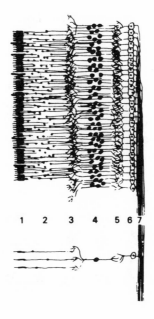

Fɪɢ. 15

where the axons of the receptors synapse with the dendritic ramifications of the "bipolar cells" (layer 4) which, in turn, synapse in layer 5 with the dendrites of the "ganglion cells" (layer 6), whose activity is transmitted to deeper regions of the brain via their axons, which are bundled together to form the optic nerve (layer 7). Computation takes place within the two layers labeled 3 and 5, that is, where the synapses are located. As Maturana has shown (Maturana 1968) it is there where the sensation of color and some clues as to form are computed.

Form computation: take the two-layered periodic network of figure 16, the upper layer representing receptor cells sensitive to, say, "light." Each of these receptors is connected to three neurons in the lower (computing) layer, with two excitatory synapses on the neuron directly below (symbolized by buttons attached to the body) and with one inhibitory synapse (symbolized by a loop around the tip) attached to each of the two neurons, one to the left and one to the right. It is clear that the computing layer will not respond to uniform light projected on the receptive layer, for the two excitatory stimuli on a computer neuron will be exactly compensated by the inhibitory signals coming from the two lateral receptors. This zero response will prevail under strongest and weakest stimulations as well as for slow or rapid changes of the illumination. The legitimate question may now arise, Why this complex apparatus that does not do a thing?

Consider now figure 17, in which an obstruction is placed in the light path illuminating the layer of receptors. Again all neurons of the lower layer will remain silent, except for the one at the edge of the obstruction, for it receives two excitatory signals from the receptor above, but only one inhibitory signal from the sensor to the left. We now understand the important function of this net, for it computes any spatial *variation* in the visual field of this "eye," independent of the intensity of the

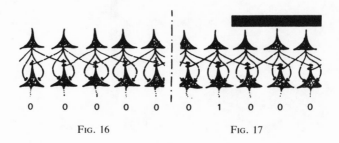

FIG. 16   FIG. 17

ambient light and its temporal variations, and independent of place and extension of the obstruction.

Although all operations involved in this computation are elementary, the organization of these operations allows us to appreciate a principle of considerable depth, namely, that of the computation of abstracts, here the notion of "edge."

I hope that this simple example is sufficient to suggest to you the possibility of generalizing this principle in the sense that "computation" can be seen on at least two levels, namely, (1) the operations actually performed and (2) the organization of these operations represented here by the structure of the nerve net. In computer language 1 would again be associated with "operations," but 2 with the "program." As we shall see later, in "biological computers" the programs themselves may be computed on. This leads to the concepts of "meta-programs," "meta-metaprograms," and so on. This, of course, is the consequence of the inherent recursive organization of those systems.

Closure. By attending to all the neurophysiological pieces, we may have lost the perspective that sees an organism as a functioning whole. In figure 18 I have put these pieces together in their functional context. The black squares labeled N represent bundles of neurons that synapse with neurons of other bundles over the (synaptic) gaps indicated by the spaces between squares. The sensory surface (SS) of the organism is to the left, its motor surface (MS) to the right, and the neuropituitary (NP), the strongly innervated master gland that regulates the entire endocrinal system, is the stippled lower boundary of the array of squares. Nerve impulses traveling horizontally (from left to right) ultimately act on the motor surface (MS) whose changes (movements) are immedi-

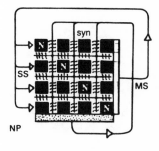

FIG. 18

ately sensed by the sensory surface (SS), as suggested by the "external" pathway following the arrows. Impulses traveling vertically (from top to bottom) stimulate the neuropituitary (NP), whose activity releases steroids into the synaptic gaps, as suggested by the wiggly terminations of the lines following the arrow, and thus modify the modus operandi of all synaptic junctures, hence the modus operandi of the system as a whole. Note the double closure of the system that now recursively operates not only on what it "sees," but on its operators as well. In order to make this twofold closure even more apparent I propose to wrap the diagram of figure 18 around its two axes of circular symmetry until the artificial boundaries disappear and the torus (doughnut) in figure 19 is obtained. Here the "synaptic gap" between the motor and sensory surfaces is the striated meridian in the front center, the neuropituitary the stippled equator. This, I submit, is the functional organization of a living organism in a (dough)nut shell.

The computations within this torus are subject to a nontrivial constraint, and this is expressed in the postulate of cognitive homeostasis:

> The nervous system is organized (or organizes itself) so that it computes a stable reality.

This postulate stipulates "autonomy," that is, "self-regulation," for every living organism. Since the semantic structure of nouns with the prefix "self-" becomes more transparent when this prefix is replaced by the noun, "autonomy" becomes synonymous with "regulation of regulation." This is precisely what the doubly closed, recursively computing torus does: it regulates its own regulation.

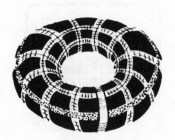

FIG. 19

Significance

It may be strange in times like these to stipulate autonomy, for autonomy implies responsibility: if I am the only one who decides how I act, then I am responsible for my action. Since the rule of the most popular game played today is to make someone else responsible for *my* acts—the name of the game is "heteronomy"—my arguments make, I understand, a most unpopular claim. One way of sweeping it under the rug is to dismiss it as just another attempt to rescue "solipsism," the view that this world is only in my imagination and the only reality is the imagining "I." Indeed, that was precisely what I was saying before, but I was talking only about a single organism. The situation is quite different when there are two, as I shall demonstrate with the aid of the gentleman with the bowler hat (fig. 20).

He insists that he is the sole reality, while everything else appears only in his imagination. However, he cannot deny that his imaginary universe is populated with apparitions that are not unlike himself. Hence he has to concede that they themselves may insist that they are the

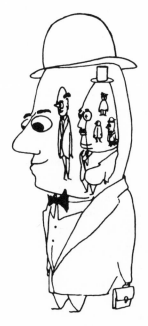

Fig. 20

93

sole reality and everything else is only a concoction of their imagination. In that case their imaginary universe will be populated with apparitions, one of which may be *he*, the gentleman with the bowler hat.

According to the principle of relativity, which rejects a hypothesis when it does not hold for two instances together, although it holds for each instance separately (Earthlings and Venusians may be consistent in claiming to be in the center of the universe, but their claims fall to pieces if they should ever get together), the solipsistic claim falls to pieces when besides me I invent another autonomous organism. However, it should be noted that since the principle of relativity is not a logical necessity—nor is it a proposition that can be proven to be either true or false—the crucial point to be recognized here is that I am free to choose either to adopt this principle or to reject it. If I reject it, I am the center of the universe, my reality is my dreams and my nightmares, my language is monologue, and my logic monologic. If I adopt it, neither I nor the other can be the center of the universe. As in the heliocentric system, there must be a third that is the central reference. It is the relation between thou and I, and this relation is *identity:*

reality = community.

What are the consequences of all this in ethics and aesthetics?

The ethical imperative.   Act always so as to increase the number of choices.

The aesthetical imperative.   If you desire to see, learn how to act.

NOTES

This article is an adaptation of an address given on April 17, 1973, to the Fourth International Environmental Design Research Association Conference at the College of Architecture, Virginia Polytechnic Institute, Blacksburg. It is reprinted here from *The Invented Reality,* edited by Paul Watzlawick (New York: Norton, 1984).

1. Literally, *con* (together), *prehendere* (to seize, grasp).

REFERENCES

Brown, G. S. 1972. *Laws of Form.* New York: Julian.
Descartes, R. 1664. *L'homme.* In *Oeuvres de Descartes,* vol. 11. Paris: Adams & Tannery, 1957.

Maturana, H. R. 1968. A biological theory of relativistic colour coding in the primate retina. *Archivos de Biología y Medicina Experimentales,* 1(suppl.): 42–51.

Maturana, H. R. 1970a. *Biology of Cognition.* Urbana: University of Illinois Press.

Maturana, H. R. 1970b. Neurophysiology of cognition. In P. Garvin, ed. *Cognition: A Multiple View.* New York: Spartan.

Naeser, M. A., and Lilly, J. C. 1971. The repeating word effect: phonetic analysis of reported alternatives. *Journal of Speech and Hearing Research:* 212–225.

Sholl, D. A. 1956. *The Organization of the Cerebral Cortex.* London: Methuen.

Skinner, B. F. 1971. *Beyond Freedom and Dignity.* New York: Knopf.

Teuber, H. L. 1961. Neuere Betrachtungen über Sehstrahlung und Sehrinde. In R. Jung and H. Kornhuber, eds. *Das Visuelle System.* Berlin: Springer.

Worden, F. G. 1959. EEG studies and conditional reflexes in man. In Mary A. B. Brazier, ed. *The Central Nervous System and Behavior.* New York: Josiah Macy, Jr., Foundation.

6 THE FRUITS OF ASYNCHRONY: A PSYCHOLOGICAL EXAMINATION OF CREATIVITY

HOWARD GARDNER AND CONSTANCE WOLF

A "Potted History" of Picasso and Cubism

The name "Pablo Picasso" and the founding of cubism are virtually synonymous. According to the widely known story, Picasso was a preternaturally gifted young artist who was drawing like a master at a young age (for biographical details, see Barr [1946], Gilot and Lake [1964], and Penrose [1958]). The sketches of his childhood, and even the scribbles in his school notebooks, showed enormous skill and imaginativeness. By early adolescence, Picasso had already exhausted the art educational resources of his native Spain. Indeed, according to the legend—and this particular legend has the ring of truth—young Pablo was so accomplished that his father, also an artist, ceased to paint after his son had reached the age of fourteen.

Visiting Paris while still a teenager, Picasso soon had mastered the various styles of Western painting that had been developed by 1900. He was able to imitate the great masters of the past with fidelity, and his paintings and drawings reflected the trends and schools that characterized *la Belle Epoque*. The periods of his art at that time merited and have come to be known by special names: the Blue Period of 1901–1904, when he concentrated on figures, using monochrome blue toning; and the Rose Period of 1904–1906, when terra-cotta tonalities brightened canvases full of circus themes or figures in a "classical" repose.

While not yet famous, Picasso was already recognized as a phenomenon. As his close friend Gertrude Stein once observed, "Picasso wrote
painting as other children wrote their a.b.c. . . . his drawings were not
of things seen but of things expressed, in short they were words for
him and drawing was his only way of talking and he talks a great deal"
(Burns 1970, p. 4).

By 1905, at age twenty-four, Picasso had clearly surpassed his contemporaries in Spain and in France. His portrait of Gertrude Stein
(1906) and his self-portrait (1906) revealed the first traces of an emerging
new style. The faces appeared masklike and reflected his growing interest in Iberian sculpture. As he himself later put it, "We were trying
to move in a direction opposite to Impressionism. That was the reason
we abandoned color, emotion, sensations and everything . . . to search
again for an architectonic basis in the composition, trying to make an
order of it" (Gilot and Lake 1964, p. 69). Then there was a landscape
painting (1907) and other portraits in which he embodied Paul Cezanne's lapidary formula, "You must see in nature the cylinder, the
sphere, the cone" (quoted in Barr 1936, p. 30). Above all, there was
his early masterpiece *Les Desmoiselles d'Avignon*, a hauntingly powerful portrait of five prostitutes. This "battlefield of trial and experiment"(Barr 1946, p. 57) portrayed figures that were fragmented in a
way never before attempted in Western painting. So iconoclastic was
this work that some of Picasso's own friends were horrified, and, for
years, Picasso hesitated to display it in public. The sketches for this
path-breaking painting were folded over in his notebook; perhaps Picasso himself was overwhelmed by his revolutionary creation.

In the next few years, Picasso saw his experiments to their logical
conclusion. In 1908–1909, analytic cubism was launched. In his works
from this period, sometimes undertaken in close collaboration with
Georges Braque, Picasso broke down familiar objects, like faces or
tableware, into their component elements so that all the facets of these
objects could be apprehended on a single canvas in a single glance. It
was said by Guillaume Apollinaire that Picasso "studies an object as
a surgeon dissects a corpse" (quoted in Penrose 1958, p. 188). Some
five years later, the synthetic cubism phase began. In this mode of
painting, the tactile aspects of the dissected objects were highlighted,
and collages were created pictorially or with parts of the actual objects
themselves. While the cubist movement as such had begun to dissipate
by 1915 or so, significant cubist canvases were painted for the rest of

the decade. Picasso continued to include cubist features in his paintings for the rest of his lengthy career; for example, they are visible in the monumental *Guernica* (1937).

What we were presented thus far is familiar to any casual observer of the arts in the twentieth century. To use a literary phrase, it is "potted history," but, we must stress, it is potted history of a definite sort. Put directly, in this history of cubism, we have focused almost exclusively on the creative genius of a single prodigious painter, Pablo Picasso. Such an account, the sort with which psychologists are traditionally most comfortable, highlights the contributions of a single individual, attributing a new movement chiefly to his efforts and thoughts. The clear implication is, Without Picasso, no cubism—or, at the very least, no cubism until many years later.

A Psychologist's Approach to Creativity

Scratch a psychologist, or turn the pages of a psychology textbook, and you encounter an account something like that just presented.[1] Individuals differ from one another in many respects, and one of the chief ones is intelligence. Some individuals are, from the first, brighter than others, and, so long as there are no drastic unexpected events, the brighter individuals will perform more successfully in this world. Intelligence tests are paper-and-pencil instruments that provide at least a rough estimate of the intelligence of a given individual.

There is at least a modest relation between intelligence and creativity. Indeed, while the intelligent person arrives at the correct answer more or less quickly, the creative individual is more likely to be fluent, to come up with many plausible answers and, perhaps, even with some answers of striking originality. The testing of creativity is not so advanced as the testing of intelligence—quite possibly because creativity is a more elusive trait. Nonetheless, by asking individuals how many uses they can think of for a brick or by requesting that they interpret a squiggle in as many ways as possible, psychologists can achieve a reasonable estimate of the creative potential of an individual.

Unfortunately, Picasso antedated creativity tests, and it is not self-evident that he would have agreed to sit for one. But any psychologist sympathetic to the account presented above would have to argue as follows: had Picasso taken a creativity test, he would have achieved an extremely high score on this measure. It was this creative trait, working in conjunction with at least reasonably high intelligence and perhaps some other talents as well, that permitted Picasso to be so innovative and that led, ultimately, to the founding of cubism.

Of course, not all psychologists would repeat exactly the same tale. Those influenced by Gestalt psychology might point to a special ability to "see" a solution to a problem, while others do not discern the crucial pattern. Those of a behaviorist persuasion would underscore a certain pattern of reinforcement (first explicit rewards from other individuals and perhaps later the anticipation of recognition or money) that drove Picasso to ever greater attainments. Those of a more contemporary cognitive bent might suggest that creative individuals are capable of a special kind of information processing, can process information with great speed, or are particularly supple at producing powerful mental models (Johnson-Laird 1983; Perkins 1981; Sternberg, in press). But all would agree that the occasion of creative output is the thought and behavior of a single individual.

Cubism as Seen through Other Lenses

There is no imperative to view cubism as the psychologist would. Indeed, just as success has a thousand parents, so, too, a movement as influential as cubism has spawned explanations drawn from a range of disciplines (N. Stahler, personal communication, 1985; see also Goldwater 1938; Gopnik 1983; and Teuber 1982). Picasso himself was skeptical of such efforts. He once declared, "Mathematics, trigonometry, chemistry, psychoanalysis, music, and whatnot have been related to Cubism to give it an easier interpretation. All this has been pure literature, not to say nonsense, which brought bad results, blinding people with theory" (quoted in Barr 1946, p. 74). But not even this caution from the founder himself has muted the efforts of researchers to discover the key to cubism.

Consider, as a start, the art historian. From his or her perspective, there was an inexorable trend away from realism at least since the mid-nineteenth century. This trend, no doubt aided by the invention of photography, gave rise first to impressionism, then to postimpressionism, and then to expressionism and fauvism. Each of these movements-in-reaction represented a further step away from faithful rendering of nature and another step toward a more direct treatment of light, emotional content, or form. Inevitably, the object itself would begin to fragment—as it did in cubism—destined eventually to disappear entirely in abstract expressionism, a movement with which Picasso never associated himself.

The art historical approach can center around individuals. In such an account, a key figure is Cezanne, who stressed the importance of ferreting out the geometric shapes that underlie familiar objects. Once Cezanne had thought and painted in this vein, the advent of cubism was inevitable. But the story can be related with a focus on other individuals as well. Some would highlight the intimate relationship between Picasso and Braque, which stretched out over several years and, as Braque said, made them feel "rather like two mountaineers roped together" (quoted in Berger 1965, p. 73). Still others would stress the artistic breakthroughs of Henri Matisse and the intense rivalry between Matisse and Picasso that followed. Once Picasso saw that his chief peer, Matisse, had turned his back on realistic portrayal in favor of the wild colors and forms characteristic of fauvism, he was determined to go even further.

Enter the anthropologist or the Africanist. From such a perspective, a decisive influence on contemporary Western painting was the accumulation, in the late nineteenth century, of many works of tribal art from Africa and the South Seas (Goldwater 1938; Rubin 1980). These masks and sculpted pieces, collected first for their scholarly interest, soon struck observers by virtue of their simplicity, elegance, directness, and expressive power. Many artists were fascinated by them, and some collected them. Picasso's fascination with Iberian sculpture led him to purchase sculptured heads. Subsequently, he visited the Louvre on many occasions and the Palais du Trocadero as well to look at African objects (Goldwater 1938). Perhaps it was just a short step from the prizing of these highly abstracted forms to the attempt to recreate them in the plastic artistic languages of Europe.

There may be no limit to the list of contributing factors. Scientists and historians of science point to the almost simultaneous emergence of the theory of relativity and the field of cubism. Musicians cite Stravinsky's flight from tonality, and literary critics note the breakdown of classic forms in the poetry of T. S. Eliot and in the novels of Virginia Woolf and James Joyce. Even scholars of childhood have their say: many (including Picasso) have commented on the childlike quality of some cubist art, and one commentator suggests that the breakdown of forms began in Picasso's high school notebooks (N. Stahler, personal communication, 1985). Finally, those involved in documentary history note the emergence of cubist forms in the popular caricatures of the late nineteenth century (Gopnik 1983) and in the geometric illusions that came to populate not only psychology textbooks but also popular magazines (Teuber 1982).

A Synthetic-Scientific Approach to Creativity

How can one make one's way among these competing definitions, particularly when it is likely that some combination of the aforementioned factors fomented the rise of cubism? Our own belief is that there is no need to favor one line of investigation to the exclusion of others and that, indeed, creative lives and creative works can come about only in the wake of numerous interacting factors. In the pages that follow, we will sketch out some of these factors and indicate the ways in which they interact. Rather than claim that all these factors must interact in a seamless manner, however, we shall suggest an alternative account. In our view, creative efforts are more likely to arise when there is a certain tension or asynchrony among the principal factors that underlie human behavior. It is this tension that ultimately gives rise to creative works.

Our working definition of creativity is rather heterodox. We view the creative individual as one who can regularly solve problems or fashion products in a domain in a way that is initially original but that ultimately is accepted in one or more cultural settings. The controversial aspects of the definition include the following. (1) To begin with, we do not see creativity as accidental; an ordinary individual will not suddenly produce a creative product. Rather, creative products or solutions can be expected with some regularity, in virtue of the kind of life led by the creative individual. (2) Just as a person is unlikely to be intelligent "across the board," so, too, individuals are not creative in all areas. Creativity tends to be domain specific. The fact that an individual may be highly creative in language predicts nothing about his or her creativity in such other domains as music, science, or social interaction. Nor does excellence in any of these other areas have any greater predictive power. (3) It is useful, and sometimes creative, to solve problems, but such solutions are, perhaps, the less compelling examples of creative capacity. It is the ability to find new problems and to fashion products of scope and power that especially marks the creative individual (Getzels and Csikszentmihalyi 1976). It is unfortunate that, because of limits of time and technology, psychologists have had to shy away from assessing the fashioning of products—for here lies the heartland of creative functioning. (4) Nearly all observers would agree that creativity combines novelty and acceptance. The question of how acceptance occurs is usually left vague, however. In our view, it is acceptance within one or more cultural settings that is crucial to a judgment of creativity. There is no time limit to such acceptance. Still, no matter how potentially creative a product may be, if it is nowhere apprehended as such, one may not consider it to be creative.

Let us mention some of the features that fail to appear in our definition. We include nothing about creativity as a trait, nothing about its being inborn (or acquired), nothing about creativity as occurring in an isolated moment or as a capacity that pervades all of an individual's activities. Whether creative potential or achievement can be assessed by a psychologist using any of the current methods is dubious, though of course one cannot ever prove that such psychometric methods are inappropriate or inadequate.

What, then, does the student of creativity do? In our view, the student's mission is to discover the rules or principles that govern the behaviors of those individuals who work productively within a domain and within a given culture. To the extent that the creative biographies of a Beethoven or a Mozart, a Rembrandt or a Picasso, a Freud, a Darwin, or an Einstein, are completely idiosyncratic, hopes for a science of creativity are misguided. If, however, one can find some principles or themes at work in disparate creative lives, there remains some hope for a science of creativity.

Two methodological guidelines are preliminary to such an undertaking. To begin with, as already suggested, the study of creativity ought to begin with unambiguous cases (Gruber 1981; John-Steiner 1985). If we can explain those individuals who most clearly merit the epithet "creative," we have some confidence that our model is apt. (Conversely, if we were to develop a model for "ordinary" creative individuals, we risk the possibility that a Freud or a Picasso may operate in a qualitatively different way from our standard case.)

The second methodological precept reflects our belief that creativity will never reveal its secrets to a single discipline. The biologist or the geneticist who claims to have discovered the "secret" of creativity is as misguided as the psychologist or anthropologist who utters a similar boast. Rather, as Medawar (1969) suggests, creativity is the discipline par excellence for an interdisciplinary or "synthetic science" approach: "The analysis of creativity in all its forms is beyond the competence of any one accepted discipline. It requires a consortium of talents: psychologists, biologists, philosophers, computer scientists, artists and poets would all expect to have their say. That 'creativity is beyond analysis' is a romantic illusion that we must now outgrow" (p. 47).

If, then, we adopt a synthetic science approach, it is necessary to indicate which disciplines ought to be brought to bear in a study of a creative individual. In our view, it is necessary to incorporate at least five different perspectives. In what follows, we introduce these five perspectives. To give a feeling for their application, we will apply them to the case of Pablo Picasso. For a contrast, we will cite evidence from another creative individual to whom we have devoted study: the psychoanalyst Sigmund Freud (see Gardner 1986).

Five Perspectives on Picasso and Freud

THE SUBPERSONAL LEVEL:
A NEUROBIOLOGICAL PERSPECTIVE

In examining creative individuals from a neurobiological perspective, one seeks to determine the influences of genetics as well as the structure and functioning of a particular nervous system (Gardner and Dudai 1985). In the cases of Picasso and Freud, it is easy, but ineffectual, to apply this perspective—for, of course, nothing is known about the neurobiology of either individual.

Still, there are two reasons for insisting on the importance of this perspective. First, there already exists considerable technical paraphernalia whereby the neurobiological features of an individual can be assessed. It is no longer in the realm of science fiction to think of a creative individual being studied in vivo, with measures being made of brain waves, cerebral blood flow activity, neuromorphological features, and so on. Of course, the brains of creative people who have died can also be examined, as has already happened in the case of Einstein (Diamond 1985; Reich 1986). To be sure, there is no guarantee that the brains of creative individuals will turn out to differ in either structure or function from those of "uncreative mortals"; but, certainly, this question deserves to be investigated.

There is another reason for invoking a neurobiological perspective. It is in the neurobehavioral laboratory that one encounters individuals with anomalous cognitive profiles (Gardner 1975; Sacks 1986). Sometimes these individuals have unusual nervous systems from birth, while at other times these anomalies are the result of brain injury. In those cases in which an unusual behavioral profile can be linked to an anomalous brain structure, one achieves powerful evidence that comparable behavior in the extraordinary individual may also be yoked to characteristic neural structure. So, for example, the incredible drawings of a single autistic child like Nadia (Selfe 1977) may yield information about the kinds of neural structures that allow facile modeling and drawing without the benefit of formal tutelage. Perhaps such studies can suggest something about the brain of a prodigious young Picasso—an individual who might be thought of as a "Nadia with concepts."

THE PERSONAL LEVEL: A COGNITIVE PERSPECTIVE

When one moves to the level of the person, or, if one likes, the psychological level, one option is to focus on the cognitive capacities of the creative individual. Indeed, as we have already observed, many, if not most, psychologists focus on the cognitive characteristics of a creative individual. Such a focus can be undertaken in many ways. For present purposes, it will suffice to comment on the kinds of distinctive mental strengths—or intelligences—displayed by our two subjects (see Gardner 1983).

In the case of Picasso, it is clear that one is dealing with an individual who had superlative spatial and bodily kinesthetic intelligence. As can be seen in his works, his notebooks, and in the movie *The Mystery of Picasso,* Picasso was able effortlessly to form visual-spatial "images in his head," to manipulate them at will, and to record every manner of transformation of probable, possible, and "impossible" forms. By the same token, thanks to virtuoso bodily ability, he was able to render these forms with rapidity and accuracy. Whatever other intelligences or combinations of intelligences may have characterized Picasso, he certainly had these two in abundance.

Paradoxically, Freud was notoriously weak in both the spatial and the bodily intelligences (Jones 1961). Moreover, he himself confessed to ineptitude in and dislike of music. However, Freud displayed a remarkable combination of three intelligences that were of much lesser import to Picasso. He possessed quite powerful abilities in the logical-mathematical areas; his knowledge of persons (both himself and others) was highly unusual for a scientist; and his linguistic genius was virtually unprecedented for a scientist. It is probably in his ability to yoke the linguistic and logical talents, which are necessary for scientific work, with superlative sensitivity to the world of other individuals that his special scientific aptitude lay.

THE PERSONAL LEVEL: PERSONALITY AND EMOTION

Creative individuals, then, seem to differ dramatically from one another in the kinds of intelligences that they possess in abundance and in the ways in which they deploy these intelligences. They prove far more similar to one another in noncognitive areas—in personality, motivation, social relationships, and emotional status. Indeed, those psychologists who claim that creative individuals exhibit common traits are on much firmer grounds in the noncognitive areas.

Like other creative individuals, both Picasso and Freud were individuals of great self-confidence; each was convinced from a young age that he knew what he was doing and that it was right. Rarely were they shaken from a course of action simply because of negative feedback. They were fantastically ambitious and hardworking, willing to neglect everyone and everything in order to accomplish their goals. Indeed, they identified quite explicitly with conquest, Picasso seeing himself as the matador taming the bull, Freud thinking of himself as a military leader, a conquistador, and an intellectual incarnation of his boyhood hero, Hannibal.

This extreme self-absorption can have its costs. Both Freud and Picasso made great demands on those about them. Both had complex relationships with both sexes, but Freud can be seen as working out much of his professional life with reference to other men in the psychiatric and medical communities, while Picasso's paintings can be viewed with reference to the many women with whom he had relations (Gedo 1980). Each man was quite capable of forming an intense relationship with another human being, exploiting it for some period of time, and then rejecting the other quite peremptorily because of an imagined wrong or because of the need for some other form of human support. On occasion, after the termination of these intense relationships, suicides followed, for which such creative individuals bore at least a tangential (or a symbolic) responsibility.

In view of our interest in asynchronous conditions, it is worth noting that both Picasso and Freud felt distinctly marginal for much of their lives. When Picasso was still very young, he left his native Spain. While he became attached to his adopted homeland of France, he always maintained extremely strong (if ambivalent) ties to Spain and was distraught by the rise of fascism there. Picasso saw himself as a Spaniard among Frenchmen, as an uneducated painter among writers and other intellectuals, and, at least initially, as a social "naïf" who painted for a Continental aristocracy. As a Jew living in Vienna, Freud always felt vulnerable; and as a maverick physician, he felt estranged from the medical profession and eventually attracted his own group of peers via the mystique of psychoanalysis. Presumably, these feelings of marginality served to motivate our two creative heroes to "prove themselves."

THE IMPERSONAL LEVEL: DOMAINS OF KNOWLEDGE

While the first three levels—subpersonal, personal cognitive, and personal noncognitive—are familiar to biologists and psychologists, the latter two levels are less well known and merit separate introduction. In explicating these concepts, we rely heavily on the works of two colleagues: David Feldman, a developmental psychologist at Tufts University, and Mihaly Csikszentmihalyi, a social psychologist at the University of Chicago.

The notion of domain is an epistemological one (see Feldman 1980). The term "domain" refers to the structure of knowledge within a particular area, craft, or discipline. Domains run the gamut from standard academic disciplines (such as physics or history) to cultural practices that are conveyed chiefly by example (such as sailing or baseball). Crucial to the existence of a domain as an end state of knowledge/ competence is a set of steps through which individuals will ordinarily pass, from novice to expert status.

While domains necessarily involve human beings, they are best thought of apart from human beings—bodies of knowledge that can be described in the abstract and that would in some sense continue to exist even if all individuals disappeared. One can think of a domain as the information that could be contained in a textbook or in a series of lessons or demonstrations.

Turning to our two creative individuals, a domain perspective yields quite different pictures. In the case of Picasso, he was involved from an early age in the domain of painting. Initially, like any young student, he was strongly influenced by the state of the domain as it existed at the end of the nineteenth century. He soon mastered the extant domain and then, in the succeeding fifty years, made a series of fresh contributions to the evolving domain. The structure of knowledge of painting—what it is—has changed appreciably, thanks to his daunting example. Picasso did make contributions to other domains as well—from sculpture to ceramics to play writing—but it is in the domain of painting that his niche is most firmly established.

Freud's life can be seen as a passage through numerous domains until he finally devised his own. He began with an attraction to philosophy—an attraction that he ruthlessly suppressed for many decades—and then turned to scientific medicine. Within medicine, he studied, and made contributions in, neurology, neuroanatomy, psychiatry, and psychology (Sulloway 1983). He also practiced clinically on the border of neurology and psychiatry. Perennially dissatisfied, however, Freud kept searching for a domain to which he could make a unique and indispensable contribution. Eventually, he invented psychoanalysis as both theory and clinical practice; so successful was this invention that it has since become a domain itself to which others can make contributions. Following the invention of psychoanalysis, Freud naturally devoted much attention to the fostering of its development—but he continued to contribute to, and exert influence on, a wide range of domains, including literary history, political science, sociology, and the visual arts. These contributions continue posthumously, as his successors continue to modify the contemporary structure of domains.

THE MULTIPERSONAL LEVEL:
THE PERSPECTIVE OF THE FIELD

While "domain" is a distinctly epistemological notion, "field" is inherently a sociological concept (Csikszentmihaly, in press; Csikszentmihalyi and Robinson 1986). The field consists of the teachers, judges, institutions, agencies, reward systems, and other entities that allow or thwart the development of a career and the production and recognition of creative works. Acknowledgment of the field entails a recognition that no individual can work in a vacuum—that, ultimately, every action must stand judged by the community.

To convey a feeling for the concepts of domain and field, it may help to offer some examples. For contrast, let us consider mathematics and the visual arts. In the case of mathematics, there is an entire discipline that has evolved over the centuries, whose contents can be summarized in textbooks and monographs. Anyone who would wish to become a mathematician must master the contents of the domain, a slowly but ever changing set of facts, concepts, and theories. However, contributions to mathematics cannot occur simply as a result of an individual intelligence wrestling with an impersonal domain. Rather, the individual must pass through an educational process during which he or she works with teachers, takes courses, discusses proofs, writes articles, has them judged by peers, and, eventually, either wins or fails to win acceptance, authority, and prizes. All these latter factors constitute the field at work. By a nice irony, the prize awarded periodically to the outstanding mathematician under the age of forty is called the Field's Medal.

If the field is obtrusive even in so apparently objective a discipline as mathematics, it is overwhelmingly evident in the visual arts. There, the envelope within which individual creation occurs consists of gallery owners and gallery spaces, curators and museums, newspaper and magazine reviewers, collectors and other "art lovers," agents, publicity experts, and the like. Some skeptics would even claim that, in the current climate in the visual arts, only the field is evident. This would be an exaggeration, however. Any artist creates with reference to— even if in reaction to—the works and the methods that have been developed by predecessors, and this is the point at which the impersonal domain exerts its effect.

Books have been written about the fields within which Picasso and Freud worked, over roughly the same historical epoch. It is difficult to think of Freud apart from the scintillating but somewhat decadent atmosphere of Vienna at the turn of the century (see Janik and Toulmin 1974; Schorske 1973). While Picasso retained much of the Spaniard within him, the environment of Paris at the turn of the century was certainly critical in his formation and his innovation. So crucial were these milieus, in fact, that one cannot readily conceive of cubism emanating from Tokyo or Los Angeles or of psychoanalysis being born in London.

The field, however, extends far beyond the city or the country in which an artist or a scientist happens to work. Field factors begin with one's family, friends, and relatives. Ultimately, they extend to the educational institutions or apprenticeships, to the set of peers with whom one begins one's career, and, in the end, to one's relationships with the leaders of a discipline, the opinion makers, the general public, and posterity.

Both Picasso and Freud lived long lives, during which they were subjected to many field forces and exerted their own force on fields. In Picasso's case, he had an intimate relationship with Braque but also a somewhat wider support system among the artists and intellectuals of Paris. Having achieved worldwide fame while still young, he spent much of his life in a kind of flirtation with many fields, alternatively teasing, tormenting, and embracing his wide public. By the end, he had isolated himself almost entirely from the rest of the world, seeking satisfaction from solitary creation. In Freud's case, the field was once as small as his correspondence with a single friend, Wilhelm Fliess. For many years, he felt alone and isolated, bitterly disposed toward the medical community of Vienna, which did not appreciate his accomplishments. Ultimately, this situation changed dramatically; fields that he had invented came to encompass much of the civilized world.

Synthesizing the Five Perspectives

We have described five different vantage points from which one can (and, in our opinion, should) view the creative lives of outstanding individuals. These cover a wide range, from the gene and the neuron to the community and, indeed, the world of ideas. While such a catholic approach may seem comprehensive, it is not immediately evident how such a range of perspectives could usefully be combined; nor is it evident how one proceeds from individual case studies to the construction of a science.

We would suggest the following investigative strategy. To begin with, it is important to carry out detailed case studies of many individuals and to determine how our several levels of analysis help to illuminate the careers and products of the individuals under investigation. Only if we have carried out studies—and ones far more detailed than those adumbrated here—can we begin to determine which factors seem to characterize all creative individuals, which characterize some set (either within or across a discipline), and which seem either idiosyncratic to a few or unique to a given individual. For instance, even our extremely modest comparison here indicates that blends of intelligence can differ widely across creative individuals; that aspects of personality and motivation may be more similar across persons, at least within a given epoch and a given civilization; and that there were certain pockets within turn-of-the-century Europe where radical departures from earlier practice were to be expected.

One ally in this line of study is the potential for pointed comparisons. It should be possible to compare unambiguous cases of creativity—the Picassos and the Freuds—with other individuals of their epoch who were drawn from the same "general population" but who differed from them in an instructive way. For example, in the case of Picasso, one could compare his life course with that of Georges Braque or Juan Gris, two other early cubists. For a more radical comparison, one could contrast his life with that of his much less successful father or with a more recent and still largely unrecognized artist such as Harold Shapinsky (Weschler 1985). Freud could be contrasted with the dominant French psychiatrist of his era, Pierre Janet, a man who had anticipated some of Freud's major discoveries but is now largely forgotten outside the French-speaking world (Ellenberger 1970). Again, for a more radical comparison, Freud could be contrasted with his contemporaries Josef Breuer or Wilhelm Fliess, who are remembered chiefly because of their early associations with Freud.

One must still ask, however, about the ways in which the various levels of analysis come together, in a description of lives and in the lives of the individuals themselves. Do the genes, the intelligences, the personality, the structure of the discipline, and the surrounding field exist as five separate entities, united only in a scientific taxonomy— or are there important and systematic interactions among and conjunctions of these analytic levels?

A promising beginning on this issue comes from the work of Csikszentmihalyi (in press). Raising questions about the classical formulation, "What is creativity?" Csikszentmihalyi suggests instead the felicitous rewording, "Where is creativity?" In his reformulation, he locates the possibility for creativity in an interaction among a number of these factors. In particular, he envisages a three-way dialectic obtaining among the personal level (individual talents), the impersonal level (various domains of knowledge), and the multipersonal level (the surrounding fields within which careers and lives unfold).

Again, a concretization can be helpful. Consider, for example, the operation of a discipline like physics. One has as a point of departure a collection of talented individuals, gifted in logical-mathematical thinking, who begin to study the physical world itself as well as the ways in which earlier scientists have thought about it. This collection of individuals in 1900 included not only the likes of Albert Einstein and Niels Bohr but also many others whose names are known only to specialists or who are completely forgotten.

These talented individuals mastered the knowledge in the domain as it existed in 1900 and attempted to add to the body of knowledge called "physics." They proposed various schemes, and these were, in turn, examined by the "high priests" of the field—those who edit journals, make appointments, publish critiques and refutations, and award prizes. A small set of individuals emerged in a single generation as worthy of special attention, and, of these, an even smaller number actually came to change the delineation of the domain. (It is said that over half the Nobel Prize winners in physics have received the accolade for work executed in subdisciplines that did not even exist when they were in graduate school.)

The cycle continues, for, in the next generation, students confront a revised physics, one that has changed fundamentally because of the work of Einstein, Bohr, Heisenberg, and other exceptional scientists. Indeed, the field may also change, as factors other than those that were important around 1900 may become relevant to the shape of a career. Also, while the individual intelligences of human beings do not themselves change, those relevant to physics may. It has been said (A. Miller, personal communication, 1985) that, before 1927, possession of strong visual-spatial skills was an important prerequisite for contributing to physics but that thereafter such skills were no longer at a premium and might even have interfered with a physics that became more purely mathematical and posited entities that were difficult to envisage.

On the Csikszentmihalyi analysis, then, it no longer makes sense to think of creativity as a process that occurs in a lone individual's head. There cannot be a hermit creator. Instead, creativity is more properly thought of as a process in which individual minds struggle to master and, ultimately, change a domain; in which field forces determine which individuals are picked out and recognized; in which, over time, certain contributions come to affect the actual definition of the domain (and, perhaps, of the field as well); and in which succeeding generations of students must master a somewhat different domain and be prepared to face a somewhat altered field.

So far, we have spoken chiefly about the ways in which a multilevel perspective should change the study of creativity. But can this new perspective also affect the ways in which we think of creative lives themselves?

One possibility is that the creative individual is the one in which all these levels work together in perfect harmony, in complete synchrony. On this analysis, it is the individual whose genetic inheritance, neurobiological functioning, blend of intelligences, and type of personality match perfectly with one another and, moreover, are ideally suited to a domain within his society. Such an individual is most likely to master the domain, to conceive of new contributions, and to be recognized as innovative by the caretakers of the field.

This is a credible story and, in fact, probably the correct one for certain cases—but not for the cases that we are considering here. In his studies of prodigies, Feldman (1986) proposes the concept of "coincidence"—a simultaneous coming together of a whole range of factors that allow a few individuals to become prodigies. Indeed, a prodigy—a youngster performing in a domain at the level of a competent adult—is virtually unthinkable in the absence of exemplary synchronies among a genetic inheritance, a highly supportive family, an excellent collection of teachers and mentors, a domain that is ready to be absorbed by a young mind, and a surrounding culture that chooses to honor gifted youngsters—at least so long as they are young.

But prodigiousness is not creativity. Indeed, as Bamberger (1982) has suggested, precocious superiority may ultimately cause difficulties and get in the way of ultimate achievement. Hector Berlioz quipped of the precocious Camille Saint-Saëns, "He knows everything but he lacks inexperience" (Schonberg 1969, p. 17). If all factors are unfolding and interacting too smoothly, there may be enormously rapid growth, but the ultimate level of achievement may be unimpressive or even nonexistent (Wallace 1986).

We are, therefore, stimulated to propose an alternative hypothesis. On this rival account, the creative individual is marked, not by synchrony, but by asynchrony—not by a perfect match within or across levels, but rather by strategic mismatches or asynchronies. Only through such asynchronies does the possibility arise of new creations, of new visions, ones that may initially be seen as aberrant or idiosyncratic but that ultimately come to be accepted in one or more cultural settings— our definition of creativity.

It is easy to find support for this "asynchrony hypothesis." We can begin with the two cases on which we have been focusing. Both Picasso and Freud exhibited unusual blends of intelligence. Picasso had uniquely powerful visual-spatial skills but was unremarkable in most other intelligences and was reportedly not even able to master his numbers in school. Freud complained of his inferior spatial and bodily intelligence but was able to yoke extraordinary personal intelligences to the linguistic and logical intelligences more typically associated with scientific work. Surely, it is plausible that these uneven cognitive profiles helped our heroes to see the world in an unaccustomed way.

Even as their own intellectual profiles were unusual, so, too, both Picasso and Freud failed to blend in easily with the communities in which they lived. Picasso was too talented and too driven to remain in his native Spain, so he somehow found his way to Paris. (One may well ask how so many young talents found their way to Paris in 1900 or to New York in 1940.) He remained on the margins of the French and Spanish cultures for the remainder of his life. Freud lived in Vienna for most of his life (he seemed to hate other locales even more) but was never comfortable there. As a Jew in the medical profession, he felt estranged; in fact, his ambition seems to have been fueled by his consistent clashes with the gentile establishment.

Numerous instances of asynchrony can be found within these two lives. Moreover, the literature of creativity abounds with other classic asynchronies: the homosexuality of many artists; the clashes of Mozart and of Beethoven with members of their families; Einstein's and Churchill's early difficulties in school; the childhoods of sickness and loneliness that seem almost de rigueur for writers of the Romantic era.

But here, of course, is the problem. Asynchrony is too easy to find. Given a complex life, and even a minimally competent biographer, one can dredge up multiple instances of asynchrony. What is needed are definite objective ways in which to assess asynchrony, to ascertain whether there are certain kinds of asynchronies that stand out and which are particularly likely to mark the lives of creative individuals.

At the same time, it is important to document the lack of asynchrony in those who do not attain the same level of creativity.

Coming up with a metric of synchrony, asynchrony, and (perhaps) productive and unproductive asynchrony is by no means a straightforward task. How much must a youth clash with a parent, a young worker with his peers, an ambitious researcher with his community, before the requisite level of asynchrony is reached? When does asynchrony become counterproductive? Should these measures be pursued primarily in a case-study manner (as we have proposed here), or is it better to use statistics drawn from large populations, as Simonton (1984) has done in his studies of eminent individuals? These and many other questions need to be tackled if our asynchrony hypothesis is to be reasonably assessed.

Even if we do find convincing support for the asynchrony hypothesis, a further troubling consideration arises. Perhaps creative individuals are marked by asynchrony not because it plagues them but rather—and precisely—because they seek it. Perhaps their temperament is such that, constitutionally dissatisfied with the status quo, they are perennially predisposed to up the ante, to stir up troubles, to convert comfortable synchrony to tension-producing asynchrony. Should this be the case, the asynchrony hypothesis would be confirmed but for an unanticipated reason—certain individuals seek asynchrony, and, if they do not readily find it in sufficient quantity, they create it or exacerbate it.

Perhaps, indeed, creative individuals find asynchrony where others detect only harmony. It is told that, when Freud returned to Vienna after his only trip to the United States, his then associate Carl Jung remained in the States. Jung had a wonderful time touring the salons of the Eastern seaboard and finally sent back to his mentor an enthusiastic telegram—"Psychoanalysis great success." Ever vigilant and perhaps searching again for asynchrony, Freud immediately wired back—"What did you leave out?"

Conclusions: The Inevitability of the Field

From a psychological perspective, it is bracing, but somewhat distressing, to conclude that creativity can no longer be thought of, at least exclusively, as the purview of the individual. There may come to be an individual of the greatest potential in one or more domains, but, if he or she fails to come into contact with that domain, misconstrues the domain too radically, or fashions products that cannot be assimilated by the field, such work will not be considered creative by our definition. Enlarging the disciplinary realm within which one must consider creativity may be scientifically necessary, but, for those researchers accustomed to working at the level of the person, it makes the task much more difficult. Still, it is useful, at least as an exercise, to consider creative processes in the absence of the field. Is it possible to create in the absence of the field, and, if so, what form does such creativity assume?

We may consider three instances of apparently "fieldless" creativity. There is, first of all, the accomplished master—say, a Picasso—who continues to engage in creative work while paying little or no attention to the reactions of the field. This instance proves not to be problematic from the point of view of our analysis. In the course of his development, Picasso internalized the standards of the field and could, even in the privacy of his atelier, bring to bear the kinds of considerations that others had earlier presented to him in a more direct manner. Actual contact with the field was for him no longer necessary. Of course, in the long run, the field will still determine the merit of Picasso's work. In fact, in the case of his later works, those produced in virtual isolation from the rest of the artistic world, there is at present considerable controversy. Perhaps Picasso would have done well, in his later years, to remain in closer contact with his various publics.

Picasso and the field were inevitably intertwined. But what of the solitary individual, the one who continues to work in an area in apparent ignorance of, or indifference to, the external field? There is Emily Dickinson, unpublished in her lifetime but afterward discovered to be a major poet. There is the aforementioned Harold Shapinsky, who painted in total obscurity for thirty years but who has recently been promoted as a significant abstract expressionist of the second generation and whose canvases now earn considerable sums. There are no doubt thousands of amateur writers, artists, musicians, scientists, and mathematicians who either continue to produce for their own satisfaction or have tried and failed to exert an influence on the field—or even to be noticed at all.

Are not these individuals creative as well? Is the field really necessary? As a start, it is important to point out that these individuals have not created in complete isolation from the field. They have all

115

been formed on the basis of earlier work produced in a domain/field, and, in that sense alone, they are not complete isolates. Still, it is true that the interaction has been unidirectional: they may have learned from the field, but the field has—at least so far—proved indifferent to them.

We would discern here a kind of indeterminacy principle at work. Of course, in one sense, Dickinson or Shapinsky remain the same kind of person, whether or not the field ultimately decides to award them the accolade of "creativity." But, unless the field's standards are brought to bear on their work, the status of that work remains completely indeterminate. Moreover, once the field is brought to bear, then it *has* been brought to bear. It is no longer sensible to talk of a Dickinson or a Shapinsky in the absence of the field. Thus, in a manner analogous to Heisenberg's principle in particle physics, the very act of determining whether something is creative immediately and inevitably involves the invocation of the field: to ask whether something is creative is to introduce the field irrevocably into what might hitherto have been viewed as a relatively fieldless endeavor.

Neither Picasso nor Dickinson, then, can be thought of as individuals outside a field, even if they themselves worked in splendid isolation. There are individuals who do create largely outside the field, however. These are young children. In every culture, young children play with the symbol systems of their milieu. They make graphic depictions, they sing, they tell stories, and they tinker with objects. And they undertake this activity with sublime indifference to the domain, the structure of knowledge in a particular discipline, and with equivalent indifference to the field, the roles and institutions that determine the paths of careers. To be sure, in the course of socialization, these youngsters will be introduced to the relevant domains and fields, and they will thus enter into the process—the dialectic—of creativity. But, at least at the outset, their protocreative activities occur outside the field, if not beyond the pale.

For the most part, this distancing from the field is a two-way process. The child ignores the field, and the field ignores the child. In nearly all societies, and for nearly all human history, the protocreative products of young children have been of essentially no interest to anyone except the children themselves. If the insightful developmental psychologist Piaget (1962) is to be believed, children themselves would never think to raise such questions. Only in our time, and in no small measure because of the rise of such fields as child psychology and psychoanalysis, the works of young children have begun to arouse interest and to be assessed in terms of the criteria of creativity. To the extent that this trend continues, the field of artistic production will have entered the realm of childhood creativity and may even be transformed by it.

This coming together of childhood activity and the study of creativity is appropriate. Even if, in the final analysis, creativity cannot be assessed apart from the Csikszentmihalyi dialectic, there remains a sense in which it begins in the activities of young children (Gardner, Phelps, and Wolf, in press). Here, we believe, children first begin to toy with the boundaries around them, to engage in novel activities, to gain pleasure from the manipulation of symbolic forms. It is this activity—often long suppressed during latency years—that resurfaces in the more competent hands of the master and seems to constitute an important part of the thrill of the creative life. Childhood creativity is not equivalent to the creativity of the master—but it is difficult to envisage the possibility of adult creativity without the experience of childhood. In this sense, it is fitting that our modest study of creativity has focused on two individuals who have helped to form the sensibility of our time: Sigmund Freud, who first underscored the extent to which later mental life is dictated by the experiences of childhood, and Pablo Picasso, whose work had such deep links to the simple forms favored in childhood and who recognized the deep truth, "Once I drew like Raphael but it has taken me a whole life to learn to draw like a child" (quoted in de Meredieu 1974, p. 13).

NOTES

This paper has been adapted from oral remarks presented to the Conference on Creativity and Adolescence, American Society for Adolescent Psychiatry, Philadelphia, September 1986. Some of the work described in this chapter was supported by the MacArthur Foundation and the Spencer Foundation.

1. For a representative set of readings in the psychology of creativity, see Vernon (1970).

REFERENCES

Bamberger, J. 1982. Growing up prodigies: the midlife crisis. In D. H. Feldman, ed. *New Directions for Child Development,* vol. 17. San Francisco: Jossey-Bass.

Barr, A. 1936. *Cubism and Abstract Art.* Cambridge, Mass.: Harvard University Press, 1986.

Barr, A. 1946. *Picasso: Fifty Years of His Art.* New York: Museum of Modern Art, 1974.

Berger, J. 1965. *The Success and Failure of Picasso.* New York: Pantheon.

Burns, E. 1970. *Gertrude Stein on Picasso.* New York: Liveright.

Csikszentmihalyi, M. In press. Society, culture and person: a systems view of creativity. In R. Sternberg, ed. *The Nature of Creativity.* New York: Cambridge University Press.

Csikszentmihalyi, M., and Robinson, R. 1986. Culture, time, and the development of talent. In R. Sternberg and J. Davidson, eds. *Conceptions of Giftedness.* New York: Cambridge University Press.

de Meredieu, F. 1974. *Le dessin d'enfant.* Paris: Editions Universitaires Jean-Pierre de Large.

Diamond, M. 1985. On the brain of the scientist: Albert Einstein. *Experimental Neurology* 88:198–204.

Ellenberger, H. 1970. *The Discovery of the Unconscious.* New York: Basic.

Feldman, D. H. 1980. *Beyond Universals in Cognitive Development.* Norwood, N.J.: Ablex.

Feldman, D. H. 1986. *Nature's Gambit.* New York: Basic.

Gardner, H. 1975. *The Shattered Mind.* New York: Knopf.

Gardner, H. 1983. *Frames of Mind: The Theory of Multiple Intelligences.* New York: Basic.

Gardner, H. 1986. Freud in three frames. *Daedalus* 115 (Summer): 105–134.

Gardner, H., and Dudai, Y. 1985. Biology and giftedness. *Items* 39:1–6.

Gardner, H.; Phelps, E.; and Wolf, D. In press. The roots of creativity in children's symbolic products. In C. Alexander and E. Langer, eds. *Beyond Formal Operations.* New York: Oxford University Press.

Gedo, M. 1980. *Picasso—Art as Autobiography.* Chicago: University of Chicago Press.

Getzels, J., and Csikszentmihalyi, M. 1976. *The Creative Vision*. New York: Wiley.

Gilot, F., and Lake, C. 1964. *Life with Picasso*. New York: McGraw-Hill.

Goldwater, R. 1938. *Primitivism in Modern Art*. Cambridge, Mass.: Harvard University Press, 1986.

Gopnik, A. 1983. High and low: caricature, primitivism and the cubist portrait. *Art Journal* (Winter), pp. 371–376.

Gruber, H. 1981. *Darwin on Man*. Chicago: University of Chicago Press.

Janik, A., and Toulmin, S. 1974. *Wittgenstein's Vienna*. New York: Simon & Schuster.

Johnson-Laird, P. N. 1983. *Mental Models*. Cambridge, Mass.: Harvard University Press.

John-Steiner, V. 1985. *Notebooks of the Mind*. Albuquerque: University of New Mexico Press.

Jones, E. 1961. *The Life and Work of Sigmund Freud*. Edited and abridged by Lionel Trilling and Steven Marcus. New York: Basic.

Medawar, P. 1969. *Induction and Intuition*. Philadelphia: American Philosophical Society.

Penrose, R. 1958. *Picasso: His Life and Work*. 3d ed. Berkeley and Los Angeles: University of California Press, 1981.

Perkins, D. N. 1981. *The Mind's Best Work*. Cambridge, Mass.: Harvard University Press.

Piaget, J. 1962. *Play, Dreams and Imitation*. New York: Norton.

Reich, W. 1986. The stuff of genius. *New York Times Magazine* (July 25), pp. 23–25.

Rubin, W. 1980. *Pablo Picasso: A Retrospective*. New York: Museum of Modern Art.

Sacks, O. 1986. *The Man Who Mistook His Wife for a Hat and Other Clinical Tales*. New York: Summit.

Schonberg, H. 1969. It all came too easily for Camille Saint-Saëns. *New York Times* (January 12).

Schorske, C. 1973. *Fin-de-Siècle Vienna*. New York: Knopf.

Selfe, L. 1977. *Nadia*. London: Academic Press.

Simonton, D. K. 1984. *Genius, Creativity, and Leadership*. Cambridge, Mass.: Harvard University Press.

Sternberg, R., ed. In press. *The Nature of Creativity*. New York: Cambridge University Press.

Sulloway, F. 1983. *Freud: Biologist of the Mind.* New York: Basic.

Teuber, M. 1982. *Formvorstellung und Kubismus oder Pablo Picasso und William James in Kubismus: Kuenstler, Themen, Werke, 1907– 1920.* Cologne: Josef-Haubrich-Kunsthalle.

Vernon, P. 1970. *Creativity.* London: Penguin.

Wallace, A. 1986. *The Prodigy: William James Sidis, America's Greatest Child Prodigy.* New York: Dutton.

Weschler, L. 1985. A strange destiny. *New Yorker* (December 16), pp. 47–48.

7   POETRY AND CONSCIOUSNESS

C. K. WILLIAMS

When I began to consider what I was going to discuss about poetry and consciousness, it occurred to me that the title of my chapter probably should be "Poetry and Emotion" or "Poetry and Feelings" because in an essential way poetry is most strictly defined by its relation to feeling. I also realized that, no matter what one were to try to speak of in relation to consciousness, one would have to deal with emotion. Our ultimate judgment of any experience is how it "feels" to us, how our emotional response to the experience has been evaluated. We also know that even the most abstract idea has some sort of feeling attached to it and that, without that feeling, an idea has no resonance for use, no meaning.

At the same time, though, I have been troubled for a long while with how our culture defines emotion, particularly in relation to mind. Certainly, our philosophical and psychological heritage offers a rich store of debate and reflection on mind. But when I actually consider my own mind—particularly the way I experience mind in relation to emotion—I find that, although I have learned a great deal from James, Freud, Ryle, and Wittgenstein, somehow the consciousness and emotional mechanism with which I live has not quite been accounted for in any of the systems with which I am familiar.

To begin with, I have been puzzled for a long time by what exactly an emotion is. I know the words for emotions: "love," "hate," "anger," "dread," and so on. But, considering the central position emotions play in our lives, we have a surprisingly small number of terms to describe or embody them, and often we find ourselves groping for modifying systems that become overcomplicated and confusing.

© 1988 by The University of Chicago. All rights reserved.
0-226-24061-4/88/0015-0005$01.00

Next, even with the terms we do have, we seem to be terribly vague and general in our dealings with emotions. If I say to you, "I am depressed," you will have, we will both think, a pretty good idea of what I am feeling. If, on the other hand, either of us wishes to be more specific—if I want to tell you more or if you want to ask more—we run into problems. Rather than being able to speak more precisely about the emotion itself, usually what we will try to do is to find out what I am depressed about.

The problem with the way we communicate our emotions and try to delve more deeply into them is that we tend to leave the emotion itself out. Mostly what we are doing when we are investigating an emotion is surrounding it, giving it a clearer background. That background can extend, in classical analysis, to the cradle, but, as for the emotion itself that we are experiencing, it can somehow not have been touched. We may both come to feel better about what we have done, but, generally, what that will have been is a sort of dissipation and distraction.

Presumably, then, we might say that at least I myself know my emotion. But do I? If I were to describe the feeling itself to myself, what would I say? Much the same sort of thing. I am depressed about death, say, separation, isolation. But these, again, are conditions of the emotion, frames, even causes; the emotion itself will often remain vague, uncertain, and transitory. Often it seems that, by the time we are into the investigation of an emotion, that emotion has been frus-tratingly replaced by the one attached to the investigation. If we push ourselves to ask, "What am I really feeling?" we will probably begin to refer to the body. We will say, "I am feeling this in my gut, in my heart, in my genitals." But this, too, tends to be rather crude. In our culture, we feel fear in the pit of the stomach, but we also feel some components of "truth" there and of true love.

Yet, with all this apparent imprecision and reflective uncertainty, we know that, when we are feeling something, it is anything but crude, vague, and approximate. We know that we are feeling this exact feeling at this exact time. We know we will never feel this precise feeling again, and, what is more, we know exactly to what degree we are suffering from or exalting in this specific emotion. The problem seems to arise when we have to describe ourselves to ourselves. For whatever reason, human consciousness is not satisfied with experience in itself; it is our reflection on our experience that allows us to consider ourselves le-gitimate, that makes us recognize an emotion as authentic. Unless we can manage to accomplish this reflection, we feel we have been cheated and, in a radical sense, may even begin to question the reality of what we have experienced. Emotion, then, clearly must be considered in relation to the larger concepts of consciousness and of mind.

I would like now to offer a brief characterization of mind and consciousness as I experience them myself. I do not in any sense mean to revise existing psychologies or epistemologies, and I surely do not mean to assume to tell you anything that you do not already know. What I am proposing, I think, are questions of emphasis that interest me.

The mind I experience myself seems to be a much more chaotic and turbulent phenomenon than those minds that I have heard about: there is much more happening in it, much more happening at once, and much more happening in a nondetermined way. If I were to try to make a rough section of it, I would first find sense data arriving from various parts of the body—usually through the eyes and ears—bringing with them what philosophy traditionally calls "impressions." Then there are the processing systems of these impressions, which discard most of them, filing some for future reference, although not necessarily the ones one would think to have selected. Then there are the various, and more numerous, elements of consciousness that mind itself generates. Of these elements, what I will discuss first—because I think it is not only the most basic of the mind's activities but also the least remarked on—is what I call the image-making mechanism. This is a phenomenon that is hinted at but not really captured by the term "stream of consciousness." It is also the source of our access to "primary process" but differs from it in some essential ways.

Briefly, it is my observation that one of the major activities of the mind is the constant, incessant, and terrifically rapid production of image. I mean by "image" those mental pictures that exist aside from, or rather along with but as it were behind, the images received by sense. There is a kind of perception screen through which we process images that arrive from the world and a screen behind that perception screen onto which the interior images are being projected. We are always aware of which is the "real" image, but, at the same time, we are also always able, when we wish, to refer to the other image mechanism as it works or plays. I have no idea how to measure the number of images that pass out of our interior world into this portion of consciousness. When I have discussed the question with young poets in my workshops, I have mentioned at least several per second, and none of my students have found that unreasonable. These images, as I say, are rapid, incessant, irrepressible (although we do learn not to pay attention to them), and often utterly unreasonable in origin, and very often they have nothing to do with what is going on in the rest of consciousness, with the projects of our "reality." Sometimes the images arise from memory—places seen, people known. Sometimes they will have to do with words that are going through our minds at the moment. Although sometimes these images are surely the result of the action and interaction of instinctual forces, sometimes they will have no discernible genealogy, no roots whatever in anything we can account for. Sometimes the images will begin to link together—by "sometimes" I mean several times a minute, at least—and sometimes these linkages, fragments of narrative, will catch the attention of other portions of mind, and the narratives will extend and become what we call "fantasy."

It is this constant flow of image and narrative, generated by consciousness in a nondetermined way, that is the key to our beginning to characterize emotion adequately. I say "characterize" purposefully, and not "embody," because the other element of my thesis is that, in fact, it is already embodied, with great precision and rigor, in poetry.

Now I want to continue with the scheme I am developing, the next element of which would be language. Language is layered over and somehow weaves in and out of the flow of image and narrative-fantasy. Usually, it seems to exist apart, but, at the same time, it is constantly referring to the image world, recuperating portions of it for its own use and feeding back into the image world material that would not otherwise be there. Language, as we know, is an enormously complex phenomenon in itself. We know amazingly little about it; we are not even sure whether we teach ourselves to learn language or whether, figuratively at least, it teaches us to learn it.

The way we generally experience language in consciousness is of itself of interest in terms of our emotional life. Language seems to come to us through what we might call the voice of the mind. There is a voice within us, certainly. Sometimes we hear it rather vaguely, sometimes surprisingly sharply. Sometimes it seems to speak to and for our conceived identity, sometimes it conducts a dialogue with that identity, and sometimes it is sharply critical. Usually, it speaks in our everyday voice, but sometimes we can be surprised to hear someone else's voice within us. Sometimes it seems to be telling us what we had in mind to say but did not know how. Sometimes it refuses us utterly, denying us what we know is on the tip of the tongue. When it speaks out into the world, it sometimes does so with our concurrence, satisfying our pre-meditations. But sometimes it can seem to have a perversely contra-dictory program of its own, hardly consulting with us, producing one of the more interesting of the mind-body syndromes: the foot in the mouth.

Language and the voice of mind are deeply involved in but do not entirely determine what we call "sentiments," that is, our feeling about the general tone of the proceedings, short term and long, in conscious-ness and in the world. Out of these sentiments arise our grander notions of mortality and ethics and our social and political beliefs and attitudes.

Beyond all this, there is what we call "thought," what is known as discursive thinking, something presumably similar to what I am at-tempting here. In this activity, the mind picks its way through all the littered landscapes I have been describing, making what we call "ra-tional sense," acting as though all these detourings and blind alleys did not exist.

The capacity of consciousness to juggle these elements of itself is, one might say, mind-boggling. What I want to emphasize most sharply in the characterization I am offering, though, are what I have referred to as the nondetermined, apparently arbitrary phenomena generated by mind by way of both image and language, for I feel that these arbitrary aspects of mind are what, in fact, are at the foundation of imagination. I seem to be coming into conflict here with the whole universe of psychology, particularly Freudian psychology. As we know, part of Freud's genius was to dissect, as it were, the soul into its historical components, showing how these small histories determine us. Freud's theoretical models were, of course, necessarily of his time. He proposed a sort of geology of consciousness that, as has been remarked, was similar to the earth science that had been elaborated in the nineteenth century. He also proposed a vision of consciousness that we might say was Darwinian. More than that, though, the universe in which Freud situated mind was a Newtonian universe in which phenomena could be accounted for with calculus and, by extension, in a cause and effect relation, however complicated this relation would have to be. The products of consciousness itself—fantasy and dream primarily—were, for Freud, the products of tensions in the past, pre-sumably repressed tensions. Consciousness could be accounted for, and possibly redeemed, by a scrupulous attention to these pastnesses, and part of that scrupulousness was the proposition that nothing in consciousness was arbitrary, that the mind had a Newtonian coherence.

The universe in which we find our models is quite different. It is the universe of quanta, of events that bear a quality in themselves of a kind of indeterminateness. The curves of experience that our physics deals with are larger and are describable only by attention to their larger activities. Necessity becomes statistical rather than calculable, and the possibly arbitrary nature of the individual event becomes something that must be taken into account.

The events of consciousness that I am describing seem to me to partake of a universe of possibility in which the arbitrary, unpredictable, undetermined event has a remarkable metaphoric similarity to that of a quantum. I believe that, in order for us to make our consciousness appear to be the neat Freudian, Newtonian mechanisms we have conceived them to be, we must do a remarkable amount of disattending, disregarding, something like what the word "repression" indicated, but probably something that is in some ways more radical.

Simultaneity is a thorny problem in epistemology, but I hold that there is something in the potential of our mind that can and does as a matter of course entertain simultaneously a startling range of content. As I was composing the sentence I am starting now, for instance—it was written in my mind late at night in bed a month or so ago in Paris— I was also thinking about what this room would look like today, what you would look like before me, of what my friend Loren would look like as he sat among you listening, of what he would think of this, of Loren's new house, of the evening I spent there with my wife, then of a street somewhere in Italy (why it came to me I had no idea), then of another friend, then another landscape totally unknown to me. There were also the words more or less as they are of this sentence, plus my remarking to myself how remarkable what I was doing really was. Beyond all that I was humming under my breath a Robert Burns song that I had been memorizing the day before, "For A' That and A' That," and, of course, I was paying enough attention to all this to be able to report it, at the same time being aware that a number of images and bits of narrative had occurred that I was too preoccupied to attend to.

My point here is that I do not feel that this was an unusual moment of consciousness, at least in its complexity. Clearly, we do not generally pay such meticulous attention to ourselves for very long; we would not be able to go on with the business of living. We learn to disregard most of these obscure goings on, and how successful we are at it might be a measure of what we call "sanity."

I am sure this has all seemed a very crude, oversimplified depiction of consciousness. I imagine I have omitted much that I would find on further reflection even in my own mind. But I think I have given some notion of what we must take into account when we speak of something as complex and crucial to us as emotion. An emotion clearly is in direct relation to all the elements of mind that I have been discussing. Whatever the experience the emotion arises from, the mind will have to process it. During this processing, there will also be images generated into consciousness, some dictated by the experience itself, some with very little or nothing to do with it. There will also be the participation of the senses, of language, as it comments, criticizes, and reflects. There will also be an awareness that the equation that all this makes, the emotion, is something that is not a normal moment of passing consciousness. In our everyday experience, all this will be dealt with by the mind's various components, including that one that we call "self." A sort of majority vote will be taken, and the experience will then be denoted with one of the names for feeling we have received and learned to apply. Once so named, the feeling will generate another series of phenomena of its own as well as interpretations of these events that will in turn be voted on and, possibly, named again. There will also be a sort of checking-in process between votes to keep the mind up on what is happening on the longer term.

We can certainly say that an emotion is not a simple thing, yet it is the odd conceit of our culture that an emotion is the only thing in our mental lives that we do not have to doubt. We are taught that there is within us something uncontaminated, pure, something that is to be the base to which all the rest of our confusing existence is to refer: our feelings. We are somehow given to assume, even more strangely, that emotions are the one thing for which we do not have to be educated. Even in the various psychotherapy systems, there often seems to be the assumption that one is to get back, somehow, through all the storm and "thrust" of the rest of the mind to these islands of purity, spontaneity, and clarity.

Emotions, I hold, are, in and of themselves, neither pure, spontaneous, nor very clear. They require a stringent attentiveness, and, if the soul is to do justice to their turbulence and furor without belittling itself, it must indeed be educated, and rigorously so. It is my thesis that the most useful method we have devised for that education is poetry.

A poem is a wonderfully complicated instrument. It is as complicated, as an emotion, maybe more so. It also shares many characteristics with emotion. It is composed of sensation, image, language, a voice, perception, bodily reference, sentiment, morality, thought, and experience. It, like existence itself, concerns itself crucially with the arbitrary and the determined. The forms of poetry, for instance, are in a large sense totally arbitrary. What we call a convention is a system of the arbitrary and the necessary. That the most common rhythmic convention in English poetic history, iambic pentameter, has ten syllables, five stressed and five unstressed, is determined to some extent by the nature of the language itself, but, in another sense, it has nothing to do with it. The line might have easily had six feet or been syllabically determined. The fact that the line—and the other conventions of poetry—are arbitrarily determined is of the utmost importance because it is in the tension between the artificially determined conventions and the necessities of language and experience that the music of poetry arises. The music of poetry—that is, of consciousness at play in the fields of necessity and crisis—is one of the most important informing elements of poetry. So, too, do what we call "figuration," "simile," "metaphor," and so on have to do with the arbitrary and the necessary. We are taught that it is associative necessity that determines metaphor, but this is not the case. It is actually the ability of the poet to dissociate, to reach into the realm of chance, to fuse the unlikely with the undeniable, that determines the intensity of metaphor. So, the German poet Rilke, for instance, in contemplating the tombs of ancient Roman courtesans, trying to find their imaginative identity, ends up comparing the women to, of all unlikely things, rivers:

> over them in brief, impetuous waves
> (and wanting to prolong itself, forever)
> the bodies of countless adolescents surged;
> and in them roared the currents of grown men.
> And sometimes boys would burst forth from the mountains
> of childhood, and would descend in timid streams
> and play with what they found on the river's bottom,
> until the steep slope gripped their consciousness.

[Rilke 1982]

The tensions of poetry are, of course, most evident and most crucial in their direct relation to experience. Poetry deals with the most difficult of our experiences and emotions, and these dealings are dictated by the sharpest necessities. Poetry confronts in the most clear-eyed way just those emotions that consciousness most wishes to slide by. It deals with them in their greatest profundity, with the most refined moral sensibility. What is more, it does justice to just the sorts of complexities and simultaneities I have been sketching here.

At the beginning of this chapter, I proposed a situation in which I would say to you, "I am depressed," and I tried to point out how vague and uncertain this statement really is, whether spoken to others or to the self. I hinted that my depression had to do with death, separation, isolation. What I would like to do now is to offer you two poems by Emily Dickinson, both having to do with depression and with death. Each incorporates a specific emotion, elaborates it, analyzes it, and, in a deep sense, redeems it. For poetry ultimately has to do most with that, the redemption of our experiences from the temporal and the trivial.

The first poem is about depression. It is the most complete depiction and embodiment I know of depression, of the actual emotion of depression, the emotion that, I pointed out, in our normal experience is surrounded, backgrounded, but rarely articulated directly. In this poem, Dickinson uses the imagery of death, figures of death, actual apprehensions of death, to work with the emotion, but never tells us what her depression is about. Perhaps that would be a trivialization of it.

> I felt a Funeral, in my Brain,
> And Mourners to and fro
> Kept treading—treading—till it seemed
> That Sense was breaking through—
>
> And when they all were seated,
> A Service, like a Drum—
> Kept beating—beating—till I thought
> My Mind was going numb—
>
> And then I heard them lift a Box
> and creak across my Soul
> With those same Boots of Lead, again,
> Then Space—began to toll,

As all the Heavens were a Bell,
And Being, but an Ear,
And I, and Silence, some strange Race
Wrecked, solitary, here—

And then a Plank in Reason, broke,
And I dropped down, and down—
And hit a World, at every plunge,
And Finished knowing—then—

[Dickinson 1961]

What it is that Dickinson knows, and finishes knowing, at the end of the poem is almost too frightening to consider. She has confronted, in her investigation of that single emotion, the annihilation of consciousness, the loss of reason in its harrowing proximities to nothingness. She has enacted the terrifying closed system of depression in which content, sense, reality, all become functions of that closure. The images that occur—once the system has been impelled, after the vehicle of the funeral has been established—still partake of the kind of arbitrary mental event that I tried to sketch before, but their apparent arbitrariness only contributes to the tensions and despair of the mental experience. A "Service, like a Drum—"—there is no drum in the funerals of life, only in the rituals of depression, in which the heart itself seems to become the enemy of the organism and of consciousness. The "Boots of Lead" are heavier and more excruciating than any we know. The "Heavens" become a "Bell": all of infinite space is emptied of its possible divinities, of its potential solace, so that all of "Being," all the being of the individual and all the creatures of existence, can do nothing but listen to that divine space, now encapsulated and captured in the bell of skull and of emotion. As for the "Plank," is it the plank that a pirate's victim must walk or a plank covering a dry well, the well of inexistence? The ambiguities are as crucial as the precisions: the laying of meaning and potential meaning in the poem are the very layers of consciousness. That this dire experience could be put into words, that the voice of the mind could make it cohere, that the language of the experience could, moreover, be organized into rhythm patterns, that there could even be rhyme, all the while upholding the dark integrities of the experience itself—this is not the product of mind; this is mind and emotion and the human soul alive to itself.

The second poem is very similar in some ways. It is a poem that occupies itself with death, but this time death is not being used to incorporate another emotion. Rather, it is death itself that is being confronted—our fear of death, our apprehensions at how the mind deals and will deal with death. You will notice again that the poem works by using imagery and sensations that surround the experience of human dying, but, in this case, the theme of the poem is the subtraction of the imagery of the soul by death. Note that the poem is in the past tense, although, clearly, the events it speculates about are in an imagined future. At the same time, our reading of the poem must take place in a narrative present. Hence, even as the poem launches itself, we are in a mind situation of complexity and tension:

> I heard a Fly buzz—when I died—
> The Stillness in the Room
> Was like the Stillness in the Air—
> Between the Heaves of Storm—
>
> The Eyes around—had wrung them dry—
> And Breaths were gathering firm
> For that last Onset—when the King
> Be witnessed—in the Room
>
> I willed my Keepsakes—Signed away
> What portion of me be
> Assignable—and then it was
> There interposed a Fly—
>
> With Blue—uncertain stumbling Buzz—
> Between the light—and me—
> And then the Windows failed—and then
> I could not see to see—
>
> [Dickinson 1961]

Someone is dying, a someone who is called "I," a name with which we are all familiar. The room the "I" is in is quiet, so quiet that a single fly can be heard, but the quiet is ominous, promising to give way to great violence, as of a storm, a violence that finally occurs in a stillness yet deeper. The "I" of the poem is surrounded by other people, who have cried and who now, in the face of the enormities of death, can do nothing but wait. The one who is dying speaks her testament, and then the fly is there again. Suddenly we realize that everything in the room has become the fearful function now of mind itself. The other human beings become equal to the fly; then the fly becomes equal to the dying self, and to light itself, and to existence itself.

"And then the Windows failed—and then / I could not see to see—." The loss of actual subjecthood has been imagined, apprehended, and redeemed. The poem struggles with resignation, with all the resignations we try to teach ourselves, and it accomplishes these resignations with wisdom and grace: "I . . . Signed away / What portion of me be / Assignable. . . ," the portion of me that had to do with you, with us, with all of us, all the other subjects that are our consolation, but a consolation that no longer will operate, that we must renounce. Then that wise renunciation itself has no more reality than the fly, which still intrudes, insists, equating our time with its own; and then the fly, the tiny morsel of eternity, is gone; and then the light in which it swam is gone; "the Windows failed," the windows of sense, of soul, of self, of subject, but, too, the windows even of our attempt to contemplate the unendurable fact of death. Only the voice is left now, only the voice of mind, as it enacts, no longer with horror, no longer with fear, because there is nothing left to be horrified or fearful of, the going out of not only sight but also the sight behind sight, the very vision of the mind and soul. When the poem ends, when that voice stops, the silence that falls on us is the silence of death and inexistence.

Conclusions

It is thus that poetry speaks its emotion, its consciousness. It is thus that it teaches us the limits of the elements of consciousness that we value so—our reason, our discursive language, our notion that we can analyze the substances of being. Perhaps the real matter of the human soul is poetry itself; perhaps it is in the community that is established between the speaking soul of the poet and the attending soul of the listener that our consciousness, our culture, and our selves find their ways of being saved from the awful deaths that we imagine and die, the awful ephemeralities of our passage through eternity, and the awful disattendings to what we have of that passage.

REFERENCES

Dickinson, E. 1961. *Emily Dickinson's Poems*. Edited by Thomas H. Johnson. Boston: Little, Brown.

Rilke, R. M. 1982. *The Selected Poetry of Rainer Maria Rilke*. Translated by Stephen Mitchell. New York: Random House.

FRANK GALUSZKA

When I look at a painting, I can feel something or feel nothing at all. Actually, I only feel like I feel nothing at all. My impression is slight and hazy. It hardly dents my consciousness, which is preoccupied with other things. The painting has put me off, left me cold. The idea or point may seem so remote as to be intangible and irrelevant.

If I want to get to know such a thing, it is up to me to break the ice. I ask myself the simplest question I can ask. How is the experience of looking at this painting different from the experience of looking at just the wall? How would things be different if this painting was not here? Responses come to mind quickly. There is an overall impression: darkness, for instance, or detail, or brilliance, or vagueness, whatever. I am looking at the outcome of something, of someone else's experience. And, by the way, that someone is recommending to an imaginary audience that what I am looking at can be meaningful.

When looking at work done in other times or places, I know I am not a member of the imaginary audience of the artist. I must seek a transcultural human-to-human response—a different and perhaps deeper response than the artist intended. If I look carefully, like an archaeologist, at simple overlaps of painted edges, and if I look through translucent layers to what shows from underneath, I can gather a lot of evidence. Evidence of what? All paintings reveal something of the sequence of their production. Sometimes an artist intentionally covers his tracks, but this is hard to do completely. After following the steps of production backward, I can reverse the process and follow the decision-making sequence forward. Revisions, modifications, and pre-

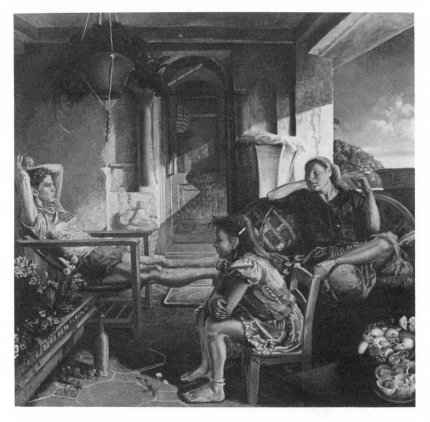

Fig. 1.—Galuszka, "Continuous Afternoon," 1986

meditated process are revealed. In revisions and modifications, we can tell what might have been, what was decided against. The dialogue between what might have been and what is represents a dialogue between lesser and greater satisfaction. From such scattered clues, aspects of a painter's aesthetic goals can be extrapolated.

Decisions

An artwork is an accumulation of decisions. There are decisions about everything. In a black-and-white drawing, the decisions are relatively digitized—to make a mark in an area or not to make a mark, how hard to press to make the mark more or less emphatic. But, in a painting, multiple options crop up everywhere. Every mark, color, form, or shape could be altered this way or that.

An artist may marshal decisions under a code or under intuitive judgment. For the sake of convenience, I would like to refer to the followers of a code as systems artists and to the followers of intuitive judgment as expressionists—although most artists combine a little of one with a lot of the other in their unique strategies. I am more interested in the expressionists than in the systems artists and count myself among them. While I intend to contrast the two, it is not my intention here to argue one side against the other.

Catalog

In order to make decisions, each artist carries in his or her mind a catalog of alternative possibilities. No catalog is comprehensive. Each artist's stock of choices has limitations intentionally or unintentionally enforced by this mental book.

In the catalog are sections on forms, images, texture, handling, line, color, symbolism, historical references, and so on. Every variant of every hue imaginable could potentially be present in each artist's color catalog. But usually artists settle into a narrow repertoire of colors. This is because the catalog, as a problem-solving device, tends to be efficient and to suggest the familiar solution before the exotic. Or, as an instrument of a code, as in Mondrian's case, in which the colors of the palette interact symbolically, the catalog itself becomes communicated as subject matter.

The depth of our appreciation of an artwork can be enhanced by our knowledge of the artist's catalog. If we are familiar enough with his "style," we can look around in his catalog and choose with him and see for ourselves how, in the case of most artworks, certain choices are inevitable.

We can appreciate not only artists whose catalogs seek to be vast but also artists whose catalogs have been consciously reduced. We can also see how artists get into trouble—how vast catalogs can get out of control, making choices arbitrary or valueless, and how narrow catalogs can become cages that close artists off from fresh possibilities and, eventually, from meaningful dialogue with life.

In art schools, students are not only educated—they are trained. They are familiarized with materials and ideas; they are also drilled in ways of translating observed phenomena. Controlled exercises that emphasize different aspects of the observable world are used to challenge clichés. Defeated clichés are replaced by strategies—ends orientation yields to means orientation. The general objective is to empower students to create for themselves functional, original, and personally satisfying catalogs of possibilities.

How does the catalog operate? While I can imagine others, the only one I know for sure is my own. I imagine that I have an unfinished painting of a figure seated in a room. There is a tabletop in the lower-right-hand corner of the painting. As the eye moves over the painting, it flows with a certain rhythm and achieves a certain frequency as it bounces from incident to incident. Only, the tabletop is a dead spot in the circuit. The eye hesitates unpleasantly at its location. I think I should put something on the table that would correct this problem. Good, I might think, this can give me some other opportunities too. Or bad, I might think, this painting already has too much in it. If my reaction is bad, I will ask myself how much it is worth to fix this spot or how I might do it with minimum obtrusiveness—say, by changing the color of the tabletop, or by putting a pattern of wood grain on it, or by showing a few knicks and scratches, or maybe by rounding off the corner so the eye does not get as pinched as it passes by and is freed to bounce off the framing edge back into the composition.

But what if the answer is good and not bad? The next thought is, Does anything naturally come to mind? Let us say that it does not. Then the question is, What might a single compact image provide for me? My mind draws up a list (all this happens as quick as thought). I could use some blue in that spot. Something, if small, should be gleaming, or sparkling? No, gleaming, that's for sure. It needs to have contrast to engage the eye properly. Metal would be good. What kind of object would be appropriate to the overall image? (First, to get it out of the way, I have to admit that a little devil is standing on my shoulder. He whispers in one ear the cheap solution: "Just lay a postcard on the table. Everything you want could be on it. Blue sky. Photo image of a metal object. What more could you want?" But the cheap solution has no resonance. It's poorly knit into the reality of the whole piece. It offers only second-hand tactility.) How about a knife? The blade could reflect blue walls, tying it in; the wooden handle might help it rest visually on the wooden tabletop. If angled parallel to the framing edge, it could add to the sense of structural integrity of that whole area of the painting. If angled another way, it would enhance the perspective. But it might look morbid given the depressed look on the face of the woman in the painting; it might make her seem to be thinking about killing herself. Too simple anyway, that line, kind of flat and bland as an image and a form. I want her to look sad, not desperate—something still compact but more complex. Why not put an apple near the knife, suggesting a more upbeat function for the knife as utensil rather than weapon. Maybe. Still, the two things next to one another tend to close up, put on a little act together to the exclusion of everything else. Besides, how trite! I'm stuck. But wait—a green apple would be more unusual (no, the debt to Magritte is too evident). A half apple already cut or bitten? That might be mysteriously redundant with the knife present, freeing the knife from its apple connection just enough to shed a small measure of threat onto the figure. Or maybe if the figure is related to the apple by the idea of nourishment and the symbol of temptation, why not connect the blade to the apple more obliquely so the two objects aren't functionally paired? A pair of scissors. As the apple could be made to relate specifically to the mouth by means of bite marks, the scissors could suggest the hand or fingers. Beyond that, a further, other kind of cutting, and, with the crossing blades opened, the image can both reinforce two-dimensionality by positioning one blade parallel to the framing edge and still promote three-dimensionality by allowing the other blade to line up with a vanishing point. And so on.

All this goes on with less than complete conscious awareness. Thoughts fly into each other rapidly, suggestions rise and fall, alter, adjust, come back in different form. This kind of process goes on in the minds of most artists I talk to. Each artist would, of course, have a different way of expressing movement toward solution. This process may continue for long stretches without committing anything to canvas. The artist does not confine this parade of imagery to the mind; he projects some kind of visualization of what he wants on canvas, changing the projected image as suggestions flow, measuring potential relations with other elements in the picture.

Visualization

How real is this projected image? It could not be mistaken for reality, but, while visually faint, it is present. With eyes closed, it becomes more vivid.

This vision is akin to another that is stronger—the persistence of patterns after long-term concentration or exposure. This is common enough. Anyone who has watched three football games in a row on New Year's Day can close his eyes to sleep and see the lines of the gridiron continue to pass as if a camera remains fixed on a ballcarrier. Bricklaying, painting a fence, or working on an assembly line should produce similar results. When, after painting stones, grass, drapery, or any kind of pattern, I step into a shower and close my eyes, I immediately see vividly the pattern I have been working on. Even as I work from a model, I see weak projections ahead of me—not a whole image, but the line or smudge I am about to make. Altering swiftly, it becomes satisfactory, and I follow it with a brush.

Giorgio de Chirico has said, "What I hear is valueless; only what I see is living, and when I close my eyes my vision is even more powerful" (Goldwater 1945, p. 439). In this statement, the great metaphysical painter emphasizes the vividness of his inner vision. It transforms the natural world as the artist looks on it, but there is a reciprocal weakening. Only when the eyes are closed is this vision fulfilled. Objective reality loses as personal reality gains.

When de Chirico says that what he hears is valueless, he is aware of a double meaning. What people say is valueless. This refers to critics and teachers; by extension, it refers to the whole body of available knowledge. It is a declaration of intuitive independence. Also, however, he is talking about sound; the intensified visual life has diminished the audio. The vision of visual art is something that has been distilled from the whole world of experience, from what all the senses have to offer. To those who create self-sufficient visual worlds, these worlds must exclude what they do not contain. De Chirico's metaphysical painting functioned for him as a kind of mediumistic device for entering into another world. He believed this other world was real.

Salvador Dali (1935) saw painting as an opportunity to conquer the irrational and "bring it back alive" to challenge the "cultural reality" of this world, which he, like de Chirico, considered both arbitrary and pathetic: "I believe the moment is at hand when, by a paranoiac and active advance of the mind, it will be possible (simultaneously with automatism and other passive states) to systematize confusion and thus to help discredit completely the world of reality" (quoted in Protter 1963, p. 240).

When Dali entered the Surrealist group, it had already been in existence long enough for him to be considered a second-generation member. It favored accessing subconscious information through strategies that allowed its members to drift out of critical wakefulness into what Dali calls "passive states." Dali proposed creating a lunatic alter ego within himself, a kind of cohabitating pet monster that would feed incoming delirious material to a form-giving, critical, theoretically sane artist. Dali's strategy was an aggressive and risky experiment. While André Breton was at first delighted, the Surrealist group was not always pleased by the results. Dali's eagerness to pursue taboo sexual and political subjects brought about his eventual dismissal from the group.

Dali's shaky mental health of the mid-1920s had been transformed through complex and unique circumstances into great mental strength with wide-ranging powers and such energy that Picasso exclaimed he had a mind "like an outboard motor." In this period, Dali developed his most convincing works, among them the famous painting of melted watches, *The Persistence of Memory*. In his *Secret Life*, Dali (1942, p. 317) describes how he painted this remarkable work:

It was on an evening when I felt tired, and had a slight headache, which is extremely rare with me. We were to go to a moving picture with some friends, and at the last moment I decided not to go. Gala would go off with them, and I would stay home and go to bed early. We had topped off our meal with a very strong Camembert, and after everyone had gone I remained for a long time seated at the table meditating on the philosophic problems of the "super-soft" which the cheese presented to my mind. I got up and went into my studio, where I lit the light in order to cast a final glance, as is my habit, at the picture I was in the midst of painting. This picture represented a landscape, near Port Lligat, whose rocks were lighted by a transparent and melancholy twilight; in the foreground an olive tree with its branches cut and without leaves. I knew that the atmosphere which I had succeeded in creating with this landscape was to serve as a setting for some idea, for some surprising image, but I did not in the least know what it was going to be. I was about to turn out the light, when instantaneously I "saw" the solution. I saw two soft watches, one of them hanging lamentably on the branch of the olive tree. In spite of the fact that my headache had increased to the point of becoming very painful, I avidly prepared my palette and set to work. When Gala returned from the theater two hours later, the picture, which was to be one of my most famous, was complete.

This is projected vision carried on at a nearly hallucinatory level. It is also "pure inspiration." It is unusual that an artist begins a painting without an idea. Yet here Dali only set a stage, an aesthetic trap, and captured the irrational prey he sought.

Inspiration

Such sudden and conclusive examples of inspiration are rare, so rare that stories such as Dali's attract attention and are appreciated with nearly religious mystification. Inspiration also has a day-to-day life. The artist is happiest when inspiration is kept continuously alive. As a part of the self, inspiration is so surprising in its spontaneous wisdom that—to many artists of the past, as well as to many artists today— when encountered it seems an emanation from an external entity, an invisible companion, a muse: "When I begin a picture, there is somebody who works with me. Toward the end, I get the impression that I have been working alone—without a collaborator" (Protter 1963, p. 203). Picasso here describes a change in consciousness during the creation of an artwork. The work of inspiration concludes before the painting is done. Intuitive openness closes down into conscious self-reliance.

Continuous inspiration is a function of creative consciousness, a habit of mind that is reinforced by use and weakened by neglect. It is best maintained by daily practice. The highly creative artist speculates about all he sees. His environment becomes, after a time, a visual and conceptual playground. Observed relations stimulate the imagination. The mind mechanically tests imagery against the catalog, which assesses potential for realization. Passed imagery is placed where it might be retrieved. Depending on the impression it makes, rejected imagery may be held onto as pending or discarded altogether.

This speculation goes on consciously and unconsciously. While making a painting, an artist is subject to intense and continuous feedback that may jell into whole images of other paintings. Suggestions may appear spontaneously at other times of the day. Dreams may test colors against each other, may present textures and compositions. New techniques may be divulged. Imagery, of course, is there in abundance, for the taking.

I have the impression of a continuous flow of imagery that streaks through the mind, all the time. Thought and sensory experience suppress this other vision and interrupt it. Unlike dreams, which may develop plot and direction, this other vision presents disjointed scenes in random sequence, like so many animated flash cards being turned over.

All this suggests life knee-deep in chaos. How does the artist survive this continuous storm of images and suggestions? He develops a tolerance for input based on the output of work. A day-to-day involvement with art making is easier to maintain than an involvement that stops and starts. Amateurs and beginning art students often say they work only when they are "in the mood." This implies a low level of creative consciousness. Only a small fraction from general experience is being absorbed as creative input; much time goes by before enough accumulates to be unloaded as art. To such people, art making is carefree and recreational.

As the amateur gets serious, as the art student develops, things change. Expectations rise; new territory must be faced; creativity must appear on demand. Instead of relieving tension, art creates it. It becomes hard to get started.

Blocks

Visual artists often suffer from creative blocks. Most face some resistance every day. The threshold of active creation is often preceded by ceremonial procrastination: cigarettes, coffee, radios on, cleaning up the studio, reading the mail. It can get worse. Instead of getting closer, the moment of actual beginning seems more and more distant.

It is important to identify what is going on. The student often does not know anything is going on. He may not see art and a pattern of avoidance as connected. Many things may just need to be done, from his point of view, before he can get to work—he may need a better pencil, something, anything. Inveterate artists may be more familiar with the situation, but too often they regard it as something that must be personally suffered through rather than as a fundamental part of creative experience.

We should consult an expert on this matter, a highly productive artist, with unbroken stretches of daily creativity. Picasso had the key. The key is continuity. He advised that it was useful at the day's end to leave a task half finished. If you are painting a sky blue, mix up a pot of paint, paint half the sky, and stop. He understood that two distinct consciousnesses alternate in the artist. The art consciousness gives way to the day-to-day consciousness. These are so different that one offers little help in moving toward the other. In fact, they seem to want only to perpetuate themselves.

Creative blocks do not strike suddenly in the middle of a healthy day's work. While it goes less noticed, an artist who has firmly entered active creativity can also have some difficulty in breaking it off. Picasso's scheme eases the transition in. It makes getting out less satisfactory than it would be if the day's end were marked by a closing accomplishment. The discipline to leave things unfinished needs to be learned. On the following day, instead of having to start with a decision of some kind, a decision that, because of its coming from the day-to-day mind, is likely to be misguided or irrelevant, the artist simply fulfills an earlier, trusted decision. By the time the sky is painted in, sheer intimacy with the artwork has spawned the next act, the next idea, and, through the rest of the session, one thing leads to another.

In a recent show of Picasso sketchbooks, a similar device for maintaining continuity showed itself. In some cases, his sketches are so carefully numbered and dated that we can follow his daily progress. When these drawings are variations on a theme, the format and even the actual configuration of lines and forms may vary only slightly from drawing to drawing. A whole figure duplicated from one day's last drawing may appear in the first drawing of the following day. Clearly, this is a method of getting a day started.

Art school classes often begin with *croquis,* fast drawings of the model. Each pose is under a minute's duration. The purpose of this activity is ostensibly to "loosen the student up," but its main function is to create a bridge from one consciousness to another by means of low-pressure exercises that are not meant to be art or contain thought. Each of these starting techniques is mechanical and intentionally transitional. They work to break down resistance and attach today's activity to yesterday's. But, if an artist who has been productive becomes unproductive, it becomes harder to connect. Time away causes input to build up to a point that puts greater strain on judgment to choose wisely among possibilities. Strain on judgment and need for commitment are likely to worsen an existing block. If this goes on for long, art-relative input begins to diminish for the sake of self-preservation, and the artist drops to a lower level of creativity from which he can build upward again over time.

Without the inertia of ongoing physical art making, ideas can become wide ranging; the desire for their fulfillment can become daydreamy and wishlike. As the habit of painting is restored, ideas become more focused and practical. Still, for every workable synthesis and conclusion, there are many faulty syntheses and half-baked conclusions.

Keys and Locks

The unfeasible and inappropriate are inspirations as well. It is not success that makes an inspiration inspirational. Inspirations are only proposals. It is a power of discrimination that allows an artist to recognize an inspiration as fitting a problem like a key to a lock. A serious inspiration may originate beyond conscious awareness, but it is nevertheless the result of floating configurations of catalog possibilities past the problem. The artist attentively follows the flyby, measuring interaction between problem and solution. Friction draws attention. The friction-producing element is tinkered with until it becomes a hook. Consciousness floods the situation. The response to the problem is monitored until a key is made. When the artist begins to realize this "key" on the site of the artwork, he is usually surprised to find that it does not fit the lock. The actual artwork had contained more variables than the mental model of the problem had accounted for.

At this point, systems artists are inclined to retool the key. Expressionist artists get to work changing the lock. The systems view seems to imagine art as a force of mind over void or a force of mind against physical matter. Systems artists have a strong sense of power over the creative situation and a sense of conscious responsibility for its outcome. Expressionists see themselves as working among unseen, unknowable forces. They act as arbitrators and conduits, relying heavily on intuitive judgment. The systems artist hopes to communicate through logical exposition. Expressionists try to communicate through empathy. The systems artist approaches art making with a plan. The expressionist approaches with a sensibility. Either can have a stunning inspiration. Such an inspiration is both rare and inevitable. Statistics favor the intensely creative artist who aims countless ideas at targets daily. Inspirations happen on every level of the decision-making process. There are big decisions, small decisions, and middle-sized decisions. There are also mysterious solutions.

Large and Small

The big decision is the basic idea for the work of art. For the systems artist, the big decision has absolute power. For the expressionist, the big decision is provisional, for the idea, more than anything, is to set up an arena, a set of circumstances within which unexpected and valuable things are likely to happen. The systems artist foresees; the expressionist prepares for the unforeseen.

There are many kinds of systems artists. Minimalists usually fall into this category, as do earthworks artists, academic realists, and photorealists. These artists often work in series to accommodate ideas that are too big to be contained in a single work. Each work becomes a participant in a huge decision and draws some importance from that fact. As each work coordinates variables and constants differently, a sense of "formula" emerges by which the viewer can project works beyond the series. The big decision is found to operate poignantly in photorealism, where an artist makes the commitment to copy a particular photograph. By doing so, he sets it up so that middle-sized decisions never take place as there are no alterations of the program. Ultra-small decisions take place by the thousands, mostly in the form of matching and approving things—color for color, shape for shape, edge for edge. Small decisions occur on the run, so to speak, as the artist works continuously, instinctively expressing intentions or following a plan of repetition/variation.

Middle-sized decisions fill in the space between large and small. Consciously relating localities to the whole or creating areas of individuality, the artist chooses from the catalog of possibilities. My earlier description of movement toward solution is a sample of middle-sized decision making at work. The systems artist uses middle-sized decisions to realize the foreseen. The expressionist uses middle-sized decisions to court the unforeseen objective.

Turnabout

Conscious decisions have their limitations. Even instinctive decisions go only so far. As the expressionist's big decision to create a promising circumstance pans out, problems start to occur. These problems can take the form of inconsistencies, compositional awkwardness, misleading imagery, or spatial or stylistic anomalies. While these may be solved by a leveling-out kind of compromise, they also offer the challenge of being solved by "quantum leap"–type solutions. By this time, the total accumulation of decisions has become huge, and, since these decisions, if good, are interconnected well into a single mass, the artist suddenly finds himself smaller than the work. Added small and middle-sized decisions amount only to chasing one's own tail. It is at this point that a common occurrence takes place; there is a major turnabout in the work. Instead of the artist continuing to impose his will on the work, the work of art begins to dictate to the artist. The artist resists for a while but is wise to become servant to the will of the work. He crosses a frightening threshold to a deeply satisfying experience of a kind of ego-free, pure creativity. From this moment, the artwork behaves like a sphinx. It seems to know its own destiny. The artist can only have faith that this is true. The artist sees this new destiny (completely different from the original idea for the work) only dimly and fleetingly. He believes, without evidence, that solutions to further problems exist. It is in this territory that art making loses touch with the rational. The proven and the provable disappear. There is a general sense of power and clairvoyance.

Testimony

In this phase, an artwork can reach conclusion very rapidly. Or it can be brought to a new level at which a fresh cycle of conscious and intuitive decisions can be made. This period of creative activity is piled high with benefits. The artwork "finds itself." As far as the artist's personal life is concerned, things could not be better: the problems of the world are forgotten as they shrink into inconsequence; heightened vision spills over into the natural world; and inspiration for future work is found in abundance.

In my experience, this state lasts for no more than a few days at a time. It subsides gently. The greatest benefit of art is to the consciousness of the artist.

I have tried to avoid naked testimony as much as possible in this chapter, but I find myself, over and over, wanting to speak from very personal experience. None of it is uncorroborated by the experience of others. Yet the internal creative life is like the dream life. It is a world, vivid and whole, witnessed by one person. It is exclusive territory.

FRANK GALUSZKA

Conclusions: A Picture in Nature

It is possible to think all sorts of things about works of art. But the interpreter eventually encounters the same problem as the artist who looks for a key to a lock. The artwork may provide considerable support for one theory or another, and the theory may look convincing in the mind. But any theory results from the interpretation of only a fraction of the total evidence. It cannot be extended to account for the whole. The thoughtful interpreter finds himself qualifying statements, accepting contradictions, and growing doubtful as he sees his theory teeter like a house of cards.

Works of art are not ideas. They are not even like ideas. They are models of realities; they are samples of mind. Like natural objects, artworks can be appreciated and investigated without becoming exhausted by being understood. Yet, as an artwork escapes the grasp of ideas and settles into the fabric of reality among the constituents of the natural world, it retains a special allure. Every dab and stroke of paint, every incident and expanse of color, continuously proclaims, A human consciousness has been here.

REFERENCES

Dali, S. 1935. *The Conquest of the Irrational*. New York: Julian Levy.
Dali, S. 1942. *The Secret Life of Salvador Dali*. New York: Dial.
Goldwater, R. 1945. *Artists on Art*. New York: Pantheon.
Protter, E. 1963. *Painters on Painting*. New York: Grosset & Dunlap.

ELLEN WINNER

Although artistic behavior has no obvious survival value, all known human societies have engaged in some form of artistry. Art has existed from the very beginning of human existence. Our earliest indisputably Homo sapiens ancestors, Cro-Magnon humans, engaged in painting and possibly even music, dance, and drama. Using natural dyes from plants, these first humans covered the walls of their caves with paintings of the animals that they hunted. The depiction of masks in the paintings suggests that the germs of theater may also have existed at that time. And the discovery of flutes in the caves, carved out of the bones of animals, tells of the early invention of music. Moreover, the prevalence of all forms of art in contemporary hunting-and-gathering societies provides indirect, converging support for the view that Cro-Magnon humans sang and danced as well as painted.

In contemporary, industrialized societies, only a handful of people are professionally engaged in making art. However, if popular forms of artistic activity are included under the rubric of "art," almost all of us are involved in some form of artistic creation: we adorn our bodies with jewelry, plant roses in our gardens, redecorate our living rooms, and arrange food on platters in colorful, balanced patterns. Moreover, almost all of us participate in the arts as audience members: we visit museums, read novels, listen to music, take in television dramas, and watch Olympic acrobatics. Artistic activity is not simply a luxury available to the leisure classes but a fundamental aspect of the human repertoire. Indeed, the production of art is not abandoned even in situations in which the greater part of a person's energy must be expended in the sheer struggle for survival, as the art of concentration camp inmates startlingly testifies.

In an effort to understand universal aspects of human beings, social scientists have studied such forms of behavior as language, tool use, aggression, and sexuality. Despite the universality of art, less effort has been spent in explaining artistic activity. Artistic behavior raises many puzzling questions. Why, for example, is there such a powerful urge to engage in behavior that does not contribute to our material survival? Is this urge related to what motivates us to play, fantasize, or dream? Or is it more akin to what drives us to solve a mathematical equation? And why do we experience such powerful emotions when we contemplate works of art?

These are psychological questions. Essential to them all is the underlying question of the meaning of the term "art" itself. Although we all know how to apply the term, the criteria that are used to classify something as a work of art prove extremely difficult to formulate.

Traditional Definitions of Art

We have little trouble supplying clear-cut examples of works of art and contrasting these to instances that plainly do not qualify as art. In normal contexts, a painting, but not a map, counts as a work of art; a Mozart concerto, but not the sound of a car honking, and a poem, but not a newspaper article, qualify as art. Because we use a common word to refer to a Leonardo da Vinci painting, a Shakespeare sonnet, a Mahler symphony, and a Greek vase, we assume that, if we can list their shared properties, we will come up with the necessary and sufficient features of art—those features that are common to all works of art and absent in all nonart objects.

Consider an indisputable example of a work of art, Leonardo da Vinci's *Mona Lisa*. By determining the characteristics of this painting, perhaps we can discover the defining features of any work of art. The *Mona Lisa* is an artifact. It was made by a human. It was made deliberately and with skill. It has no obvious utilitarian function but is intended to be contemplated. It expresses emotion, although the emotion conveyed by the smile is ambiguous. Presumably, it served as a vehicle of self-expression for Leonardo. And it is beautiful and pleasing to look at.

These properties, however, are not defining features of art. First, no single one of these properties is itself sufficient to make an object qualify as a work of art, for each of these properties is also common to objects that are clearly not works of art. A toothbrush is as much an artifact as a piece of sculpture. Many things besides art works are made by humans, deliberately and with skill. Not only works of art but many other things lack a utilitarian function (snapshots, knick-knacks). Many things express emotion (a newspaper photograph of an angry crowd, a weeping willow) and also serve as vehicles of self-expression (a political speech). Finally, nature as well as art is beautiful to behold.

Second, no single one of these properties is necessary to a work of art, for any one of them may be missing in an art object. "Found art," such as a piece of driftwood mounted on a pedestal in an art museum, is not an artifact. A finger painting by a chimpanzee may be classified as art despite its nonhuman source. A pleasing pattern created by accidentally spilled paint may be considered art, yet the pattern was made neither deliberately nor with skill. Indeed, the nineteenth-century Romantics believed that deliberation is often antithetical to art. In Shelley's "To a Skylark," the poet pours forth his soul in "unpre-meditated art." And the Surrealists espoused what they called "automatic writing," in which authors surrender all conscious control of their craft so that a supernatural medium may work through them.

Works of art surely may serve utilitarian functions. There is speculation that the cave paintings, for instance, were painted not simply to be contemplated but to engender luck and bravery among hunters. Some art, such as twentieth-century "minimal art," may not express emotion in any ordinary sense. As for self-expression, it is questionable whether artists working within a strict tradition, such as that of ancient Egypt, are expressing themselves in any way similar to the ways artists do in a more modern, individualistic tradition, in which "norm violation" is prized. Finally, if aesthetic appeal and beauty are necessary, this leaves out Marcel DuChamp's *Urinal,* which one would be hard pressed to call "aesthetic," or Edvard Munch's *The Scream,* which is not "beautiful" in any ordinary sense of the term.

Given the difficulty of discovering a set of either necessary or sufficient features of a work of art, the attempt to define art has had a long and turbulent history. Throughout the centuries, many thinkers have tried to set out the necessary and sufficient properties of art. And each new theory has repudiated those that went before. Definitions have been criticized either for incompleteness, when they exclude some forms of art, or for overinclusiveness, when they do not clearly dis-

150

tinguish art from nonart. But the attempt to define art has never ceased, perhaps in part because of the unshakable notion that we cannot talk sensibly about art unless we know what all art objects share and what distinguishes them from all nonart (Bell 1913). Two attempts to define art, the formalist and the emotionalist, exemplify the difficulty of the question.

The English aesthetician Clive Bell (1913) argued that works of art achieve their status as art not because of their content but only because of their form. In a work of art, elements are combined in certain ways to create "significant form," and the effect of this form is to arouse "aesthetic emotions" in the observer. Only art possesses significant form, and only significant form elicits aesthetic emotion.

This definition has the advantage of including as art those abstract twentieth-century works in which the traditional, narrative, representational function has been discarded. It thus directs attention away from representation to the importance of design. Nevertheless, there are some serious problems with the definition. First, significant form, the determining property of art, is defined as that which evokes aesthetic emotion, while aesthetic emotion is defined as that which is evoked by significant form. Such a circular definition is immune to verification or falsification. Moreover, the problem of defining "aesthetic emotion" is as fraught with difficulties as is that of defining art itself.

A second problem is that the definition excludes art that fails to evoke an aesthetic response. Such a "poor" work would lack significant form and thus not qualify as art. Hence, the definition can comprehend only "good" art. It conflates evaluative terms (those that distinguish good art from bad) and descriptive ones (those that distinguish art from nonart). Thus, the definition is incomplete.

Whereas Bell regarded the formal aspects of art as critical, others, such as Leo Tolstoy (1930) and the aesthetician R. G. Collingwood (1938), focused on the emotional effect of art. The truly essential property of art, Tolstoy maintained, was not form but rather the expression of emotion in a sensuous public medium. In art, emotion is transmitted to the perceiver like a spreading infection. The more potent the infection, the better the art. That which does not infect others with emotion fails to qualify as art.

This definition too is problematic. One shortcoming is its breadth. While art works typically express emotion, so do many other things.

151

A scream of terror or a sob of despair is an expression of emotion in the sensuous public medium of sound no less than is a piece of music. What is needed is some way to distinguish between emotion expressed through the invented, fictional world of art and emotion expressed quite literally by a human scream or sob. A second problem is that the status of an object as a work of art is not, in fact, determined by its degree of emotional expressiveness. The geometric lines of Mondrian's paintings do not express emotion in any obvious sense. Yet surely they are works of art.

These formalist and emotionalist theories are only two of numerous philosophical attempts to define the characteristics of art. To try to resolve this hopelessly vexed issue, contemporary philosophers have taken a radical new approach. To ask what is the essence of art, it is claimed—or, for that matter, to ask this with respect to a concept as ordinary as furniture or food—is to ask the wrong question.

New Definitions of Art

The traditional approach to definition, since the time of Socrates, has been to search for the necessary and sufficient properties of the term in question. This approach has permeated not only aesthetics but all fields of philosophical inquiry. Philosophers of mind have sought the defining properties of knowledge; moral philosophers have sought the defining properties of the good life; and philosophers of art have sought to discover the defining properties of art, beauty, and the aesthetic response.

This traditional notion of definition was challenged by the philosopher Ludwig Wittgenstein (1953). Wittgenstein argued that most concepts or categories do not possess a set of characteristics shared by all members of the category. Rather, category members are united by strands of similarity or what are called "family resemblances." The concept of games, for instance, includes board games, card games, ball games, Olympic games, ring around the rosie, and games played by oneself, such as throwing a ball against a wall. There are no features common to all these games. Skill, competition, and amusement are part of some, but not all, games. One game shares properties with some games, and another game shares a different set of properties with yet another group of games. The classification of a new activity as a game is made by judging its similarity to something already established as a game, not by asking whether it is similar to all games in the same way. Concepts such as "game" are open concepts, which possess no set of necessary and sufficient properties but are held together by a network of overlapping and crisscrossing similarities. Many common concepts are thus open ones, as opposed to the closed concepts of math and logic (e.g., as the class of prime numbers).

Art has since been defined as an open concept lacking any necessary or sufficient properties. The boundaries of art must be infinitely expandable in order to encompass new and previously undreamed of forms of art (Weitz 1956). Because art is expansive, adventurous, and never static, unforeseeable and entirely novel forms of art are always possible. Because the concept of art must remain infinitely expandable, the defining features of art cannot be listed. Such a list would close the concept. Accordingly, there is no way, in principle, to define a work of art.

A more useful approach has been taken by the philosopher Nelson Goodman (1976, 1978). While acknowledging that art cannot be defined in terms of necessary and sufficient features, Goodman proposed that art works tend to possess certain properties. Underlying this approach is the assumption that all art works contain symbols and are themselves symbols. Viewed in this way, art is a manifestation of the most characteristic activity of human beings, the construction of symbols. But to state that all art works are symbols does not solve the definitional problem. Many things that are clearly not works of art are also symbols, such as maps, diagrams, traffic lights, and numbers. Moreover, all words are symbols, but not all language is artistic language. The difficulty of distinguishing aesthetic from nonaesthetic symbols—say a painting from a traffic light or a poem from a newspaper article—brings us right back to the problem of determining the defining properties of art.

To avoid this problem, Goodman argued that the question, *What* is art? should be replaced with the question, *When* is an object a work of art? He gave the example of a stone lying in a driveway. This object is not a work of art, nor is it a symbol of any kind. The same stone in a geological museum is also not a work of art, but, because it is a sample of some of the properties of stones of a given period, it functions as a symbol. Put this same stone in an art museum, and it may begin to function as a work of art. Like the stone in a geological museum, the stone in an art museum is a symbol—but it is a sample of other properties than is the stone in the geological museum. The stone in the art museum exemplifies a certain shape, size, color, and texture. It may even metaphorically exemplify a mood. When people view the stone in an art museum, they attend to all these properties, and thus the stone can be said to be functioning as a work of art.

This example demonstrates that one and the same object can function as a symbol in certain contexts but not in others and as an aesthetic symbol in certain contexts and a nonaesthetic symbol in others. What distinguishes an object when it is functioning as an aesthetic symbol is that it tends to possess certain symptoms. These aesthetic symptoms are not necessary and sufficient properties of works of art; they are more like clues or like the symptoms of a disease. A disease such as influenza is usually accompanied by the symptoms of sore throat, cough, and fever. But one may have the flu and not have the symptoms, and one can have one or more of these symptoms and not have the flu. In the presence of these symptoms, it is simply a fairly safe bet that a case of the flu is indicated. So also, the presence or absence of one or more aesthetic symptoms does not qualify or disqualify a work as aesthetic. One or more of these symptoms simply tend to be present in works of art. This approach is a probabilistic one: if something has one or more aesthetic symptoms, it probably is a work of art.

One of the symptoms that works of art usually possess is "relative syntactic repleteness." Art works tend to be replete because, when an object functions as a work of art, relatively more of its physical properties are important than when it is not functioning as a work of art. Consider a zigzag line (fig. 1). If we are told that the line is an electrocardiogram, all that is important to note are the dips and peaks of the line. But if we are told that this same line is the outline of a mountain

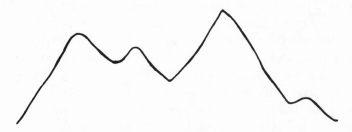

Fig. 1.—Zigzag line illustrating repleteness

in a landscape painting, we turn our attention to more of the properties of the line, such as its thickness, brightness, or color. Similarly, if a stone is placed in an art museum, we attend to its size, shape, color, and texture. When a symbol functions aesthetically, more of its properties are relevant than when this same symbol functions outside of the arts.

Another symptom of the aesthetic is "metaphorical exemplification," also called "expression," which refers to one of the ways in which art works typically symbolize. Works of art express moods: a painting may be described as sad, a symphony as elated, or a poem as gloomy. But it is not only moods that are expressed: a painting can express loudness, a symphony can express heat, or a poem can express smoothness. Though the way in which a particular property is expressed may vary from culture to culture, art of all cultures expresses moods or other qualities through formal properties, such as line, color, and rhythm. Art works typically symbolize through expression; nonaesthetic symbols do not. Only paintings, but not maps and graphs, can be sad, loud, heated, or calm. Moreover, the properties that a work of art expresses are different from those that a work literally possesses. A painting can be literally blue but only metaphorically sad.

The presence of aesthetic symptoms such as these requires us to do more than look through the symbol to what it represents, as we do with nonaesthetic symbols such as maps, graphs, and traffic lights. Their presence compels us to attend to the symbol itself. Thus, works of art are nontransparent.

A work of art may lack any one of these symptoms, and any one symptom may also be found outside a work of art. Moreover, these symptoms are differently distributed across the various art forms. If all the symptoms are found in an object, it is most certainly a work of art. If none of the symptoms is found in an object, it cannot be a work of art. But no one of these symptoms must be present for an object to qualify as a work of art.

Such a probabilistic or symptomatic definition of art makes it easier to deal with borderline cases of art. A scribble produced by a chimpanzee may function as a work of art if the observer realizes that all the physical properties of the lines are relevant (repleteness). But the work may not have functioned as a work of art for the chimpanzee: the precise variations in line and color may have been produced quite accidentally, and the chimpanzee may have paid these subtle variations little or no attention. Thus, a work may function as art for the observer but not for the maker, or vice versa. Works that are usually considered borderline cases of art, such as creations by children, chimpanzees, and brain-damaged or psychotic people, are potentially aesthetic objects, and a symptomatic approach may be applied in order to decide whether the object is functioning as art for either the maker or the perceiver.

Defining the Psychology of Art

The psychology of art focuses on questions related to the participants in the artistic process—namely, the artist, the performer, the perceiver, and the critic. Of these, the roles of artist and perceiver have received the most attention. A psychologist of art is interested primarily in the psychological processes that make possible the creation of and response to art. Two broad questions have guided the psychological study of the artist. What motivates the artist to create? What cognitive processes are involved in creating art? Two parallel questions have guided the investigation of the perceiver. What psychological factors motivate a person to contemplate works of art? What kinds of cognitive skills are required to understand a work of art? These major questions provide an organizing framework for understanding the psychology of art (see table 1).

The philosophers of ancient Greece were the first to grapple with these overarching questions. Plato developed a theory of what drives the artist to create as well as a view of the process of artistic creation. The poet was said to be possessed by divine inspiration, and the process

TABLE 1
QUESTIONS GUIDING PSYCHOLOGICAL STUDIES OF THE ARTS

	Artist	Perceiver
Motivation—the "why" of art. . . .	What motivates the artist to create?	What motivates humans to contemplate a work of art?
Cognition—the "how" of art. . . .	What cognitive processes are involved in artistic creation?	What cognitive skills are necessary to understand a work of art?

of creation was one in which the poet's rational faculties yield to irrational frenzy. Aristotle proposed a less Dionysian view of artistic creation, stressing instead the careful, controlled workmanship involved. These two divergent views—art as uncontrolled madness and art as careful craft—have surfaced time and again, even today polarizing psychologists.

Plato and Aristotle also formulated theories to explain why audience members are drawn to the arts. Plato believed that the arts exert a powerful effect on the soul. Because of the potent influence of art, Plato argued that certain forms of art were dangerous and should be censored. Aristotle believed that members of the audience are attracted to dramatic tragedy enacted on stage because of its cathartic, purging effect.

From the time of the ancient Greeks, not only philosophers but artists have continued to grapple with the puzzles of artistic creation and response. Nineteenth-century poets, for example, echoed Plato in their attempt to come to terms with the mystery of artistic creation. Writers such as Wordsworth, Blake, Shelley, Coleridge, Baudelaire, and Rimbaud glorified the imagination, the emotions, and the irrational—in contrast to reason—as the source of art. Art, they believed, cannot be produced by rational rules or mere "skill." Rather, it is created by irrational means. Not only was the conscious, rational mind viewed as irrelevant to artistic creation, but artistic creation was believed to be actually threatened by the intervention of reason.

In some sense, the Romantic position constituted a return to Plato's stance. Both the Greeks and the nineteenth-century Romantics believed that creation can be explained only by forces independent of the rational self. But while Plato viewed artistic creation as having an external source, divine inspiration, the Romantics believed artistic creation to have an internal source, the unconscious. For this reason, the roots of creativity in dreams, drug-induced fantasies, and psychoses, as well as physical illness, were sometimes stressed. While the Greeks believed in inspiration from above, nineteenth-century artists believed in inspiration from below (Arnheim 1962). The nineteenth-century insistence on the importance of the irrational not only echoes Plato but also anticipates Freud's emphasis on the role of the unconscious in artistic creation. The problem of inspiration remains a key and unsolved puzzle in the psychology of art today.

The way in which psychologists have grappled with fundamental questions about art differs from the approach of both philosophers and artists. What distinguishes psychologists' studies of the arts is not the questions asked but rather the way in which the questions are answered. Whereas the arguments of philosophers and artists are based on introspection and logical analysis, psychologists found their answers on an empirical, sometimes experimental base.

Conclusions

The psychology of art lags considerably behind the psychology of other human activities. While psychologists have devoted a great deal of attention to the type of reasoning demanded by participation in the sciences, relatively little attention has been paid to the arts. Yet, over the course of human history, the arts have occupied a much more central position than the sciences. Logical, scientific thought is an invention of Western, post-Renaissance culture, and it remains restricted to a small enclave of individuals. Participation in the arts, in contrast, has been widespread for thousands of years.

The reasons for the relative dearth of investigations into the psychology of art are at least twofold. First, because the arts are often considered mysterious, investigators have assumed that they are not open to empirical study. Second, most psychologists have been relatively unfamiliar with the arts and thus unwilling to investigate them. Indeed, there is no area of psychology in which a greater distance prevails between what should be known and what has been established.

NOTE

Presented at the Conference on Creativity and Adolescence, American Society for Adolescent Psychiatry, Philadelphia, September 1986. This chapter was first published as "The Puzzle of Art" in *Invented Worlds: The Psychology of the Arts* (Cambridge, Mass.: Harvard University Press, 1982), chap. 1.

REFERENCES

Arnheim, R. 1962. *The Genesis of a Painting: Picasso's Guernica.* Berkeley: University of California Press.

Bell, C. 1913. *Art*. New York: Stoke.

Collingwood, R. G. 1938. *The Principles of Art*. Oxford: Clarendon.

Goodman, N. 1976. *Languages of Art*. Indianapolis: Hackett.

Goodman, N. 1978. *Ways of World Making*. Indianapolis: Hackett.

Tolstoy, L. 1930. *What Is Art?* Oxford: Oxford University Press.

Weitz, M. 1956. The role of theory in aesthetics. *Journal of Aesthetics and Art Criticism* 15:27–35.

Wittgenstein, L. 1953. *Philosophical Investigations*. New York: Macmillan.

10   ART AND PSYCHOPATHOLOGY: THE MESSAGE OF "OUTSIDER" ART

AARON H. ESMAN

The relation between art and psychopathology has been a staple of discussion and controversy for over 2,000 years. As with many such perennial issues, opinions have moved in cycles over the centuries. To Plato, the artist was one of those gifted by the gods with a "divine madness." Aristotle connected creativity with melancholia, but, according to Zilboorg (1941), he also cited "the case of a poet by the name of Marascos who, when well, was rather a poor or mediocre poet; whenever Marascos had an attack of mania he wrote excellent poetry" (p. 56). In the Middle Ages, the mentally ill were thought to be instruments or victims of the devil. Those we consider to be artists, such as the monks who produced the illuminations that are the glory of medieval art, were regarded rather as artisans or craftsmen. The individual as a creative figure did not reappear until the late medieval and Renaissance periods. The Romantic movement of the later eighteenth and nineteenth centuries again linked genius with madness, and, in fact, many of the major creative figures of this era manifested striking psychopathology that has made them favored subjects for psychoanalytic speculations about creativity. Kernan (1979) has shown that Romantic aesthetics and Freudian psychoanalysis sprang from the same intellectual roots (see also Trosman 1985). Thus, Freud and the pathographers who followed him equated the artist with the patient and the artwork with a dream or symptom, seeking to reveal the wish or complex that was expressed.

More recently, under the influence of ego psychology, psychoanalytic emphasis has shifted to the role of nonconflictual "autonomous" factors in creativity. Kubie (1958), for instance, speaks of "neurotic distortions" of the creative process, and Gedo (1983) refers to the nonconflictual origins of artistic style. Rothenberg (1983) emphasizes the nonpathological and preconscious character of the cognitive styles of Janusian and homospatial thinking, which he regards as central to the creative capacity. Others, however, consider creativity, in the sense of the production of works of imaginative art, to be self-healing efforts on the part of persons who, deprived of this restitutive activity, would fall ill. Usually, the premised illness is of a depressive nature, as with the Kleinians in particular. Andreasen and Powers (1975) report a significant correlation between literary creativity and affective disorder both in the writers they have studied and in those writers' primary relatives. They found that, contrary to their expectations, the writers' cognitive styles were close to those of manics rather than those of schizophrenics (although Andreasen [1973] considers Joyce to have been "schizoid").

Of obvious interest in this connection are those major artists who have, in the course of their creative careers, suffered psychotic episodes—artists such as van Gogh, Munch, Robert Schumann, Strindberg. Here, too, opinions differ as to the effect of their illness on their creative products. In the case of van Gogh, for instance, some see in his last paintings, created in the throes of his suicidal disintegration, a loosening and deterioration of formal structure, while others see an intensification of expressiveness. Indeed, the Expressionist movement in German art in the first two decades of this century and the neo-Expressionists of the 1980s could be seen as the heirs to van Gogh's last paintings.

I should like to approach this complex question from another standpoint, that of the so-called outsider artist. The outsider artist is often, though not always, a psychotic or at least an eccentric person who, in the words of one student, operates outside the "norms" of art and the world of art. I speak here primarily of persons who are untrained and minimally, if at all, aware of the canons of "official" art. At some time in their lives—often at times of intense psychic crisis—they begin to draw or paint (occasionally to sculpt) in ways that, though highly personal and idiosyncratic, often tend to conform to certain formal criteria that characterize what Jean Dubuffet designated as "Art Brut"—"raw art."

The first serious attempt at a scientific study of the artistry of the psychotic was that of the German psychiatrist Hans Prinzhorn, published in 1922. Prinzhorn, previously trained as an art historian, became interested in the spontaneous productions of some of the patients in the University Clinic at Heidelberg and undertook to collect material from hospitals all over Europe. His collection of some 5,000 pieces languished after his departure from Heidelberg shortly before his book actually appeared and has only recently been rescued from oblivion, restored, and rehoused.[1]

Although some of the psychotic "artists" whose work Prinzhorn studied had some training in such areas as architectural draftsmanship, most demonstrated an interest in art only long after they entered the hospital, usually after the acute phase of their psychosis had subsided. In no case was the work directed or interpreted—art therapy did not exist as a discipline at that time. Perhaps the best known of Prinzhorn's artists was Karl Brendel, one of the rare sculptors—in this case wood-carver—in his collection. Brendel was hospitalized at thirty-five, after ten or twelve years of violent and increasingly paranoid behavior, and began making figures after he had been in the hospital for about six years. An outstanding example of his work can be seen in figure 1.

Many of the works in Prinzhorn's collection are of an extraordinarily haunting quality, exploiting formal devices akin in many ways to those of modernist artists of whom these patients could not have been aware or whom they actually predated. A small watercolor by the psychotic watchmaker Hermann Mebes (fig. 2), created in the late nineteenth century, powerfully evokes images from the work of Paul Klee, who was active a generation later. Klee acknowledged that his work had been powerfully influenced by Prinzhorn's book, which was greeted with enormous enthusiasm and excitement by many avant-garde artists of the period, such as Jean Arp, Max Ernst, and Alfred Kubin. At least one, Hans Bellmer, described it as the most important educational experience of his life. In a drawing of social life in a hospital (fig. 3), the psychotic artist Gustav Sievers used bodily distortions akin to those of the American sculptor Lachaise (fig. 4) and the expressionists, several of whom also acknowledged their indebtedness to Prinzhorn and his "artists." Similarly, the chronically unemployed London truck driver Albert Louden (fig. 5) uses bodily distortions not unlike those of Picasso (fig. 6), whose work he had, until recently, never seen. In each case, the distortions seem aimed at emphasizing the awesome and seductive power of women. What is striking is the definition and pres-

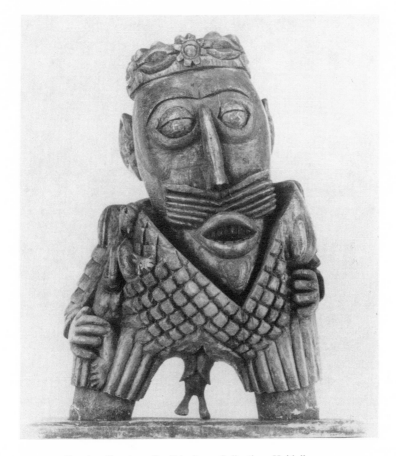

FIG. 1.—Courtesy the Prinzhorn Collection, Heidelberg

ervation by each of these "outsiders" of a distinctive personal style even in the face of severe psychological disturbance.

Like most of us, Prinzhorn had some idea about what such works as these implied for a theory of creativity. Many of these ideas were derived from the speculations of the then-influential German philosopher Ludwig Klages. In Prinzhorn's view, a creative urge, an innate drive for "configuration," is a human universal. Training may superimpose certain cultural constraints on this urge, but it does not create it. Accordingly, sharp distinctions between "psychotic art" and "fine

163

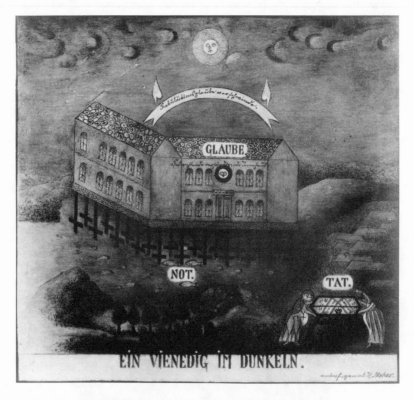

FIG. 2.—Courtesy the Prinzhorn Collection, Heidelberg

art" are "arbitrary" and "dogmatic" since the same internal impulses are responsible for both.

In his study of the drawings of a schizophrenic architect, Ernst Kris (1952) defined the difference in terms of the work's communicative functions: "The artist proceeds through trial and error; he learns and his modes of expression change, or his style changes. The psychotic artist creates in order to transform the real world; he seeks no audience and his modes of expression remain unchanged once the psychotic process has reached a certain intensity" (p. 169). He thus identified one of the defining stylistic characteristics of such psychotic art—its rigid repetitive quality. Kris linked the aesthetic—and thus the social— aspect of art with ego intactness, implying that the psychotic artist is engaged in an essentially solipsistic, noncommunicative act. One might well question this idea, particularly in the light of work on the com-

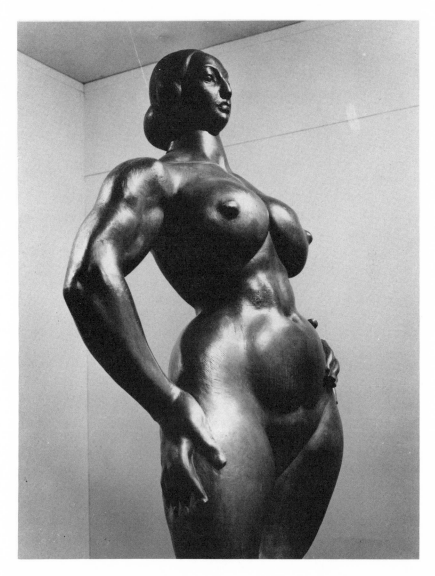

Fig. 3.—Courtesy the Prinzhorn Collection, Heidelberg

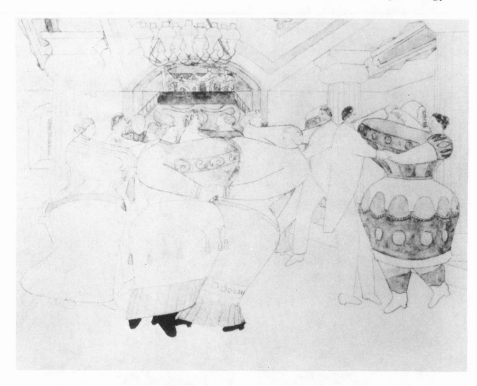

Fig. 4.—Courtesy the Museum of Modern Art, New York, Mrs. Simon Guggenheim Fund.

municative function of schizophrenic speech and language. There is good reason to believe that the psychotic artist, like the "normal" one, is addressing an audience—though it is an audience of primitive, internal object representations and the communicative "language" involved is an arcane one incorporating symbols whose private meaning can often be inferred only with difficulty by the outside observer. It is this that accounts for the uncanny feeling induced by much outsider art.

Because of his training as an art historian, Kris was, of course, committed to the canons of what Dubuffet called the "cultural art" of post-Renaissance Europe. Like Kris, and in contrast to Prinzhorn, Billig and Burton-Bradley state categorically, "The psychotic cannot produce significant art" (1978, p. 231). Apart from its excommunication from the realm of the elect of such figures as van Gogh, Munch, and others who produced art during psychotic states, this statement raises

166

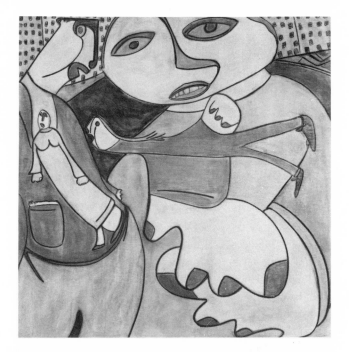

FIG. 5.—Courtesy the Rosa Esman Gallery, New York

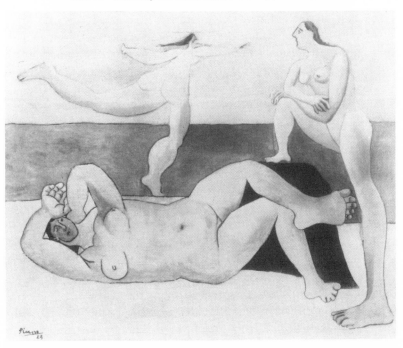

FIG. 6.—Courtesy Stephen Hahn, New York

the crucial and thorny question of just what is significant art. Such judgments are notoriously subject to change from time to time, from culture to culture, and from critic to critic. Certainly, Dubuffet, who knew a thing or two about "significant" art, differed seriously with them; like Prinzhorn, he rejected out of hand any qualitative distinction between "Art Brut" and what he called "the art of culture." "They [works of Art Brut] are charged . . . with everything that can be asked of a work of art: burning mental tension, uncurbed invention, an ecstasy of intoxication, complete liberty. Mad? Of course. Can you conceive of art which is not mad? . . . there is no art of the insane any more than there is an art of dyspeptics or an art of people with knee complaints" (1959). Of course, the Nazis disagreed; they defined "psychotic art" as "degenerate," along with the art of the avant-garde, and consigned it to cultural ghettos like the physical ghettos into which they herded the Jews. The Prinzhorn collection itself was barely saved from the terror of the Nazis, who almost consigned it, as they did everything and everyone they regarded as outsiders, to the flames.

Despite the fact that the efforts of Prinzhorn and others to define specific formal characteristics of psychotic art were unsuccessful, there are certain features that do characterize a good deal of the art of outsiders, including psychotics. One of these is the use of unusual and untraditional materials—often whatever is at hand. Brendel, for instance, before he began his wood carvings, constructed figures out of bread crumbs in a manner similar to that of some peasant artisans and prisoners, like the so-called Prisoner of Basel (fig. 7). The paranoid French secondhand dealer, Maisonneuve, never hospitalized, began in his sixties to create satirical portraits out of sea shells (fig. 8). The eccentric English mystic Madge Gill produced endless ink drawings, many on long rolls of muslin rigged up in a special contraption by her son—drawings that were, she maintained, actually the creation of the spirit she called Myrninerest, of which she was only the mediumistic vehicle.

Gill's drawings (fig. 9) reveal certain other features that are often characteristic of outsider art. Most typical, perhaps, is the compulsive tendency to fill every inch of space on the sheet—the *horror vacui*. Another is the extraordinary sureness of line through which incredibly complex graphic structures are created without correction and with a sense of intense determination, as in the paranoid-appearing portraits of the San Francisco hospital worker Ted Gordon (fig. 10). The pre-

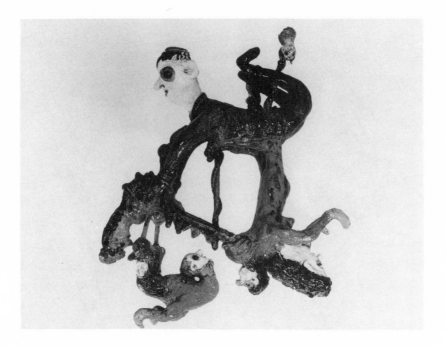

FIG. 7.—Courtesy Collection de l'Art Brut, Lausanne

cision and goal directedness of the graphic effort in these works (Gill produced hundreds, even thousands of them) is both impressive and bewildering. Another instance of this remarkable graphic precision is the work of the illiterate Scottish odd-job man Scottie Wilson. In Wilson's early work, at least, there is a quality of automaticity combined with a characteristic sureness of line, formal ingenuity, and disturbing content (fig. 11).

Another frequent feature of such work is what both Prinzhorn and the Viennese psychiatrist Leo Navratil (1983) called "physiognomization"—the tendency to assign human facial features to nonhuman and inanimate objects. A very graphic instance of this tendency is the extraordinary drawing from Prinzhorn's collection by one August Natterer (fig. 12) in which a landscape is "physiognomized," suggesting both a regressive dedifferentiation of animate and inanimate objects and the attribution to the inanimate world of the frightening aspect of persons. Natterer was a mechanic who, in 1907 at age thirty-nine, became psychotic with a highly elaborated, grandiose delusional sys-

169

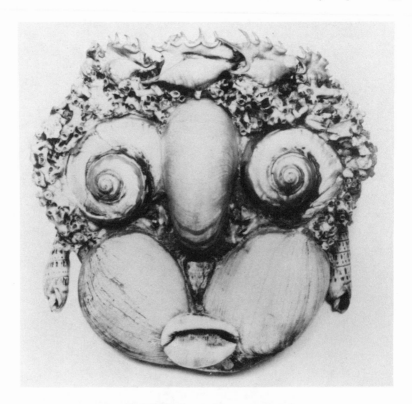

Fig. 8.—Courtesy Collection de l'Art Brut, Lausanne

tem. He was diagnosed as schizophrenic then, but, from the limited data available now, he would probably be called manic-depressive by current criteria.

It is perhaps in the works of the best known of all outsiders, the Swiss child molester and paranoid Adolf Wölfli, that these characteristics can most clearly be seen. Wölfli, who lived from 1864 to 1930, was hospitalized at age thirty after his third episode of child molestation. He was so violent and assaultive that he spent almost twenty years in solitary confinement, and it was in that setting, after about four years, that he began to draw, ultimately devoting all his waking hours to creating drawings accompanied by lengthy and incomprehensible "texts" and to composing music in a notation nobody has ever been able to decipher. Wölfli's remarkable drawings (fig. 13) demon-

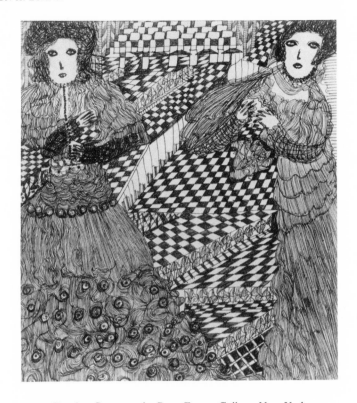

Fig. 9.—Courtesy the Rosa Esman Gallery, New York

strate his extraordinary gifts and technical skills. To quote Cardinal (1972), "The quality of monstrous exactitude may also be found in the drawings. Wölfli never planned in advance, and never hesitated. Normally he would begin drawing at the edge of the sheet, and having drawn the border device would add successive layers moving inward toward the center and stopping only when the whole space was filled in—at which he would turn over and start his commentary. What Morgenthaler calls his 'horror vacui' means that he left not a single empty space, if necessary adding disjointed sentences in the gaps in the picture" (p. 59). When Wölfli, who was probably also a manic depressive, died, the pile of drawings next to his bed was six feet high. His work illustrates yet another common feature, the use of words as plastic elements without their usual communicative function.

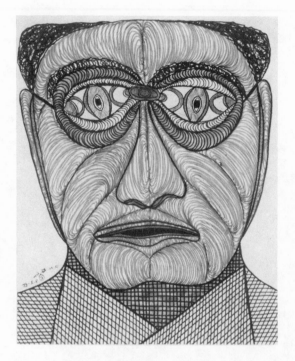

Fig. 10.—Courtesy the Rosa Esman Gallery, New York

What are the theoretical issues that emerge from this brief survey of outsider art? First and broadest is the old question, Does severe psychopathology or "madness" enhance or impair creativity? Given the estimate that perhaps 2 percent of hospitalized patients spontaneously undertake such plastic efforts, it does not appear that psychiatric illness per se generates creative urges or unharnesses creative capacities. It does appear, however, that for a small number of psychotic or marginal persons—or, as Laing, Foucault, and Dubuffet would say, those defined by society as markedly deviant—the creation of plastic forms contributes to their efforts at integration and restructuring of the personality and at ordering their chaotic and frightening experience of the world. The subject matter of these efforts at form creation may, of course, and often does, reflect the patient's delusional thinking and system building. The Swiss woman Aloise Corbaz, permanently hospitalized in 1918 at thirty-two, after years of bizarre religiosity and

172

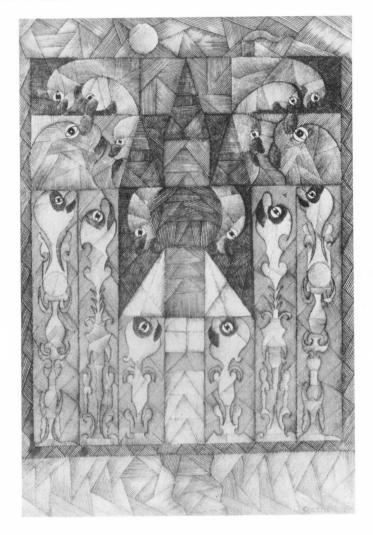

Fig. 11.—Courtesy the Rosa Esman Gallery, New York

erotomanic delusions, rendered both in her remarkable drawings in which erotically tinged, buxom, deminude women are often combined with religious messages (fig. 14). Similarly, the Austrian schizophrenic August Walla, continually in terror of both evil spirits and persons, was preoccupied with both God and persecutory political systems, and his richly detailed drawings incorporate all these elements (fig. 15).

173

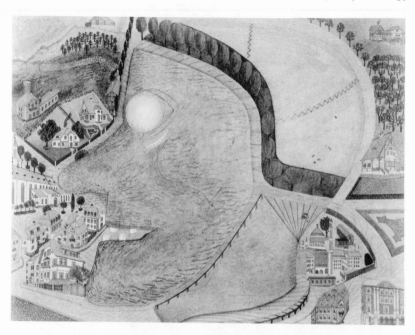

Fig. 12.—Courtesy the Prinzhorn Collection, Heidelberg

This effort at system building derives in its own way from the same integrative function, miscarried—or at least did so in the days before neuroleptics interrupted this course of events and deprived us of the opportunity to observe this restitutive process in its full flowering.

In this respect, Glick (1984) had said, "Antipsychotics appear not to affect performance; they clearly help the illness and therefore the creative process" (p. 11). I know of no evidence to support this contention. He quotes Killian, Holzman, Davis, and Gibbons (1984) to the effect that "the chemical compounds apparently derive their effect by making it possible for patients to attend their environment" (p. 68). Unfortunately, creativity derives not from "attention to the environment" but from the ability to respond to and utilize internal cues and, in the case of graphic art, to maintain good hand and eye coordination. Navratil (1983), who from his clinic outside Vienna has been a long-time student and promoter of Art Brut, describes the effect of a single injection of five milligrams of perphenazine on the drawing of one of the psychotic artists in his hospital. As shown in figure 16, the preinjection drawing

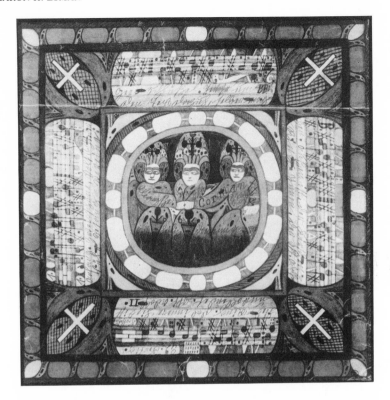

FIG. 13.—Courtesy Collection de l'Art Brut, Lausanne

on the left is far the more forceful and more elaborated. The postin-
jection drawing on the right is constricted, more conventional, lacking
in animation. Whatever the effect on the illness, it seems clear, from
this illustration at least, that neuroleptics may have a deadening effect
on creativity—a conclusion supported by artists with whom I have
spoken who have worked with psychotic patients in hospitals in recent
years.

On the other hand, the existence of so substantial a body of work,
as represented in such collections as those of Prinzhorn, the Collection
de l'Art Brut in Lausanne, the Galerie l'Aracine outside Paris, and
others, testifies to the fact that psychosis need not preclude creative
achievement, often achievement of a remarkably high order despite its
deviation from the formulas of cultural art. Further, it is often difficult
to distinguish the work of psychotic artists from that of other outsiders,

175

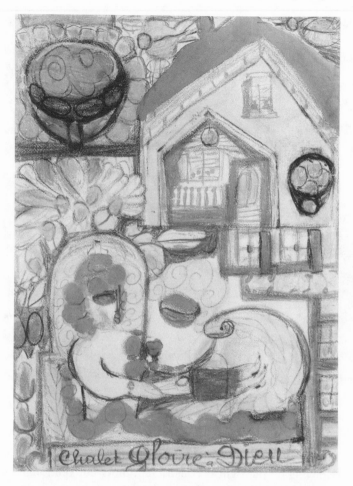

Fig. 14.—Courtesy the Rosa Esman Gallery, New York

who may share their obsessive style and their penchant for unusual materials—for example, the tile setter Simon Rodia of the famous Watts Towers in Los Angeles. Plokker (1965), a Dutch student of psychotic art, has said, "Professional artists and trained amateurs who become the victims of the schizophrenic process continue to work in their old styles in almost all cases. They can also stick for a long time to the subject they previously painted. . . . some retain their former technical skills for a very long time" (p. 148). As Gedo (1970) has put it, "It should be recalled that artistic style is so resistant to involvement (or

176

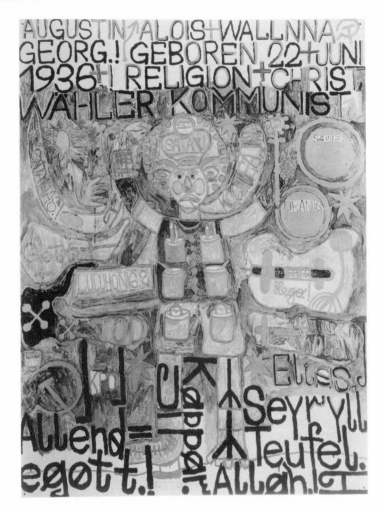

FIG. 15.—Courtesy the Rosa Esman Gallery, New York

reinvolvement) in conflict that it remains intact in the presence of severe psychotic regression'' (p. 230).

Kris's observation about the tendency of psychotic artists to repetition and stereotypy rather than stylistic development is certainly true— once having found a style, they stick to it; once having found a motif, they repeat it, often endlessly. The remarkable semi-illiterate schizophrenic Martin Ramirez, for instance, produced dozens of ''Caballeros'' (fig. 17) among the hundreds of drawings he created during his

177

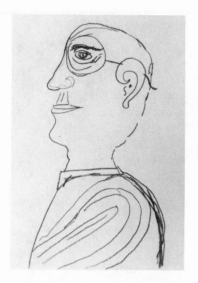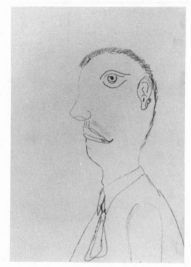

FIG. 16.—Courtesy Dr. Leo Navratil, Vienna

many years in a California state hospital. But, as Plokker points out, the same is true of most "naive," "folk," or tribal artists—of all, that is, who work outside the framework of the art of the museums. What is remarkable is the extent of variation and nuance of subject elements; they rarely repeat themselves.

Conclusions

This raises the question of the nature of creativity itself. Is it, as Kris and others have proposed, based on some sort of "controlled" regression or "regression in the service of the ego"? In the classical psychoanalytic view as enunciated by Freud (1908) and as argued more recently by Noy (1978) and others, the motive force for the "normal" artist's creative act comes from a drive derivative or unconscious wish, which is then "tamed," "disguised," or "sublimated" by the ego so as to achieve acceptable representation and gratifying discharge. The psychotic artist, however, like his noncreative fellows, suffers, by definition, from massively uncontrolled regression in a wide range of his ego functions. It would seem, therefore, that the motive force for the artistry of the mentally ill derives from the operation of certain intact

178

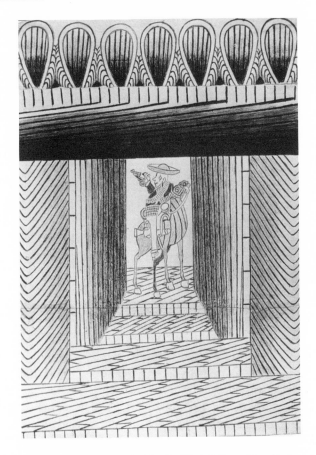

Fig. 17.—Courtesy the Phyllis Kind Gallery, New York

areas of the ego—areas that are concerned, as Navratil (1965) has suggested, with the ordering of experience, with symbolization, and with formalization. Unconscious wishes, "id" content, drive derivatives, appear to be exploited by the residual ego for purposes of representation, but the creative effort itself seems to be more restorative than expressive in its purposes. As Cardinal (1972) suggests, it is precisely this role of the individual ego that accounts for the diversity of personal styles that characterizes the art of psychotics and other outsiders. As to what differentiates the psychotic artist from his noncreative fellow sufferers—that is as great a mystery as is that which

179

differentiates most of us from the artists in our (ostensibly) nonpsychotic world.

As to the status of the "artistry of the mentally ill" as "Art" (with a capital *A*), Navratil (1983) said, "Creativity is a psychological phenomenon; art is a historico-sociological one" (p. 398). The definition of art is elusive, shaped not only by social forces but by the activities of artists themselves. It was Marcel Duchamp who, through his determined iconoclasm, succeeded in having a bathroom urinal enshrined as one of the crucial icons of twentieth-century art. It is largely through the interest and attention of Picasso, Derain, and Matisse that African tribal sculpture became identified as "significant" art in the early years of this century. In any case, to quote Cardinal again, "What one should seek is not to analyze the product so much as to attune oneself to the creative process; not to spot masterpieces but to respond to the vitality of the expressive act itself" (1972, p. 53). By establishing a museum for Art Brut, Dubuffet has achieved, perhaps, the ultimate irony—the incorporation of outsider art, including the art of psychotic patients, into the international system of cultural institutions.

NOTE

1. A selection from these works was recently exhibited at a number of university museums in the United States. The exhibition catalog contains a brilliant historical essay by Gilman (1984), to which I am much indebted.

REFERENCES

Andreasen, N. 1973. James Joyce: a portrait of the artist as a schizoid. *Journal of the American Medical Association* 224:67–71.

Andreasen, N., and Powers, P. 1975. Creativity and psychosis. *Archives of General Psychiatry* 32:70–73.

Billig, O., and Burton-Bradley, B. 1978. *The Painted Message*. New York: Halstead/Wiley.

Cardinal, R. 1972. *Outsider Art*. New York: Praeger.

Dubuffet, J. 1959. "Art Brut." In *Catalogue, Collection de L'Art Brut*. Lausanne, 1976.

Freud, S. 1908. Creative writers and day-dreaming. *Standard Edition* 9:141–156. London: Hogarth, 1959.

Gedo, J. 1970. Thoughts on art in the age of Freud. *Journal of the American Psychoanalytic Association* 18:219–245.

Gedo, J. 1983. *Portraits of the Artist*. New York: Guilford.

Gilman, S. 1984. Madness and representation: Hans Prinzhorn's study of madness and art in its historical context. In *The Prinzhorn Collection*. Champaign: University of Illinois Press.

Glick, I. 1984. Creativity and madness. Typescript.

Kernan, A. 1979. Romantic aesthetics and Freudian analysis. *International Review of Psycho-Analysis* 6:209–216.

Killian, G., Holzman, P., Davis, J., and Gibbons, R. 1984. Effects of psychotropic medication on selected cognitive and perceptual measures. *Journal of Abnormal Psychology* 93:58–70.

Kris, E. 1952. The creative spell in a schizophrenic artist. In *Psychoanalytic Explorations in Art*. New York: International Universities Press.

Kubie, L. 1958. *Neurotic Distortion of the Creative Process*. Lawrence: University of Kansas Press.

Navratil, L. 1965. *Schizophrenie und Kunst*. Reprint. Munich: Deutscher Taschenbuch Verlag, 1976.

Navratil, L. 1983. *Die Künstler aus Gugging*. Vienna: Medusa Verlag.

Noy, P. 1978. Form creation in art: an ego-psychological approach to creativity. *Psychoanalytic Quarterly* 48:229–256.

Plokker, J. H. 1965. *Art from the Mentally Disturbed*. Boston: Little, Brown.

Prinzhorn, H. 1922. *Artistry of the Mentally Ill*. Reprint. New York: Springer, 1972.

Rothenberg, A. 1983. Psychopathology and creative cognition. *Archives of General Psychiatry* 40:937–942.

Trosman, H. 1985. *Freud and the Imaginative World*. Hillsdale, N.J.: Analytic Press.

Zilboorg, G., and Henry, G. 1941. *A History of Medical Psychology*. New York: Norton.

11 THE CREATIVE MOMENT: IMPROVISING IN JAZZ AND PSYCHOTHERAPY

RUSSELL E. PHILLIPS

The conviction that direct deed is the most meaningful reflection
. . . has prompted the evolution of the extremely severe and unique
disciplines of the jazz or improvising musician. [Bill Evans, from
the notes to Miles Davis's *Kind of Blue*]

An interviewer once asked Leonard Bernstein's father why he had not
offered Leonard music lessons until his son was nearly an adolescent.
"How did I know he would grow up to be Leonard Bernstein?" he
replied.

When it exists, true genius asserts itself. There is a limit, however,
to how much we can learn about the creative process itself by distantly
analyzing the lives, motives, and talents of creative geniuses. As psychotherapists, we do not have to look that far to study creative individuals; we merely have to look more carefully at ourselves.

The effective psychotherapist works creatively in every session. Faced
with a new patient, a therapist cannot fall back on the responses he
has uttered to other patients in the past. A new set of spontaneous
reactions is required in every session; a fresh combination of therapeutic ideas and behaviors is always needed. Patients so often rework
the same themes during the course of their psychotherapy that, even
with the same patient, the therapist continuously is challenged to restate
old ideas in new ways.

Several years ago, while studying jazz inprovisation, I began to explore the analogy between the tasks of the jazz improviser and the

creative psychotherapist. Improvisation, a mysterious process to many, means the simultaneous creation and execution of ideas. Just as the jazz player performs new melodies extemporaneously, the active psychotherapist renders original melodies of his own in the form of spontaneous therapeutic responses. When a patient presents himself and his problems, the therapist must react *now*. He or she cannot go home, mull things over until the next session, and then respond to the patient. Even when the therapist does reflect on a particular problem, a patient, or an interaction in the time between sessions, his face-to-face work with a patient must convey immediacy to have a therapeutic effect.

Seasoned psychotherapists do not repeat such stock phrases as, "Tell me more about that," or, "Tell me how you feel about that," over and over again. Instead, they draw from the wellsprings of their own lives to listen and respond to every phase of a patient's therapy in a new way. They associate patients' problems with their own experiences. They observe their own inner emotional reactions, and they express their ideas in ways that reflect their own personalities and their own personal histories. Psychotherapists use their preferred theories and methods as guidelines, but the actual conduct of a given session is highly individualized and, thus, improvisational. To be otherwise, to be mechanized and predictable, could never be therapeutic. The capacity to improvise, to adapt to every patient and every session in a unique way, is one of the factors that distinguishes psychotherapists from computers that are programmed to give "therapeutic responses."

Prerequisites of the Improviser

The word "improvise" is related to French and Italian words meaning unprepared, but true improvisers know that, without preparation, creative activity is impossible. Whether the improviser is a jazz player or a psychotherapist, he must be well schooled and disciplined in the skills of his trade. A masterful improviser is a technical master. Without expertise, his art cannot become a medium of self-expression.

Nowadays, aspiring jazz musicians attend fine music schools, where they spend years in preparing for their careers. After graduation, they continue to "pay their dues" in lengthy apprenticeships with more established players, as studio musicians, and as opening acts for better-known players. Likewise, young psychotherapists attend professional training programs, study exhaustively, endure field placements, internships, and residencies, and then struggle to get started in practice. In jazz or psychotherapy, many years pass before the novice becomes a master of the tools and techniques that will enable him to become a virtuoso.

Technical expertise, of course, does not lead automatically to creative depth. Once the techniques and structures of the profession have been mastered, the would-be improviser must meet four psychological conditions in order to use his skills creatively. The improviser must (1) have access to his past, (2) be able to focus his attention intensely on the present, (3) be comfortable giving up enough control over the outcome of his task to experiment as he performs, and (4) recognize the significance of accidental experience.

The first of these conditions, psychological access to one's past, permits the musician or the therapist to draw his ideas and responses from his entire range of life experiences. Fragments of the improviser's past are recombined in novel ways as the creative process unfolds.

Jazz musicians play in personally distinctive styles, recognizable because of the musical ideas common to many of their performances, just the way certain colors, shapes, or textures define the style of a given visual artist. Jazz performers do not always play new ideas, but in each performance they will at least recombine old ideas in new ways. Psychotherapists also develop personal styles, and, in large measure, the individuality of each therapist derives from his own life experience and how he utilizes it in relating to his patients. A therapist working with an adolescent patient, for instance, ought to have access to memories and feelings from his own adolescence. Such memories are a rich source of understanding for the therapist, and they help shape his unique, creative therapeutic reactions. Permitting fragments of past experience to become conscious is one of the keys to the mystery of improvisation.

The second psychological necessity for the improviser is the ability to focus his attention intensely on the present. One's associations to past events, as important as they are for improvisation, are useful only if they are stimulated by the content or process of the present task. The past filters into the improviser's awareness, but a dual awareness of both past and present permits old memories and feelings to attach to current events in unfamiliar ways. Preconceptions and stale reactions are thus shed since every moment bears the potential for a new discovery. The improviser must be immersed in all the stimulation of the present, including the ideas of others, nonverbal social cues, and his own spontaneous sensory and motor reactions. With this kind of full and deep participation in the proverbial "here and now," the merger of one's immediate task and one's history begins to yield the process we recognize as creativity.

The third psychological set required of the improviser involves the capacity to relinquish total control over one's task and to experiment. Both psychotherapists and musicians spend an enormous amount of time learning to be in control of their therapeutic or musical tasks. Paradoxically, it is this training that permits the therapist or player to give up just enough conscious control to permit a creative, improvisational experience to take place.

To use a musical example, suppose a jazz player is familiar with a certain five-note riff, which he usually starts on the third degree of a particular scale. Let us say that he has played that riff hundreds of times, and he knows just where it will take him, how it will end, and to what it will lead. But what will happen if, in the midst of a performance, he spontaneously begins that riff on the fifth of the scale or on the seventh? That little experiment will take him into new, uncharted territory. He will end in a new and unfamiliar place on the scale, and the ideas that follow will be unplanned, unpracticed, and unpredicted. The new melodic ideas suggested by this experiment probably will not depart radically from ideas played before; yet neither will the ideas be under completely conscious control. Likewise, a psychotherapist must allow himself to be led onto new ground where his responses to patients will differ from those of past interactions. Willingness to enter new turf spontaneously creates therapeutic excitement. Without this kind of risk taking, psychotherapy becomes boring, lifeless, and, usually, useless.

Finally, the improviser must be attuned to the significance of accidental experience. Accidents differ from experiments in that the latter are at least semicontrolled. The experimenter purposely alters some parameters while holding others constant in order to observe the effects of his actions. Surpassing the mere experimenter, the improviser also grasps the importance of events outside the bounds of his direct actions and predictions, events that creatively suppressed individuals define as trivial or fail to see altogether. Sir Alexander Fleming, for example, realized that the mold that contaminated his cultures was more important than the bacteria with which he was experimenting; he "accidentally" discovered penicillin.

How often do a jazz pianist's fingers accidentally strike a "wrong" note that leads to the creation of a beautiful melody? How often does an accident in psychotherapy (e.g., the therapist unexpectedly sees his patient in a restaurant, cancels an appointment at the last minute because of a personal emergency, shows a previously hidden feeling, or makes an uncharacteristic value judgment on a day when he is tired and his guard is down) arouse intense affect in a patient and provoke new material that bears immense therapeutic benefit?

Improvisation is born of the interplay among one's technical mastery, one's past experiences, one's present activity, an experimental attitude, and an openness to the accidental. If all a therapist or musician does is draw from his past, he may be competent, but he will not be creative. If all a therapist or artist does is open himself to new experiences, he may be exciting and spontaneous, but he also will be impulsive and chaotic. But if the improvising therapist or performer blends all he has been with what he is doing now, if he can relinquish some of his control and be aware of the importance of what he has not anticipated, his work will be vigorous and unique.

Describing the Creative Moment

On his television series devoted to masters of modern jazz, Oscar Peterson, the great jazz pianist, recently interviewed Toots Thielemans, a performer and composer best known for his innovative harmonica playing (Peterson 1980). Thielemans revealed the way his creative process combines his technical expertise, his personal history, and his intense concentration with an experimental attitude and an openness to accidental experience.

Asked how he conceived the idea of playing jazz harmonica, Thielemans explained that, as a child growing up in Belgium, he played the accordion. He had always wanted to improvise, but his only medium then was the French musette waltz. "Later on," he said, "I got turned on to the blues, and I bought a harmonica . . . and just tried to express myself. It was a hobby from the start. It still is a hobby."

While a student at Brussels University during the early 1940s, Toots often brought his harmonica along when going out dancing with his friends. The harmonica helped him become popular, but when he played with other musicians, they did not take him seriously, advising him instead to "play a real instrument." Thielemans soon took up the guitar to acquire "the keyboard knowledge . . . the vision of the complete spectrum, not just the top note melody." After mastering the guitar, he returned to his old harmonica. "Automatically, the road became clear," he told Peterson. "I knew which note not to play too often, which notes to skip . . . how to play more selectively."

Thielemans went on to describe how he came to write the jazz classic "Blusette," his best-known composition. The creative moment occurred while he was warming up for a concert in Brussels with jazz violinist Stephane Grappelli. He explained that the piece has a blues form and yet does not have a single blues note or a syncopated beat. "It's purely French, really. It can be traced to the musette waltz. . . . I didn't look for it, but it happened. . . . I was strumming the guitar . . . the chords are Charlie Parker chords. . . . I hummed the piece. Stephane said, 'Oh that's pretty.' Then I wrote it down. . . . I knew I had something."

All the elements of improvisational creativity are present in Thieleman's story: the acquisition of technical knowledge and skill on the guitar; the transfer of that expertise to the instrument of his adolescence, the harmonica; further contact with his past, the French musette waltz; the focus on the present, the Charlie Parker chords, the blues form, and warming up before a concert; the conscious experimentation involved in combining all these elements; and recognizing the significance of the accidental, the tune itself.

To study the improvisational processes of psychotherapists in their day-to-day work, I interviewed forty-three therapists about what goes on in their minds as they listen and respond to patients. A psychiatrist of ten years' experience provided this artful example from an actual session:[1]

A seventeen-year-old girl I had seen weekly for six months came in for her session one day obviously upset. She told me of a blowup the day before between her and her stepmother that she had provoked by making a hurtful, spiteful, thoughtless remark after her stepmother had spent hours helping her with her college application essay. She loves her stepmother, who has been the most emotionally giving figure in her adolescence, for which she is grateful. Her guilt seems boundless, and she chastises herself for the comment she made: "I hate myself when I do things like this."

Many things go through my mind as she speaks. Some of them? My memory of her psychodynamic conflicts and her family constellation; an intellectual awareness of her tendency to alienate others and punish herself; her feeling of not expecting or deserving real love and concern; my emotional awareness of her pain; a book I read a few months ago about adolescent girls and psychotherapy; a novel I read in college; a play I saw five years ago; an article I read in *Newsweek* last week about depression and suicide in adolescence; lyrics from a bunch of songs of the "you always hurt the one you love" genre; wanting to help her feel better; seeing her right leg double twisted around her left calf, locked at the ankles; awareness of fidgiting in my seat and tension in my forehead; wondering what to say to her.

After she's stopped and we've shared a brief moment of quiet, I begin to speak. I'm surprised by what I tell her.

I tell her a story of my own adolescence, a story of an offhand remark I once made to my own father when I was sixteen years old that offended and hurt him. I remembered him screaming at me, confronting me with my own narcissism and adolescent self-absorption at an age when my struggle for independence from him tended to take precedence over my concern about inflicting pain on him. What I also told her, though, was that my father was right. I had been thoughtless and selfish, and I had hurt someone I loved. Beyond that, had he not shown me so violently his hurt, I never would have understood my impact on him. I felt terribly guilty that day, but that episode was an important lesson in relatedness for me. It helped me grow up.

That story seemed to make an impression on her. It helped relieve her guilt because I had done something just like she had when I was her age, and, since she had a positive image of and relationship with me, it meant that she could not have been that bad after all. Neither did the story relieve her of responsibility for being selfish and provocative. Instead, it defined her behavior as something to outgrow.

"It's funny, but I'm sure I've never shared that story with anyone before. I don't even think I had thought of it in over twenty years."

This psychiatrist's vignette describes a truly creative moment. His training (he thinks first of psychodynamic and family issues), his engagement with his patient and his task, his own personal history, and his ability to give up conscious control all set the stage for his complex reaction. In the end, an improvised response carries his therapeutic message.

Creativity and the Personal Metaphor

My interviews revealed that, just as I apply the metaphor of jazz to psychotherapy, many therapists keep a personal, extratherapeutic model in mind as they work with patients. Some of the metaphors psychotherapists described included the Asian martial arts, dancing, painting, sculpturing, gardening, playing tennis or basketball, understanding fine literature, acting, and learning a spiritual discipline.

The particular model applied by a given psychotherapist should not be confused with the process of improvisation so clearly present among all creative therapists. Freud (1913) drew an analogy between chess and psychotherapy, writing that the possible opening and closing moves of a game are easy to describe but that all the intervening steps must be carried out intuitively. Yalom (1980) opens his book on existential psychotherapy with a description of a gourmet cooking class he once took with an Armenian matriarch and her servant. The students tried but never could duplicate the dishes of their teacher. Finally, they realized that, as the carefully prepared dishes were being carried to the oven, the servant surreptitiously threw in handfuls of assorted spices and condiments. Yalom writes, "That cooking class often comes to mind when I think about psychotherapy, especially when I think about the critical ingredients of successful therapy. Formal texts, journal articles, and lectures portray therapy as precise and systematic . . . , yet I believe deeply that, when no one is looking, the therapist throws in the 'real thing' " (p. 3).

An episode from early in my treatment of an adolescent boy illustrates how one's personal metaphor can be used improvisationally in the therapeutic process. The model here is one of my jazz heroes, Duke Ellington. Ellington's orchestral arrangements were carefully composed; yet they allowed plenty of room for improvisation by his individual musicians. Unlike composers or arrangers who wrote for anonymous players, his pieces were tailored to the potentials and proclivities of specific members of his band. One of the features of his arranging, unique in his day, is called "scoring" or "voicing across sections." Whereas, in other bands, instrumental sections were played off against each other—saxophones against brass, for example—Ellington pitted unusual combinations of instruments against each other.

My patient, a seventeen-year-old high school dropout, was hospitalized because of his violence. Just before admission, L lost control of his rage and hurled a chair through a picture window at home. The psychodynamic and familial origins of his problems were obvious: five operations for hypospadius before the age of five, an overbearing and overprotective mother, and an uninvolved and aloof father. The parents had serious difficulties throughout their marriage and finally separated when L was thirteen. Not only did L have a defective penis, but he was also a puny child who was picked on mercilessly by bigger boys as he grew up. His anger and violence in the home clearly was in reaction to all these conflicts, as was his omnipresent daydream of becoming a Mafia hit man.

While in the hospital, L decided to open a business. His idea was to place advertisements in newspapers and magazines saying that, if customers would send him fifteen dollars, he would send them instructions on how to make $30,000 in just one month. The instructions would state, "Put an ad in the newspaper just like mine, and 2,000 people are sure to send you fifteen dollars apiece. You'll be rich in a month!" He proposed to use the hospital as his mailing address.

Now, L was talking about committing mail fraud, and the administrators on the adolescent unit were not about to aid and abet a teenager in the commission of a federal crime. Most of the staff on the unit became stuck in an unproductive, moralistic/legalistic power struggle with the patient. They treated him as a sociopath who needed control and limits. Even his individual psychotherapy became bogged down. Session after session, all L could talk about was how the staff was holding him back, how he knew he could be a success if they would only let him try out his business, and how unfairly the world always treated him.

At this point, I decided to try an Ellington technique, voicing an arrangement across the sections of the staff. One psychiatric technician and one activities therapist seemed much more interested in working with the patient's need for mastery than harping on his superego deficits. I joined forces with them and the patient against the authoritarian position of the rest of the staff.

The psychiatric technician taught L to box, giving him a new sense of physical control and a chance to channel his aggression less destructively. The patient was eager to learn this manly art; after all, a Mafia hit man had to know how to defend himself. The activities therapist started talking to L about work skills, always framing her advice in terms of the self-discipline he would need to run his "mail-order" business. I started talking to L about the practical aspects of his business, like how to write an appealing advertisement, how to manage money, and how to obtain a post office box since the hospital address could not be used.

L suddenly realized that he would need a way to deposit the checks his customers would send him, so he decided to open a bank account. I gladly helped out by driving him to the bank one afternoon. When we got to the bank, L seemed confused. "I've never opened a bank account before. . . . What do I do?" he asked. I directed him to the bank officer behind a desk and drifted over to a couch to wait while he opened his account. A few minutes later, I heard his panic-stricken voice scream my name. "He says I need more identification," L cried. Pathetically, all he had to identify himself was a Nautilus ID from his hometown.

"Where's your driver's license?" I asked.

"I lost it a few months ago, and I never got around to writing for a duplicate," he sheepishly replied.

We returned to the hospital. For the first time, L realized that he was held back, not by other people, but by his own lack of realism, his lack of education and social skills, his impulsivity, and his anger. He began to take his education at the hospital's high school seriously. He stopped resisting people's efforts to help him, and he started to make good use of his psychotherapy. He became insightful about himself, and he tried hard to free himself of the destructive patterns of his past behavior. After discharge from the hospital, he completed his high school education and went on to college. Recently, he wrote to me that he had been listed in *Who's Who in American Colleges and Universities*.

The "Ellington" intervention arose in my mind as a musical idea applicable to a clinical impasse. Actually, it was a joining technique, a reframing of the patient's interests, strengths, and weaknesses in a way that permitted a therapeutic alliance to develop. This kind of maneuver occurs often in creative psychotherapy, although seldom as publicly or dramatically. That interventions like this one are common should not obscure their improvisational nature.

As the primary therapist and architect of L's overall treatment, I met all the criteria needed for an improvisational performance. I had access to my past—not only to my musical background but also, and more important, to my own adolescence. I understood what it was like to be a boy in need of autonomy, personal power, and mastery. My intense, daily immersion in the task of this patient's psychotherapy helped set the stage for all that happened as treatment unfolded.

The entire intervention was experimental, complete with an opposing faction of the adolescent unit staff who helped control the experiment. Mutual respect between me and the staff members who saw my patient and his needs differently was essential to the success of the process. We all had to be comfortable with less than total control over the outcome.

Finally, some of the key elements of the process seemed accidental at the time. I believed in advance that, by allying with my patient in pursuit of his fantasy, I would force him to confront his limitations and give up his grandiose ideas. I did not predict that he would panic in the bank. I did not know that the maneuver would help him to accept his ineptitude or that the episode would crystallize his motivation to learn. Once these unexpected results occurred, it was up to me and the treatment team to recognize their importance and use them therapeutically on the patient's behalf.

Conclusions

The key to improvising in music, psychotherapy, or any creative endeavor is the artist's capacity to draw on all of himself in the service of his task. With the proper perspective, models from outside one's profession can inspire uncommonly inventive solutions to difficult problems. James Levine, musical director of the Metropolitan Opera, spoke about the relation between his musical and extramusical activities in a recent television broadcast ("American Masters" 1985). Where Levine speaks of musicians and music, insert therapists and psychotherapy:

> I think musicians are awfully fortunate that our work is so all consuming. By that, I mean virtually everything I really love to

do is essential to my musical work. I like to study history and cultures and languages, everything that relates to other arts and to drama and poetry and the human emotions and human conflicts. So no matter what I'm doing, whether I take a trip to somewhere I haven't been before, or read a novel, or have a conversation with someone in a completely different profession, it all helps my experience. . . . It helps my perception so that I can achieve a stronger rapport with a specific composer and apply it to the details of a specific piece. And there's never a feeling that one kind of thing is work and another kind is play. It all flows in such a way that it's a really unified life.

As psychotherapists, we too can lead unified lives by availing ourselves of the whole spectrum of our personalities and of all our life experiences in our daily work. With preparation, discipline, and openness, everything we have done and been as individuals can help us help our patients, one creative moment at a time.

NOTE

1. The clinical example quoted was obtained during research for a book, in progress, concerning the origins and functions of individuality among psychotherapists. All psychotherapists interviewed in the study were guaranteed anonymity.

REFERENCES

American masters: James Levine. 1985. Newark, N.J.: Public Broadcasting System, WNET-13; Munich: Unitel.

Freud, S. 1913. On beginning treatment (further recommendations on the technique of psychoanalysis). *Standard Edition* 12:121–144. London: Hogarth, 1958.

Peterson, O. 1980. Oscar Peterson and friends. Toronto: Canadian Broadcasting Corp., Toronto/5.

Yalom, I. 1980. *Existential psychotherapy*. New York: Basic.

12 THE CREATIVE THERAPEUTIC ENCOUNTER AT ADOLESCENCE

E. JAMES ANTHONY

The adolescents that I know best, a precious few, are those who have elected to become intensively engaged with me in a long-term psychotherapeutic allliance carried out within a psychoanalytic framework. As a sample, they clearly provide a limited perspective on the wide psychosocial world of adolescence. But, at the same time, they have been able to furnish me with unusual insights into the so-called intermediate area of experience (Winnicott 1958). The patients did not choose me since they knew nothing about me or about the field in which I worked. I was selected by parents who had exalted notions of the latent potential of their offspring and, having researched my professional reputation, had concluded that I was skilled in releasing the creativities and thwarted talents underlying the manifest disturbances.

An avowed interest in giftedness tends to bring this type of clientele to the office. At this point, the adolescents were chosen by me because of therapeutically oriented qualities they possessed—more specifically, a self-reflective propensity, an avid curiosity about their environment, an openness to novel experiences, a fluency of communication, a flexibility of frames and boundaries, a zest for exploring relationships, and an altogether refreshing spontaneity. This constellation of characteristics is not as rare at this time of life as it is later in the established adult since the adolescent process itself tends to reinforce such inherent or acquired proclivities. At this stage, there is an extraordinary upsurge of new cognitive mechanisms that allow for the abstract thinking needed for the construction of theoretical systems. Speculation is rife during these years that have been termed "the metaphysical age." From the point of view of psychological therapy, the adolescent, unlike the child, becomes introspective, self-critical, and capable of scrutinizing reactions and interactions with a shrewdness and directness that is often disconcerting for the clinician.

The Gifted Adolescent Patient

Having formulated some of the qualities of the gifted patient, one can next examine the types of exchanges that may occur with those therapists who fail to live up to the capacities of such patients and attempt to treat them stereotypically. Occasionally, they may misuse theory and interpret inappropriately and even wildly.

CASE EXAMPLE 1

A fifteen-year-old adolescent girl confronts her male therapist with what she perceives as being his air of smugness and superiority. Without the necessary prior work on her defenses, he tells her without much ado that she is suffering from "penis envy." Her response is properly scathing. "You men are so scared of loosing your dicks that you treat them like bullions of gold, preserved securely in the vaults of a bank. You assume that women are equally entranced with them and that they can think of nothing better than of stealing them and sticking these ugly pieces of flesh grotesquely between their legs. Doesn't this strike you as being a lot of sexist hogwash? If you want to know what I really envy, it's someone who uses her mind wonderfully like Emily Dickinson; not someone who just thinks with his crotch. I don't blame Freud for getting this idea because women were put down in those days as a matter of tradition. Now it occurs when they become patients. You're taking advantage of me and you shouldn't. Besides, how can you divide this world of creatures into haves and have-nots when each side has so much to give and to share." Here then is a fifteen-year-old who refused to accept a deprecating psychological idea dogmatically administered to her. She is a gifted adolescent who, despite her psychosocial disorder, is becoming aware of the intellectual and creative forces operating within her at this phase of her development. She reaches out excitedly beyond the limits of what seem to her to be restricted and small versions of reality and is obviously aware, in this encounter, of the discrepancy between her fertile explorations of herself and the therapist's trite use of a theoretical construct. She makes it clear that she is not just another patient but an adolescent in a state of creative ferment who is searching for a self, for a place to be, and for an object to relate to and love. Within this context, she finds the interchange with the therapist meaningless and, consequently, walks out on him. If he, like Freud in the case of Dora (1905), can now reexamine the abrupt termination, he may well be able to learn something about the mysterious workings of transference and countertransference, or, failing a tremendous discovery, he might, perhaps, gain at least a new realization in the area of therapeutic tact.

One cannot think of therapy as continuously creative since this is not in the nature of human creativity, which is often climactic against a background of relative quiescence. Gifted patients enter the therapeutic situation without being aware at first of its generative possibilities, but, because of the assimilative powers, the openness and freedom involved soon engage their attention and interest. The urge to solve a specific emotional problem is not their immediate concern since the encounter with an unknown individual will often take precedence and, in some cases, lead to the production of psychological noise purposefully and artfully directed at distraction. The therapist must wait for quiet before the imperative underlying needs make themselves evident. It can be quite effective to mitigate this introductory storm with the help of therapeutic commonplaces that have the backing of universal emollients—the "good morning and how are you" approaches of everyday life.

CASE EXAMPLE 2

In this next vignette, the therapist waits until the turbulence subsides before he makes effective contact with the patient. It is only when this has been done that the gifted patient becomes able to make creative use of the situation. A tempestuous seventeen-year-old girl, looking confident but belligerent, comes in for her first session, seats herself in my chair, takes up a pad and pencil from the desk, and stares contemptuously at me. She is manifestly about to conduct an interview. I smile, wish her good day, and inquire, very neutrally, how do you do. She dismisses this overture. "And you, what have you got to say for yourself today?" she asks, with her voice taking on a mock British accent. "You're silent? You have difficulty expressing yourself, have you? Let's see what we can do for you. Would you like me to hold your hand? No, not ethical? What does it matter? We are alone here. No one will ever know. If you seduce me, I'll tell people that you did it just out of nervousness." She stares at me quizzically, but I can sense the glowing hostility in the look. I am taken aback with her approach and uncertain how to respond. Eventually, I bring myself to say to her, "Perhaps you're teasing me like this because you're nervous and don't quite know how to begin." She is properly sarcastic. "Now there's a clever therapist for you. Always knows what's going on in his patient's mind. Top marks for you. You're going to make good grades in therapy one day. Trust me to get a beginner." I wait this out, hoping she will run out of ammunition. For a while, we stare at each other. Her eyes are still angry, but her fingers have begun to drum the table as if she too was at a loss. "If *you* don't know where to begin, I better start. What do you want to hear about first? My bitch of a mother or my sot of a father?" I say to her with as much calm as I can muster, "Just tell me what's upsetting you most at the present time and then we can take it from there." She glares at me. "Christ! You're such a gentleman. You sound so prissy. I wonder if you're really male. Are all therapists castrated before they're allowed to work with girls?" I find no ready comment to this. We stare silently at each other, but there is no amusement in her eyes. After a while, she says, "Christ! I can't stand being in here. I want to start throwing things around and smashing things up." I find myself at the beginning of some understanding, some recognition of the logic of her reactions, and I find myself saying to her, "I feel your anger, and I feel some anger in myself in response to it, even though I realize that you are trying to make me angry. But I also feel that not all your anger is at me. I feel a lot of anger left over for others." This is followed by a long period of silence, during which I half expected her to begin another tirade, but, to my surprise, she says, "You're right, Anthony. My fucking mother tried to strangle me today and I just had to give her a black eye. She wanted to ground me and I told her to fuck herself. Christ! That pleased me to see her smashed up." She looks at me defiantly, and then her voice once again takes on a mincing, British quality. "And now tell me all your troubles. What's wrong with your saintly life?" I say to her, "It's very hard to attack one's mother without feeling bad about it, but I expect that feeling bad about her is making you even more angry with her. How can you make

197

it right that you hurt her?'' She answers without sarcasm. ''You've hit the nail on the head, Anthony. Christ! She looked so pathetic. I felt like crying, even though I hated her. I want to kill her but I also want her to remain alive and live with me and love me. I'm crazy. I wish I knew what to do. What can anyone do with a dumbo like me?'' She gets up, goes to the window, and looks out. Neither of us says anything, as if we have nothing to say, and the minutes pass. Finally, she turns her head very slowly toward me and says, ''You know, it's very quiet in here. Is it always so quiet?'' I smile and shake my head. ''Only when there is too much to say.'' She smiles back, and I sense her receptiveness and the lowering of barriers. I was emboldened to say to her, ''It is quiet, so quiet that I can now feel your sadness, and it makes me sad for you.'' She begins to cry softly, and I let her remain for a while before closing the session. In subsequent sessions, she continued to demonstrate her skill in reaching ruthlessly into the less defended portions of the therapist's psyche, but she also drove as ruthlessly into herself, despite the pain incurred. Once the destructive impulse diminished, it was replaced by an exuberant flow of creative fantasy, and, in the outside world, the storms of rage largely subsided. Perhaps the more striking outcome of the treatment was her starting to write autobiographical short stories that appeared to take off from the fantasies generated in the therapy.

The dream, sometimes referred to as everybody's creativity, is often treated as a fascinating curiosity by the gifted adolescent, who may keep records of it, carry out research on it, and even attempt to interpret it. In the therapeutic situation, when dreams begin to mirror the workings of the transference, this type of patient plays with the dream material with zestful fascination, explores the content, and is even ready to interpret the meaning. If the therapist has been engaged in this mode of activity, a certain amount of rivalry may well creep into the picture, and not only on the side of the patient.

CASE EXAMPLE 3

Fred is a gifted mid-adolescent patient with borderline qualities that verge toward the neurotic side of the spectrum. He has been in treatment for about a year. He comes into the session carrying a book but keeping its cover, and therefore the title, hidden from me. He sits down comfortably, very much at home in the situation, and maintains an easy eye contact with the therapist. He begins by saying, "I had an interesting dream last night; at least I thought you might find it interesting since you like this sort of mental garbage." I do not rise to the bait but remain silent, and, after a while, he can stand it no longer. "Don't you want to hear about it?" I tell him that I always want to hear what he has to tell me, but it is up to him to decide whether to tell. He looks disgusted. "Geez, how neutral can you get!" Again, I am silent. Eventually, he sighs deeply and then says, "Well, since we're getting nowhere, I might as well tell you in case it means anything to you, which I doubt. There is a woman outside the house, I think it's my home, in the garden. A small dog comes out and pees on her. She doesn't seem to mind, but her husband gets very angry and kicks the dog and drives it away." I ask for clarification: "Was it a male dog?" He smiles and says, "Very male." I wait for him to continue, but he is clearly wanting something from me. His frustration increases with much sighing. "Is this your technique, to do nothing? You want me to do all the work? You want me to be the therapist, but you want to get paid for it." I have nothing to say to this, and he shakes his head despairingly. Eventually, he shrugs his shoulders and says, "It's all pretty obvious. It's the old Oedipus stuff. Clearly I'm the dog and the woman's my mother. The guy does not look like my dad, but he's a jerk like him. It could be you because you sometimes behave like a jerk. Then there is the sex stuff. I suppose I'm trying to have sex with my mother, but being a small kid I can't do it. I can only pee. I remember when I was a kid I used to think that men peed into women to make babies and I thought that that was what they were telling us in sex education school. But one of the other guys told me better." There was a pause. "What do you think about my interpretation?" I say to him, "You wanted to tell me this dream very much, Freddie. I wonder why?" He is outraged. "Is that all you have to say when I bring you a beautiful dream and a beautiful explanation! Don't you like my interpretation?" I hesitate. "Well, Freddie, it's very Freudian." He shakes his head as if giving me up as a hopeless case. As if to underscore my ineptness, he holds up the book to show me its title—*The Interpretation of Dreams*. He points an admonitory finger at me. "Now *he* would have been really turned on by my dream. But then he was a genius. He appreciated his patients. He gave them credit for their understanding. You're so full of yourself that you think only your interpretations are any good. If you want to know the truth, I think I'm better at it than you. You are not God! You are not even a decent therapist." The silence between us becomes quite uncomfortable, and I begin to wonder inwardly whether there is something in what he is saying. He watches me with curiosity and then asks what I am thinking about. I tell him that I am still wondering why he had wanted so much to tell me this dream and also so much to explain the dream to me. Had he dreamed the dream for me so that we could get to know each other better? Once again he is outraged. "That remark just stinks! You've just got to have all the answers. You think you're the greatest because you're a professor, but have you thought why you're a professor? It's because you couldn't earn a living in private practice. You don't know how to treat patients. You are just an egghead." The barrage resonated within me as I struggled to maintain some semblance of therapeutic equanimity. I ask him why he thinks we are working against rather than with each other. He had come to the session with a dream that seemed like a present for me, with an interpretation that he felt was better than anything I could produce, and with a volume of Freud to back him up. This had led me to feel that he was dissatisfied with me and disillusioned, just as he was with his father, who also took advantage of his superiority and kicked him around. He hears me out and then says, "I think you are just protecting yourself and covering over. Why don't you admit that you were angry with me just as I was angry with you." I brace myself and say, "I think I was a little angry with you." He snorted with disgust: "Think? Little?" I take a breath. "You're right, I was angry with you." He smiles, reaches out to shake my hand, and says, "Now we can continue."

The gifted patient does not make things easy for the therapist. He seems to be uncannily aware of the countertransference and often pushes to work with it to the chagrin of the therapist. We did continue, and I learned a great deal from him. I had entered the situation to treat him, and, to my surprise, I occasionally found that I too was being treated. It reminded me of Freud's joke about the priest who went in to save the soul of a dying insurance agent—while the agent died unconfessed, the priest came out fully insured.

The interview described took place many years ago. Fred went on to medical school and eventually into psychiatry—more specifically, psychotherapy. He recently got in touch with me to say that he was writing a paper on my treatment of him as an adolescent. I have to admit that my stomach turned over as I listened to him on the phone,

200

wondering how I was going to come out of this disclosure. At the end of the call, I found myself saying to him, "I hope you'll be kind to me, Fred." He seemed surprised. "You didn't do so badly," he said, "I think that I benefited from the treatment, which is what I owe to you, but what I learned, I learned from myself. It was your technique and my insight that did the trick."

Over the years that I treated him, Fred's reactions often made me squirm within myself. I reminded myself that there were at least twenty-one good reasons why the "good enough" therapist sometimes hated his adolescent patient and, at times, toyed with the idea of annihilating him. That the patient is creative in no way implies that he is easy to deal with or that he follows the therapist's line rather than his own idiosyncratic path of therapeutic progression.

The Gifted Therapist

As was observed in the previous section, the gifted patient may not be associated with a gifted therapist, although such a patient may be able to upgrade the therapist and provide him with a sense of creative accomplishment. Similarly, the gifted therapist may help the average, workaday patient to blossom introspectively, insightfully, and articulately. When the gifted therapist and gifted patient occupy the same therapeutic space, as was the case with Freud and the adolescent Dora, new developments in treatment may take place. Freud was undoubtedly impressed by his young patient's "sound and incontestable train of argument" and by the connections that she made between some of her actions and the motives that presumably underlay them (Freud 1905). In this therapeutic investigation, according to Rieff (1979, p. 82), "Dora was a brilliant detective too, parrying Freud's own brilliance. Her interpretation of her situation was often so acute that Freud could not help asking himself why his was superior. As the case took its course, Dora would propose explanations of her wretchedness which Freud criticized, countering with his own; or Freud would spin out his arguments, ending with a fair challenge to his patient—'And now, what have your recollections to say to this?' " But it was not just Dora's intellectual gifts remarked by Freud that made this disputation possible. The discursive web of treatment was not spun merely to suit this precocious girl. It characterized the method long after Freud's own stated preference for intelligent patients dropped out of the canon. Regardless of the intellectual facility of the patient, psychoanalysis makes a procedural assumption that necessarily exaggerates the import of the patient's present talk and her understanding of it. That is, it equates the events of the patient's life with her verbal account of them, precisely by treating the verbalisms as telling distortions of the truth. In reading the account by Freud, we become aware of the way in which the gifted therapist functions, catching "the drift of the patient's unconscious with his own unconscious" (Freud 1905, p. 239) or, as he put it further on, bending "his own unconscious-like receptive organ toward the emerging unconscious of the patient." This unconscious mode of communication is very much at the heart of the work of the talented therapist.

Freud also spoke of the way in which the therapist directs his attention to the fantasy life of the patient, but he also pointed out that there was a path from fantasy back into reality, which is the circuit undertaken by the artist and also by the therapist (Freud 1916–1917). These dual transformations are essential to the cure of neurosis and require the exquisite sensitivity of an individual equally at home in both worlds—fantasy and reality. What the therapist interpolates between fantasy and reality, between primary and secondary process, is an imaginative capacity that is largely preconscious in its functioning. The gifted therapist, therefore, is an imaginative therapist who brings about a shift from a chaotic id content to an enriched ego (Sachs 1965).

This process sees a patient in a way that he has not been seen before. One sees a patient as Cezanne sees a tree. One is "grasped" by the patient as Cezanne was "grasped" by the tree, causing something new to be born, to come into being, something that did not exist in that particular form before. When one reads the case of Dora, one is grasped by the act of encounter between Freud and his young patient. As May (1965, p. 286) points out, symbols (like Cezanne's tree) or myths (like Oedipus) are born out of the heightened consciousness of encounter and express the relation between internal and external, fantasy and reality, subjective and objective, consciousness and unconsciousness, and one individual's present history against the background of all human history.

The gifted therapist is also "grasped" by himself, by his own inner world. He needs not only to understand his patients but also to be understood by them and to be as much in touch with his own psychic operations as he is with those of his patients. Long ago, Maimonides said, "If I were not interested in myself, what would others be able to do for me, and if I were not interested in myself, what would I be able to do for others?'' A therapist needs a workable quota of narcissism to tolerate the long, demanding hours of therapy.

It is not at all surprising that a gifted therapist like Winnicott was deeply preoccupied with two spontaneous manifestations of the human spirit, play and creativity. The gifted therapist should be able to play and create a space for playing between himself and the patient. ''Psychotherapy,'' says Winnicott (1974, p. 44), ''takes place in the overlap of two areas of playing, that of the patient and that of the therapist. (It) has to do with two people playing together. The corollary of this is that where playing is not possible, then the work done by the therapist is directed toward bringing the patient from a state of not being able to play into a state of being able to play.'' So important is this creative function that, if the therapist cannot play, he is unsuitable for carrying out this work and should undergo treatment until he can play again and, thus, become creative. He is, then, not only creative himself but also a source of creativity in the patient. He allows himself to be used as a transitional object by the patient, to be caught up in the symbolization emerging in the therapy, and he learns to caution himself against deciphering it immediately and reducing it to some arid formulation. He learns to transform silence into words when this is needed, but, even more important, he learns to transform words into silence, which can have as mutative an effect. He can accept ambiguities and ambivalences, paradoxes and contradictions, meaning and meaninglessness, creative clarity and disorder. By bracketing the contents that the patient brings, he can listen to the sounds of personality as they are manifested in different affects, experiences, and conflicts.

What he does is to set up an ongoing dialogue with the patient that is sometimes near to reality and, at other times, steeped in unrealism and primitive fantasy. It is always done quietly, and, in the first approach to the patient, use is made of the everyday language of clichés and stereotypes. In case example 2, the therapist responded to the dramatic noise of the encounter with truisms and commonplace exchanges, and, very gradually, quiet emerged. Yet, there were challenging and provocative discrepancies at work in the therapeutic situation. Two different human beings from two different cultures, representing two different sexes and two different phases of the life cycle, came together to find a mutually acceptable form of exchange without any conviction that this was going to work. The feelings of panic and persecution on the patient's side were confronted by a fair degree of steadiness on the part of the therapist, and, until the situation settled down, the creative urges of the patient were stymied. Although some degree of playfulness, albeit morbid and sardonic, was already present, truly creative playfulness did not invade the space between us until later in the treatment. The "creative dialogizing" (Hulbeck 1965, p. 318) was permeated with black humor at the beginning, but this gave place to good-humored exchanges.

CASE EXAMPLE 4

A borderline girl of seventeen years brings a ready-made symbiosis with her mother into the therapeutic situation and resists all my efforts to make her conscious of me as a separate person (Anthony 1973). For her, the process is always circulating between our minds, and she is never sure whose feelings are whose. She lets me know that she has no thoughts of her own, no will of her own, no ego of her own, and, by implication, no penis of her own; she lives on borrowed egos. She says, "Tell me what to do and I'll do it. I'll do anything that you say." My comment is that we do not understand at the present time what makes her so fearful about doing things for herself or saying things for herself but that, as we work together on the problem, this eventually will become much clearer. She should understand that there are two of us in this situation and that I need to understand her and she needs to understand me. We can help each other to get to know many things about each other. I tell her that I have pictures of her in my mind of what she had told me of being a very little girl crying in her crib and of no one coming; of clinging to her mother and of being nervous when strangers came; and of being taken to the doctor's office and of being afraid that they were going to open up her body and take everything away. She had told me all this, and this is the picture that is growing up inside me and helping me to understand her better. In response to this, she says, rather shyly, that, when she goes away from her sessions, she also has pictures of me: that I keep a very untidy desk, that she wants to tidy up for me, that my drawers are stuffed with things that she would never know about but that she wished she knew about because they would tell her about me; that my ties never match my shirts, that my pants are sometimes baggy and I should really get some new clothes. She is now smiling, but very soon her face clouds again.

"I suppose this is the end of the session. When I get home, I will think of you looking angry as if you wanted to punish me for being the bad person that I am" (Anthony 1973, pp. 42–43).

As treatment progressed, she began to break away from her self-imposed enclosure and to explore new horizons. At a late point in her treatment, she said, "I used to think that you would wave your magic wand and all my troubles would be over, but you've shown me how hard I must work myself in order to get better. It's up to me as much as it's up to you" (Anthony 1973, p. 43). Her sense of reality and responsibility increased as her belief in my omnipotence and omni-science diminished. The primitive wish to swallow me up and to be swallowed up in turn also waned. She would contrast herself with me, especially in the area of clear thinking and of not being caught between thoughts, confused and uncertain. "You never seem to be like that. When I am not sick, I get the feeling that you like me and that you don't want to eat me up or to destroy me. Sometimes when you speak, I get the feeling of your kind words entering all the dark spots of my body and making them feel light again." This is what I think of as borderline poetry, some inner, almost lyrical sense of the generative space between us. I stayed with her for as long as I thought useful in the "area of formlessness" (Winnicott 1974, p. 40). We lived together in a dream world where nothing was "cut and shaped and put together," but there was always the hope within me that something would grow out of this amorphous matrix if only I could build enough trust and confidence in me.

The apparently empty space between us gradually filled with memories, fantasies, feelings, dreams, and interactions, all increasingly permeated with transference, and, eventually, I was able to interpret them without her feeling invaded or attacked. As Beres (1965, p. 220) put it, "The analyst's role is not simply to translate to the patient the meanings of the derivatives of the unconscious. Rather, the role of the analyst is to free the patient's imagination so that he may recreate the fantasies of his childhood and communicate them to himself and to the analyst. . . . the patient then re-experiences his emotions, recollects, reconstructs, and relives; and this accomplishes the conviction that marks the true insight of the analytic experience." For all this to happen, the therapist must be capable of, in Coleridge's words, a "willing suspension of disbelief," which provides a powerful dynamic that activates an internal reverberating experience.

Where does the proclivity toward the psychotherapeutic drive originate? Searles (1965) has advanced the thesis that an essentially psychotherapeutic striving is innately present within the infant's emotional potentialities. A further postulate suggesting a rescue fantasy in relation to a depressed mother or one engaged in complicated mourning may constitute a powerful motivation for the future psychotherapist. The early exposure to depressive helplessness may either stimulate the child to undergo a process of affective attunement as a means of recovering contact with the mother or paralyze his approaches to different degrees. The child who loses his mother sets about inventing a reel-and-cotton game and eventually emerges as an adult therapist helping others to deal with loss. Sensitive patients are also incited to deal with loss inside the therapist. Winnicott (1958, p. 95) spoke of patients who felt a need to relieve their supposed depression because a transferred parental depression had been revived and, in part, may have originated within the therapist. One must distinguish between what belonged to the patient's psyche, what was produced for the therapist, and what was produced by elements within the therapist. The individual's urge to repair may lead him to become either therapist or patient or both. Reparation is the creative force at the heart of the therapeutic process.

A Creative Therapeutic Situation

I have been discussing the creative forces within the patient and within the therapist. Now I turn to the contributions made by the situation itself. This situation is sometimes referred to as a stage on which the internal representations of the patient are gradually externalized. At the beginning of treatment, the stage is relatively empty, but, under the aegis of a "creative apperception" (Winnicott 1974, p. 76), a two-way process is instituted in which self-enrichment alternates with the discovery of meaning. Within this development, the peaks of enhancement punctuate periods of compliant adaptation when the therapist experiences the treatment as futile and tedious.

Perhaps the most creative aspect of psychoanalytic psychotherapy is the way in which the past grows out of the present as if the therapist had dipped a symbolic madeleine into a therapeutic cup of tea. The past is regained not in terms of simple memories but full of Proustian sensibilities, searching for every shade of feeling and sensation (Anthony 1961).

CASE EXAMPLE 5

Lilly was a seventeen-year-old borderline schizoid girl who complained of lifelessness, emptiness, and meaninglessness. Only when she was active, eating, or being touched by boys did she lose her sense of deadness. In the therapeutic situation, she wanted to be touched and to touch, not for sexual reasons but because of the life that would flow out of me and revitalize her. At certain points in the treatment, she recovered elements of her early life with eidetic vividness, characterized by synesthesia at peak moments of the transference. She referred to them as "glorious" and ached to recapture them. At such moments, her consciousness appeared to be less than full, and she seemed to be in the throes of some primal fantasy, awaiting to be recreated and relived. The natural defenses appeared to be tangently dissolved. There would often be some stimulus arising in the therapeutic situation that precipitated a train of regressive associations. For example, "I have a drowsy feeling . . . as if I were on a cloud floating away in a wild, happy state . . . it's all blue and gold . . . lovely feelings . . . all colors . . . such nice taste . . . the blues are coming near . . . and going away . . . it's gone." She shakes her head, sits up, and looks somewhat dazed. Here is its creative counterpart: "A feeling of happiness came over me . . . a deep azure blue intoxicated my sight, impressions of coolness and dazzling light hovered near me . . . the dazzling elusive vision brushed me with its wings" (Proust 1928, p. 992). Such moments for Proust led to some of the most creative elaborations of the twentieth century; such moments for Lilly brought a new depth of experience to her treatment. For such patients, the therapeutic situation affords them novel excursions into a state of being that they would not be able to reach on their own, where id content is transformed into an enrichment of the ego and self. At such moments, also, the therapist needs to free himself of what Keats referred to as the prismatic study of the rainbow and allow himself to respond with empathy. Later, he can become inventive, as the secondary process reestablishes itself in him.

The themes that make their appearance in the therapeutic situation, as pointed out by Beres (1965), are those of the mythmakers and poets and deal with birth, death, love, hate, incest, sex, perversion, parricide, matricide, destruction, violence, castration, hunger, greed, jealousy, ambition, and dependence—all themes of the forbidden, the unattainable, and the repressed. "In the artistic act and in the analytic situation, the forbidden and the repressed are recreated" (Beres 1965, p. 216).

Hulbeck (1965) spoke of three creative phases in psychoanalysis—first the encounter, then the dialogue, and finally the process of articulation. He did not feel that creativity was inevitable in therapy, meaning by that the emergence of the true self, fully realized. This requires a process of growth that allows the individual "to see the deeper realities of life," however distorted and concealed they are. Growth, therefore, involves discovery, learning, understanding, and, finally, acting on. This is achieved through the creative work of the therapist interacting with the creative potentials of the patient. It begins with the meeting of two human beings. "The patient is simply there and the doctor is simply there." The encounter entails a collision of two different worlds, arousing in both patient and therapist a creative curiosity "not unlike the creative curiosity felt by an artist before he starts painting, writing, or composing" (pp. 315–316). The partners in this enterprise discover rapidly whether they like or dislike each other, whether the differences between them are tolerable or not, and whether the effort involved is worth the commitment. "If the patient decides to continue, he has given the first proof that he possesses a potential amount of transcending ability" (p. 316). So much of chance and so much of the irrationality of life are present in this first encounter.

Then comes the creative process, which is in the nature of a "creative vacuum, a form of emptiness that may be filled with knowing later in the process of treatment. It may be or it may not. The awareness of uncertainty surrounding the encounter, so deeply felt by both parties, makes it a creative stage in the sense that no preconceived formulas can be conceived" (Hulbeck 1965, p. 317).

The dialogue is always there, is always being generated through some mode of communication. It is a dialogue of words and silences. The therapeutic dialogue generally originates in silence, but, if it does not, silence soon finds its way into the situation and arrests the minds of both therapist and patient. The interplay of silence and words is against a common background of nonverbal activity in both participants, and both are waiting for something to happen—a regression to the past, the development of transference, the recovery of an infantile memory, or the emergence of a significant dream.

According to Hulbeck (1965), the third creative phase of articulation is aimed at understanding the human situation of the patient. It involves bracketing the contents of life and "listening to the sounds of personality" (p. 323). In all this, the analytic and the creative proceed at the same time. "The different events revealed in analytical activity are comparable to a play on the stage in which the patient plays most of the roles simultaneously" (p. 323). The therapist functioning creatively disentangles a story—the plot and its meaning. He inquires into the primary choices, how and why the patient's life was taken away from his own decisions, and why he lives a false life permeated with bad faith. In the beginning of treatment, new choices open up and become available to the patient, as he understands the wellspring of his personality. It is exquisitely creative in both purpose and process. As Nietzsche put it, "One's own self is well hidden from one's own self; of all mines of treasure, one's own is the last to be dug up" (quoted by Rieff 1979).

Hoffer (1946), in a study of the diaries of adolescent patients, described the urge of normal as well as abnormal adolescents to write down their thoughts as a restitutive activity. Judging from one particular patient, there was sometimes more to this writing than just reparation. In the words of Novalis (quoted in Rieff 1979, p. 102), "It is only through representation that a thing becomes plain. There is no easier way of understanding it than by seeing it represented. Thus, the ego is understood only as represented by the non-ego." In the case of an almost-deaf adolescent girl, the problem of representation was crucial. As long as the non-ego was not taken in, the ego itself remained bare and barren.

CASE EXAMPLE 6

Dorothy was fifteen years old when she came into treatment. From infancy on, she remained inactive, disinterested, withdrawn, and seemingly "lost." During childhood, a diagnosis of autism was considered until it was discovered that she had severe hearing loss. At first, she rejected the hearing aid and would tear it off, but, as time went on, she began to acquire a rudimentary language, although somewhat dysphonic. Whenever she resorted to speech, it was literal and concrete, and nothing of her thoughts and feelings could be communicated. With the onset of puberty, she became more remote and negativistic, remaining impenetrably silent most of the time with an enigmatic expression on her face. She could lip-read when she wanted to, but mostly she would avoid face-to-face encounters. When I got to the point of eliciting responses from her occasionally, she let me know that, if I were a good enough therapist, there would be no need for words between us because I would be thinking her thoughts and feeling her feelings. Gradually, she communicated the fact that talking was painful for her. She said that her mind had no thoughts in it, only images, and these had to be converted into words before she could speak. Transforming images into words was the big difficulty. The images would either be untranslatable or disappear before she could label them, and, when the words came, they did not seem to fit the images at all. Since she could not hear herself talk, she was unable to realize how indistinct her speech was.

At this point, with nothing at all apparently happening in her therapy, I took a chance and suggested to her that she should keep a diary about what was taking place between us. She was at first reluctant to do so, she said, since nothing in fact took place between us in this curious therapeutic situation, in which I did almost all the talking. Often, I gave up saying anything, and then we would sit together silently, occasionally looking at each other. When I felt things had come to a standstill, she reported that she was keeping a diary and that she would bring it in once a month for me to see. My first assumption was that it would contain nothing but banal references to her very restricted life since she did little but stay at home and carry out some household chores. Home was not pleasant at all since she and her mother were on very poor terms. She had felt rejected ever since she was small because her mother had wanted a boy after two girls and all she got was a damaged girl. There was truth to this since her mother had become depressed after the birth and was reluctant to have anything to do with the new baby.

During the first months of the diary, there were mainly complaints about the treatment. She wrote that the sessions did not fill her in the way that she had imagined they would. There was still a big hole inside her, and at night she would feel deeply depressed and unreal and would hit her head against the wall to try and feel more real. After reading the material, I asked, sympathetically, whether she could bear the difficult times that we were passing through together, and she wrote back, "If you can do it, I can do it." The following night, she had a dream in which her mother had beaten her up and had thrown her across the room as if she were no bigger than a baby, and she wondered whether I would ever get so exasperated with her as to attack her like that.

The following are a series of extracts from her diary written during the second half of the first year of treatment:

I hope so very much that Dr. A. can understand what I am trying to say. I know it's confusing and that it takes time, but God I hope I can get across what I feel crying out inside me. I think that I am finding the words that I have been searching for when I was speechless for so long. Please help, Dr. A., please try and understand. Leave me room, don't do all the talking, but help me to begin to talk.

I get butterflies in my stomach thinking about meeting Dr. A. tomorrow. I am becoming so involved in my relationship with him—a lot of anger and I think a lot of warmth. I don't think I have ever felt so many different things consciously for one person. The funny thing is that all the old feelings I used to have are coming out into the open for the first time—at least in my head—and not being pushed away. The next step is to verbalize them, to express them and to feel them. Even though I sometimes feel very angry with Dr. A., it is so good to have him there.

[A month later.] I hate Dr. A. so much at times that I cannot stand the pain it brings. I wish he would help me to say what I feel so deeply about everything. Toward the end of the hour yesterday, I got the funny feeling that a lot of the trouble I have in dealing with Dr. A. may have to do with my relationship with Mom.

What was astonishing to me was the facility with which she was writing and the way in which her feelings and thoughts, unsuspected by her parents and certainly by me, were coming to the forefront of the therapeutic situation. It was strange in that there would be a lag between what she had to say and when I received the communication, so that my interpretations of the material were always retrospective. I was conscious that some of the affect was dissipated in my reading aloud from her diary during the sessions. It soon became apparent to me that my recital of her material, as she read my lips intently, brought a huge satisfaction to her. Somewhat later, her face began to lose its stony appearance, and rudiments of emotional expression would break out. I began to feel her feelings in the way that she wanted, and the resonance between us slowly increased.

The intensity of the relationship both in the analytic diary and in the treatment situation made me concerned that the extratherapeutic part of the process lay outside my control, and I wondered about her ability to cope with it. About the middle of the second year, she had this to write:

> I feel like the world is coming to an end. I think I am getting closer to something very painful and there is a battle between living (getting better) and dying (not getting better). What makes it so frightening is that I cannot understand the thoughts I am having now that they are getting attached to images. It is like another part of me is coming out in the open, but it comes and it goes and I keep losing it when it comes to talk with Dr. A. Things are changing between me and Dr. A. It is amazing. I am now saying things to him in the session. He has become very important to me and I care for him and love him. It is so empty here in my apartment without him and so much more lonely. There are times when I have been very angry with him and have felt like hurting him, but I hate having him leave which he does sometimes. Then I miss him. If anything should happen to him, it would crush me. Yet, my feelings are so strange for him. One minute I feel warm toward him and feel that we can work things out together, and at the next minute I am so angry that I could kill him.

> I am really beginning to feel Dr. A. is helping me. I am getting to respect him very much. I wanted to tell him how much he means to me, but I keep holding it back. The words simply don't come. I like his shape. I love him so much that I want to hug him. I really am confused. Will I ever become a complete person.

At this juncture, something was happening in the treatment as in the world outside. She was recovering many memories from her early years, preverbal in her case around the age of six. She offered eidetically vivid images that she now began to translate directly to me in a somewhat halting speech. I told her that the diaries had served the wonderful purpose of introducing her internally to me but that there was now an important need to bring her thoughts and feelings, as they

212

occurred, in my presence. I wanted to be in touch with her here and now. What happened in this third year was an escalation of both the therapeutic and the developmental process, with occasional outbursts of spontaneously manifested creative productions. Pregenital dependencies and mergings, reminiscent of borderline patients, overlapped the primal scene imagery and belated genital urges that hovered uncertainly between me and the parental figures. Both past and present seemed to be cascading together along the same slope of consciousness. Once she said, somewhat shyly, that she had very strong sexual feelings toward me but that there was so much else to think about me that this had to wait until she was more "grown up."

Toward the end of this third year, she appeared to be experiencing the outside environment in an entirely new sort of way. She now dressed very prettily, looking, as she put it, "just like a real girl." She said that she kept feeling elated (although she never took drugs or alcohol) and wanted to do so many things that she got herself quite jumbled up. Everything seemed interesting to do. Yesterday she had wanted to go out running, to ride a bicycle, to go for a walk, to look at a particular garden, to play tennis with a friend, to get a job, or to go to the zoo and find out what the animals did when there was no one around to watch them! She was active, joyous, and curious about everything about her, eager for direct contact and excited about turning it all into words and telling me about it. I remarked to her, slyly, that she seemed to be having "a love affair with the world," and this little piece of plagiarism from Greenacre (1958) seemed to please her enormously. She said that it was a funny way to put it but that was how she actually felt. I asked her to explain all this to me, and she said, spontaneously, "I feel I've come alive."

I speculated at the time as to whether this could possibly be a late exemplar of the "practicing subphase" in the Mahlerian stage of separation-individuation (Mahler, Pine, and Bergman 1975) since it seemed to have so many of the qualities that she had missed out during her junior toddler period when she was so out of touch with both the human and the nonhuman environment. This hunch seemed to be confirmed when she went home that evening and wrote a poem entitled "Being Born":

> From the beginning, as of birth, listen;
> Just listen around and open your eyes.

Any while opening them, look around.
See what has happened to my insides.
Which I kept locked up in my shell;
And to my outsides . . .
Which is a mystery to other people;
My mind becomes confused, becomes angry,
Gets to know hurt;
No fear—then I get a cleared picture
And maybe understand.
Growing to learn the secrets of my soul.
From the beginning, as of birth, open your heart.
I am looking for someone to tell my troubles to,
Let there be time to grow forever,
Cause right now I feel small.
Learning the secrets of my soul
I am slowly finding my way . . . on the road.
From the beginning, as of birth
I have slowly opened my eyes.

My therapeutic heart leapt with pleasure when she presented this to me as a gift. It seemed like a perfect description of "psychological birth," and the creative expression emerged as an integral part of the treatment and development of the patient. Following this, further creative elements were unleashed, and she began a small, unobtrusive career of creative writing. The poem clearly represented a transference gift to someone who had struggled with her remoteness, accepted her chronic irritability, listened to her first stumbling communications, and helped her slowly to find her way on the road. It was not, in the nature of things, a transference state that could be resolved within months, and, in fact, it took a few more years until she was able, with great difficulty, to attend a local college and expose her handicap constantly to others. Her mind had found new horizons, but she was still only in the process of opening her eyes and groping her way along the developmental path.

Conclusions

Through a series of vignettes depicting encounters with gifted adolescent patients, I have tried to demonstrate the unfolding of the cre-

214

ative process in psychoanalytic psychotherapy. One begins with a frame enclosing an empty space, a crossroad where patient and therapist elect to meet; within this frame the rages and loves of a lifetime can be contained, scrutinized, experienced, and worked through. The empty area is soon populated with a dramatic potpourri of characters from childhood, events of long ago, and facts, fantasies, feelings, memories, and dreams associated with them. To some extent, the therapist directs the production, but the situation soon takes hold of him as well, and he becomes a chameleonic character drawn into the vortex of the therapeutic activity. The encounter carries within it "all Africa, and her prodigies"—would but the participants know it. Re-creation, remembering, reenactment, and realization boil together within this cauldron of creative ferment.

REFERENCES

Anthony, E. J. 1961. A study of "screen sensations." *Psychoanalytic Study of the Child* 16:211–250.
Anthony, E. J. 1973. Between yes and no. *Psychosocial Process* 3:23–46.
Beres, D. 1965. Communication in psychoanalysis and in the creative process: a parallel. In H. M. Ruitenbeek, ed. *The Creative Imagination*. Chicago: Quadrangle.
Freud, S. 1905. A case of hysteria. *Standard Edition* 7:3–122. London: Hogarth, 1953.
Freud, S. 1916–1917. Introductory lectures on psychoanalysis. *Standard Edition* 15:3–239. London: Hogarth, 1963.
Greenacre, P. 1958. The family romance of the artist. *Psychoanalytic Study of the Child* 13:9–36.
Hoffer, W. 1946. Diaries of schizophrenic adolescents. *Psychoanalytic Study of the Child* 2:293–312.
Hulbeck, C. 1965. Three creative phases in psychoanalysis: the encounter, the dialogue and the process of articulation. In H. M. Ruitenbeek, ed. *The Creative Imagination*. Chicago: Quadrangle.
Mahler, M.; Pine, F.; and Bergman, A. 1975. *The Psychological Birth of the Human Infant*. New York: Basic.
May, R. 1965. Creativity and encounter. In H. M. Ruitenbeek, ed. *The Creative Imagination*. Chicago: Quadrangle.
Proust, M. 1928. *The Past Recaptured*. Vol. 2 of *Remembrance of Things Past*. Translated by F. Blossum. New York: Modern Library.

Rieff, P. 1979. *Freud: The Mind of the Moralist.* 3d ed. Chicago: University of Chicago Press.

Sachs, H. 1965. Aesthetics and psychology of the artist. In H. M. Ruitenbeek, ed. *The Creative Imagination.* Chicago: Quadrangle.

Searles, H. 1965. *Collected Papers on Schizophrenia and Related Subjects.* New York: International Universities Press.

Winnicott, D. W. 1958. *Collected Papers: Through Pediatrics to Psychoanalysis.* London: Tavistock.

Winnicott, D. W. 1974. *Playing and Reality.* Harmondsworth: Penguin.

DYNAMIC ASPECTS OF THE CREATIVE PROCESS: OVERVIEW

HOWARD S. BAKER

Motivation, experience, and facilitation are the subjects of this section. What motivates, even compels the artist to create? What is the internal experience of artists while they are creating? What assistance is necessary for them to create? Using clinical material, biographical data, and ideas and characters in literature and film, the authors provide some useful answers to these difficult questions. Additionally, we are provided fascinating information about the ideas and lives of William Shakespeare, Wolfgang Mozart, James Joyce, and Peter O'Toole.

The internal experience of creating is a simultaneous immersion into the ridiculous and the sublime. Using *A Midsummer Night's Dream*, Elio Frattaroli states that Shakespeare found these apparently opposite elements central to his "introspective understanding of his own creativity and of a creativity immanent in the universe that is especially focused in human nature." The artist must stand with feet firmly planted in the ridiculous and the sublime, in primary and secondary process, trying blindly to commit himself fully to a stampede to express the inexplicable. It is thrilling and terrifying, invigorating and depleting, often profoundly unsettling and confusing. Heisenberg compares it to suspending all perception "over an unfathomable depth." Through this process artists create their work and in so doing also create a more substantial self. The payoff is great, but the price is high.

Carl T. Rotenberg approaches these concepts from the perspective of self psychology, leading us to see that the creative product and the creative process function as essential sustaining selfobjects for the artist. This perspective affords remarkable clarity to what many artists themselves experience when they work—that they are transformed through the self-selfobject relationship with their work. Whereas before many feel confused, isolated, disorganized, even fragmented, while working they feel complete, cohesive, and vigorous. It is not merely the content of the work but the process of doing and the involvement with the particular esthetic elements that consolidates the artists' self.

Since selfobjects accomplish this transformational process for everyone, why do some people organize their lives around the selfobject provided by creativity whereas others organize their selves around selfobjects such as family ties? Also using a self psychological perspective, Howard S. Baker offers some possibilities while considering the life of James Joyce and one of his principal characters, Stephen Dedalus. The vicissitudes of their lives led them to the conclusion that people were not reliable selfobjects, that people could often destroy the cohesion of the self-experience. Complex and anxiety provoking as the creative process might be, it proved more satisfactory for them. Joyce, however, adds a powerful addendum to that conclusion. Selfobject support from people is often essential for the artist to tolerate the creative process and actually to produce. In comparison to Dedalus, Joyce's early development was not as difficult. He was able, therefore, to open himself in a number of crucial ways, and his adult, creative life was generously filled with people who were consistently and sufficiently empathic. Joyce was able to find and use people as selfobjects, and they were essential for him to produce.

In addition to an ongoing supportive milieu, artists are involved consistently in mentoring relationships. In his discussion of this subject, David A. Halpern notes Bloom's highly influential concept that art is always produced in relation to the art of both the present and the past. This both helps and interferes with the creative process, establishing in artists what Bloom calls the anxiety of influence. Will it be possible to form genuinely new and valid art? The risk of merely repeating the work of others provokes the "anxiety of influence," which causes artists to distort others' work so that there is a creative "space" in which they are free to work. Using three films by Peter O'Toole, Halpern examines the complexities of the relationship between younger and more experienced artists. At its best, a relationship develops in which students obtain knowledge, strength, and courage through idealization of their teachers. The teachers, in turn, experience confidence and security from the positive mirroring that the students provide. Under circumstances of mature and mutual development in both, the relationship evolves to a more even balance of teacher and student

218

providing each other both idealizing and mirroring experiences that consolidate their self-experience and facilitate their artistic development. Such is often not the case, however, because narcissistic vulnerability and competitive intensity may lead the teacher to inhibit the student and the student to destroy the significance of the teacher. To the detriment of one or both, this battle may be played out on turf that is both sexual and artistic.

Internal conflicts and facilitating and mentoring relationships are all elucidated in John E. Gedo's exploration of the life of Mozart. Mozart pursued and was rejected by Aloysia Weber and accepted an unsatisfactory marriage to her sister, Constanze. As the "German Orpheus" his grandiosity was wildly overstimulated, but he knew that his acceptance was almost totally contingent on his genius. His parents, particularly his father, feasted on the fame of their son rather than delighting in his success for his own sake. These and other factors combined to create a personality that was narcissistically vulnerable and frequently consumed with disappointed misogyny. Mozart reworks these conflicts through the content of some of his greatest operas. Gedo believes that the composer's overwhelming genius kept him producing and maturing artistically throughout a life marred by personal disappointment and psychological immaturity. Still, it is undeniable that he experiences a reduction of productivity when rejected by Aloysia, and his father provided mentoring that was highly successful—particularly when the son was able to manipulate geographic distance from his father. Biographical limitations seriously limit our ability accurately to understand the role of Constanze in facilitating or inhibiting her husband's work.

In this section, the authors provide a lively opportunity to examine essential intrapsychic and interpersonal factors that combine to require, direct, facilitate, and/or inhibit the creative process. We are led to new insights in our treatment of creative blocks, and we may also find useful ways to more deeply probe those countertransferences that minimize our own creativeness as we work with all of our patients.

13 THE LUNATIC, THE LOVER, AND THE POET: A STUDY OF SHAKESPEARE'S CONCEPTION OF CREATIVITY

ELIO J. FRATTAROLI

A Midsummer Night's Dream is perhaps the single most profound and far-ranging work ever written on creativity.[1] Along with *The Tempest,* it might be said to represent Shakespeare's introspective understanding of his own creativity and of a creativity immanent in the universe that is especially focused in human nature.

I was not sure whether to make that the beginning or the end of my presentation, largely because I had trouble deciding what I could say in the middle that would justify such an assessment of the play and at the same time show its relevance to an audience of adolescent psychiatrists. I was in awe of the power of Shakespeare's conception, but time and time again, when I would try to put this conception into words other than Shakespeare's, I failed. I mulled over the problem unproductively for several days and finally decided I was at an impasse. I was tempted to let my opening statement stand as both opening and closing, invite you all to reread the play, and call it a day. Then I had a happy thought. Perhaps I could deal with this impasse the same way I deal with impasses in psychotherapy with difficult patients.

In such situations I have generally found that, if I can articulate the impasse in the form of an interpretation, the problem has a way of turning into the solution. My favorite example of this occurred with Mike, a seventeen-year-old impulse-ridden boy who, after eight very productive months of inpatient treatment, suddenly insisted on leaving the hospital, discontinuing psychotherapy, and moving 1,500 miles away to live with his older sister. This decision was so different from the treatment plan we had been working with, and he announced it in such an arrogant, peremptory, defiant way, that I was infuriated. Projective identification strikes silently and suddenly. In an instant I was ready to retaliate vengefully against this boy, whom I really liked, either by taking away his privileges and trying to force him to stay or by washing my hands of him and discharging him on the spot. Fortunately, I resisted both impulses and reflected. If I tried to force him to stay, I would be repeating the mistake of his overbearing, sometimes brutalizing father. If I let him go, I would be like his abandoning mother. Then it hit me that much of my anger stemmed from the frustrated feeling that these were my only two choices, so I said to him, "It feels like you're pushing me to be either like your father or like your mother. I think we both need a better option." It worked. First, it made me feel immensely better because my response was unlike either his father's or his mother's. Second, it made Mike feel better—for the same reason. Finally, because our shared good feeling stood out in contrast to Mike's expectations, it enabled him to gain insight into his own mistrustful, testing provocation. He stopped demanding and started talking. Very quickly, what had been a peremptory impulse became a well-thought-out discharge plan that, I regretfully had to agree, made sense. Within two weeks he was off to his sister's and, hopefully, adulthood, with my blessing.

Now this anecdote may have sounded like a digression from my stated theme or, perhaps, like a regression in the face of my difficulty in grappling with Shakespeare. Nevertheless, I am going to pursue it a bit farther, trusting that this problem too will turn into a solution and will lead me back to *A Midsummer Night's Dream* eventually. There were two kinds of creativity in the interaction between Mike and me. The most obvious was my using an articulation of the problem as a solution. But a deeper and more important kind of creativity was contained in Mike's impulsive demand to be discharged. This was the universal creativity of adolescence, by which the adolescent frees himself from the external constraints of parental authority and weltanschauung and gives birth to change in the world by articulating his own unique identity. At the same time, it was also the universal creativity of transference, by which a person frees himself from the internal constraints of unconscious fantasy, using another person for projection and projective identification, making what was internal external, what was unconscious conscious, and objectifying the unknown within. When that unknown is recognized as self, which may be sooner or later, requiring one or many transference experiences, this process too, like adolescence, leads to the articulation of new identity. Shakespeare summed it up in Prospero's closing words about Caliban: "This thing of darkness I acknowledge mine." Freud (1933) put it, "Where It was, there I shall be."[2]

I have just used the word "articulation" in two related but distinct senses: to articulate is, first, to exemplify or body forth, to express in actions, and, second, to conceptualize, to express in words. The first sense applies to Mike's impulsive, rebellious, self-assertive decision to leave the hospital. It involves an acting out of an attitude, a value, or a weltanschauung that cannot be put into words but demands expression. The second sense applies to the method of problem solving that I used in my impasse with Mike (and that I intend eventually to try out on my impasse with Shakespeare). It involves putting into words an initially nonverbal, emotionally unsettled experience. These two uses of the word "articulation" define two modes of creativity, behavioral and verbal, each characterized by an unresolved state seeking resolution through expression. In the case of behavioral articulation, the unresolved state is experienced as impulse; in the case of verbal articulation, it is experienced as feeling. The sense of verbal articulation is the one most commonly associated with creativity. For instance, the poet-scholar Ghiselin (1952) has this to say about poetic and scientific creativity: "Creation begins typically with a vague, even a confused excitement, some sort of yearning, hunch, or other preverbal intimation of approaching or potential resolution. Stephen Spender's expression is exact: 'a dim cloud of an idea which I feel must be condensed into a shower of words.' Alfred North Whitehead speaks of 'the state of imaginative muddled suspense which precedes successful inductive generalization,' and there is much other testimony to the same effect" (p. 14).

But the creativity of the artist and that of the scientist represent only two highly evolved forms of the more general process that informs the creation of words out of feeling, the creation of actions out of impulse, and the creation of dreams out of—well, out of "the stuff that dreams are made on." We will get back to dreams when we get back to Shakespeare, but here it is worth noting that, as we go from dreams to behavioral articulations to simple verbal articulations of transference to the higher-level verbal articulations of science and poetry, there is a progression from unconsciousness through several levels of consciousness to the most profound level of self-consciousness. In fact it makes sense to see this as a developmental progression, with the two modes of behavioral and verbal articulation being two phases of one creative process. For instance, we saw in the clinical vignette that Mike was able to move from acting out to talking out. The impetus for this development is inherent in adolescence and in transference, and I suspect it operates at every level of human development—ontogenetic, phylogenetic, and historical—moving through behavioral toward verbal articulation, mediated by feeling. For instance, to make an effective interpretation, I had to recapitulate in a few minutes the development of consciousness from infancy to adulthood and, perhaps, from the Stone Age to the Computer Age, moving from fantasied impulsive action through an awareness of feeling to a conceptualization (verbalization) of that feeling, then to a self-conscious understanding of its significance, and, finally, to the reworking of the verbalization into a usable interpretation. If we consider again in this light Freud's dictum, "Where It was, there I shall be," we can see in it a description not only of what happens in psychoanalysis but of what happens in life. Recall that the domain of the It is nonverbal while the domain of the I is verbal. Freud is actually describing a spontaneous creative process in human development. The It evolves into the I, in a biphasic process of creative articulation, from the behavioral to the verbal, through primary process into secondary process.

As therapists, we become aware of this creative process as an innate striving for health—a growing edge, in our patients and in ourselves. My interaction with Mike, like all effective therapy, happened at this growing edge. My intervention allowed Mike's conscious behavioral articulation to blossom into a self-conscious verbal articulation. His impulse was—to take calculated liberties with Yeats (1921, p. 187)—a rough beast slouching toward articulate self-awareness. But this is the sort of thing that generally happens in adolescence and in transference. We can see it as a thrust through action toward verbalization or as a spontaneous unfolding of the verbal from the nonverbal, depending on our perspective. Therapeutic intervention can serve as a catalyst for this process, but the process tends to happen on its own, like a chemical reaction, perhaps more slowly, perhaps less completely, or perhaps able to take advantage of more than one kind of catalyst.

Also like a chemical reaction, this creative process requires two participants. Adolescent identity formation requires parents against whom the adolescent can define himself. Transference requires a transference object who can receive one's projections and projective identifications. In both cases, the creative process is one of articulation through interaction. It is dialectical, like childbirth. For instance, we could say that Mike's behavior was pregnant with meaning and that, as transference object, I was father to that meaning. Then, as therapist, I was also midwife to the birth of that meaning. The childbirth metaphor and the idea of articulation through interaction apply to all new meanings, not only to those of adolescence and transference.

For instance, in the realm of literature, critic Harold Bloom (1973) has found what he calls the anxiety of influence at the center of poetic creativity. Bloom contends that each new poet establishes his unique voice and meaning through a combined transference distortion of and adolescent rebellion against the work of a strong poet of the past. Bloom's idea can be generalized to apply to creativity in all the arts, and it resonates as well with Kuhn's (1962) concept of paradigm clashes as the dialectical substrate out of which new ideas grow in the sciences. Every new meaning requires a mother and a father, but not necessarily a midwife. Freud did not need an analyst, nor did Shakespeare need a Fool to his Lear or an Ariel to his Prospero, but they did not create alone. They needed transference objects. Freud always wrote for someone or against someone. Without Fliess there would have been no self-analysis and no *Interpretation of Dreams*. Without Adler and Jung there would have been no *On Narcissism* and, without Rank, no *Inhibitions, Symptoms and Anxiety*. Likewise with Shakespeare. Without the Elizabethan playgoer for whom he wrote there would have been no *Midsummer Night's Dream*. In a larger sense we are all Shakespeare's transference objects, as he is ours. As he was speaking to us, we are the transference parents of the meaning he put into his play. As we are learning from him, he is the transference parent of the meaning we take out of the play.

All this brings me back to *A Midsummer Night's Dream* and the impasse I created for myself at the beginning of the presentation. It now begins to look like a transference impasse in which I am blocked from articulating the meaning I take out of the play by Bloom's anxiety of influence, a literary form of the Oedipus complex. If you remember, I found myself unable to get past the opening statement that *A Mid-*

summer Night's Dream represents Shakespeare's introspective understanding of his own creativity and of the creativity that is immanent
in human nature and the universe. My hope was that this impasse would
yield to the same method of impasse busting that works for transference
impasses, like the one I described with my patient. Let's find out. It
is time to look Oedipus in the eye and cross the beams.

Step 1. Articulate the problem. Describe the quality of the emotionally unsettled experience of impasse: anxiety. How can I do justice
to Shakespeare's genius? How can I hope to deliver on the promise of
my opening statement? How can I hope to explain the sublime without
sounding ridiculous?

Step 2. Restate the newly articulated problem in the form of an
interpretation. The thing I am preoccupied with as a problem, the
possibility of reducing the sublime to the ridiculous, is in fact the
solution, the very thing I want to explain about *A Midsummer Night's
Dream* and creativity: to articulate the sublime is necessarily to bring
it into the realm of the ridiculous.

Definition. The essence of creativity is to embody the sublime in
the ridiculous.

Well, that's intriguing, but it is not at all clear what it means. Perhaps
by trying to apply the definition to different examples of creativity we
can get a better sense of it. To embody the sublime in the ridiculous—
this could certainly apply to some of the experiences of creativity that
we have just been looking at. We have only to recall the popular songs
of our own adolescence to remember how often the adolescent's budding awareness of the sublime is expressed in ridiculous infatuations
and even worse poetry. Adolescent love is a vitally important creative
experience, an integral part of the larger creative process of identity
formation in the cauldron of adolescent turmoil—again, the sublime in
the ridiculous. The definition also applies to the creativity of transference, the expansion of consciousness through misapprehension. Now
it might be said that, in both these cases, we are dealing with the
emergence of the sublime from the ridiculous rather than the embodiment of the sublime in the ridiculous. However, these are not either/
or, true/false formulations but rather alternative perspectives on one
process, each representing a valid but incomplete articulation of it.
Another example of the same dual perspective would be the differing
religious and scientific mythologies of the creation of man. The priest
says man is the image of God embodied in dust. The evolutionary

biologist says that life and then consciousness are emergent properties of an evolving, complexifying organization. Each mythology captures and articulates a different aspect of that ineffable unitary reality, the human soul. Is the soul miraculously embodied in primordial dust (the sublime into the ridiculous), or does it miraculously emerge out of primordial soup (the ridiculous into the sublime)? Yes!

To embody the sublime in the ridiculous—this could also apply to the creativity of sexuality. As Yeats's Crazy Jane puts it (1933a, p. 259),

> . . . Love has pitched his mansion in
> The place of excrement;
> For nothing can be sole or whole
> That has not been rent.

Yeats here tells us that the wholeness of the experience of generativity is born out of the rift between sublime and ridiculous: "Love has pitched his mansion in / The place of excrement." To experience love in sexuality is to embody the sublime in the ridiculous, to make whole what was rent, to heal the split between soul and body and return us to the state of original grace.

By now it should be clear that the words "sublime" and "ridiculous" are open to many meanings, which may be thought of as either a virtue or a vice, depending on whether we feel that poetic or scientific definitions come closer to the truth. I would not presume to say that my first definition of creativity, "articulation through interaction," is rigorously scientific, any more than I would claim that the second, "to embody the sublime in the ridiculous," is good poetry. However, the two definitions do tend toward opposite ends of a spectrum from scientific to poetic. One check on the usefulness of the more poetic definition is to ask whether the more scientific one is included under its umbrella of meaning. Is the definition "articulation through interaction" consistent with the definition "to embody the sublime in the ridiculous"? It is if we think of the creative articulations, the new meanings, as the sublime and of the kinds of passionate interactions in which the articulations occur as the ridiculous. Yeats has something to say here too, in "A Dialogue of Self and Soul" (1933b, p. 236):

> I am content to live it all again
> And yet again, if it be life to pitch

Into the frog-spawn of a blind man's ditch,
A blind man battering blind men;
Or into that most fecund ditch of all,
The folly that man does
Or must suffer, if he woos
A proud woman not kindred of his soul.

I am content to follow to its source
Every event in action or in thought;
Measure the lot; forgive myself the lot!
When such as I cast out remorse
So great a sweetness flows into the breast
We must laugh and we must sing,
We are blest by everything,
Everything we look upon is blest.

As I understand it, Yeats's image of life, "to pitch / Into the frog-spawn of a blind man's ditch, / A blind man battering blind men," refers to the kinds of passionate interactions that lead to creative articulations. He suggests that, by trusting in the value of blind men battering blind men, we can follow such passionate interactions to their source in action or in thought, that is, discover their meaning by articulating it in behavior or in words. In this way vision grows out of blindness, and we find the sublime, a new level of consciousness, a state of blessedness, in the ridiculous, the frog-spawn of a blind man's ditch. Creativity is, then, the articulation of the inarticulate, a sublimation of the ridiculous. This fits my description of the interaction with Mike, and, in general, it fits my experience of how insight is attained in psychotherapy. As a therapist, I find that only after I have begun to experience countertransference and become, at least briefly, a blind doctor battering a blind patient does the light of understanding dawn, as I begin to feel and then see what all the battering is about.

On the other hand, we could turn this view of creativity as "articulation of the inarticulate" on its head by looking differently at what is articulated. Perhaps it makes more sense to say that what is articulated is the sublime while the articulation itself is the ridiculous. For instance, the creative process is the sublime. My attempt to describe it and at the same time to exemplify it in this presentation may be seen as the ridiculous, even if you are enjoying it, in the sense that it is an attempt to express the inexpressible and must inevitably fall short. What I did with Mike and what I have been doing with all of you (or at least with my transference image of you) is to analyze a unitary experience, to break it down into component perspectives that are describable in words. With Mike, I thought in terms of adolescent rebellion, projective identification, mother transference, father transference, and countertransference, each concept offering a valuable but partial focus on the unitary process, the existential moment we experienced together. With you, I have been trying to describe creativity in terms of articulation, embodiment, emergence, evolution, and dialectic. But, in each case, the creative process itself, in its wholeness, transcends any and all of these component perspectives and eludes precise description in words.

Words are always inadequate to express the wholeness of experience. To articulate a meaning is to reduce a multidimensional experience to one dimension. From this perspective, the articulation of new meaning that we initially identified with the sublime (the creative product) can now be seen as the ridiculous. The passionate interactions that give birth to these articulations we have identified with Yeats's image of the ridiculous, "the frog-spawn of a blind man's ditch," but we can equally well see them as sublime (the creative process). For instance, if we think of Winnicott's (1953) description of transitional phenomena as a model for all creativity, then the mother/child experience would be the prototype for all creative interactions, and the transitional object would be the prototype for all the articulations that grow out of these interactions. As a symbolic objectification of the magical, mysterious intersubjectivity of mother and child, the transitional object is the embodiment of the sublime in the ridiculous. Generalizing from this prototype, we can see the sublime as something that happens between people in passionate interaction and the ridiculous as the individual's attempt to articulate that transindividual experience. Creativity, from this perspective, is not the "articulation of the inarticulate" but the "articulation of the inarticulable."

It begins to appear that the sublime and the ridiculous are like the twin masks of tragedy and comedy. Whenever we try to see through one mask, we find the other mask behind it. In our definition "articulation through interaction," we have found that the articulation can appear as either sublime or ridiculous, depending on whether we focus on the evolution and discovery of new meanings or on the inadequacy of their expression. Likewise, passionate interaction has two aspects, the spirit of love and communal experience on the one hand and the drivenness of blind men battering blind men on the other. Love itself can appear as a mansion or as a place of excrement. The sublime and the ridiculous are two seemingly contradictory aspects of one reality. Which aspect we see depends on what we are looking for or how we are looking.

This kind of divided vision is familiar to most of us in the form of the psychological mechanism of splitting. Although it is generally thought of as a characteristic of borderline patients, experience with neurotics in psychoanalysis suggests that splitting is always a prominent feature of intense transference. One need only remember the centrality of war in history to realize the ubiquity of splitting in human consciousness. In war and in borderline transference, we are dealing with splitting into good and evil rather than into sublime and ridiculous, but the two dichotomies are not unrelated. The split into good and evil is the general theme of tragedy, while comedy, at least Shakespearean comedy, revolves around the split into sublime and ridiculous. Both cases are covered by the general principle that what we see depends on what kind of lenses we are looking through. To see the relevance of this principle to creativity, consider that to view reality is to interact with it and that to act on or describe one's view of reality is to articulate it. This is a generalization of "articulation through interaction" to include not only interactions between two people but also interactions between man and nature. It is a semiconstructivist position, emphasizing that our construction of reality is a creative act. To articulate the meaning of one's interaction with reality is to construct reality. I call the position "semiconstructivist" because the principle of split vision adds the important qualification that there *is* a reality independent of the observer but that all articulations of that reality, all constructions, are necessarily incomplete. They are articulations of the inarticulable, partial images of an unimaginable whole.

Some of you may have recognized that this principle of split vision is an extension of Niels Bohr's principle of complementarity, the epistemological counterpart to the Heisenberg uncertainty principle (see Bohr 1954). If we do one experiment, we can measure the position of an electron. If we do another experiment, we can measure its energy. But to do one precludes doing the other. This is simply a special case of the more general constructivist position, with the crucial added implication that by engaging in one construction we blind ourselves to another. To measure an electron or to articulate a meaning is to reduce a multidimensional whole to one dimension. The interaction of experimental apparatus and electron leads to the articulation of position or of energy, but the electron itself is inarticulable. The interaction of self and other, subject and object, leads to the articulation of good or of evil, of the sublime or of the ridiculous, but truth, like the electron, is inarticulable.

So what does all this have to do with *A Midsummer Night's Dream?* You may have been kind enough not to notice, but I have yet to show the relevance of the impasse-busting definition "to embody the sublime in the ridiculous" to *A Midsummer Night's Dream*. I have taken you on a roller coaster ride from adolescence to evolution to quantum physics, from Freud to Yeats to Genesis to Bloom to Winnicott to Bohr, but I still have not got back to Shakespeare, and by now most of you are probably a bit dizzy. Although I had not consciously intended it, it may seem I have been playing Puck to Shakespeare's Oberon and to your Athenians:

> Up and down, up and down,
> I will lead them up and down. . . .
> [3.2.396–97]

But if so, then I have succeeded in communicating indirectly the quality of my experience of *A Midsummer Night's Dream* and something about Shakespeare's meaning as well. Dizziness is an appropriate response to the giddy paradox of the sublime in the ridiculous. *A Midsummer Night's Dream* is full of both the paradox and the dizziness. The play allegorically depicts and metaphorically describes the very experience it evokes, and I have been trying to recreate the multilayered sense of that experience. So far, I have taken you from Athens and got you lost in the woods. It remains to be seen whether I can help you find the concord of any discord thus engendered.

A Midsummer Night's Dream is a play that takes place in two worlds, the human world of Athens and the fairy world of the woods. Athens represents law, work, reason, sunlight, and sanity, while the woods represent love, play, imagination, moonlight, and madness. The two worlds are related much as the ridiculous to the sublime, but it is often difficult to know which is which. Oberon and Titania, king and queen of the fairies, have come to Athens to bless the marriage of Theseus and Hippolyta. As spirits of love and generativity, they represent the sublime. However, when they first appear on stage, they are doing a good imitation of the ridiculous, locked in a petty, jealous custody battle over a changeling boy. But sublime or ridiculous, they are powerful, and their power operates at all levels of nature—human, animate, and inanimate. Titania reproaches Oberon with the fact that all of nature— the flocks, the fields, and the floods—has been shuddering to the sound of their discord. By the same token, nature will be healed in their concord.

The dizziness comes in at the human level. The main plot involves the adventures of four adolescent lovers who have arrived at an impasse reflecting the state of dissension in the fairy world. Hermia and Lysander love each other, but Hermia's father rejects Lysander in favor of Demetrius, who now loves Hermia and rejects Helena, whom he used to love and who still loves him. Theseus, duke of Athens, declares that within three days Hermia must either submit to her father's will, be put to death, or become a nun. That night Hermia and Lysander elope to the woods, pursued by Demetrius, who is pursued by Helena. In the woods, they fall under the enchantment of moonlight and the uncertain providence of Oberon and his somewhat sadistic factotum, Puck, and strange things begin to happen. Lysander rejects Hermia and falls in love with Helena. Demetrius, who had already rejected Helena and fallen in love with Hermia, now reverses field and falls back in love with Helena, so that the two who loved Hermia in Athens suddenly love Helena in the woods. Hermia feels betrayed, and Helena feels the other three are conspiring to make fun of her. Lysander and Demetrius try to settle things by killing each other, but Puck wraps them in a fog, and eventually they all fall asleep. When they wake to the sound of Theseus's hunting horn, Lysander loves Hermia, Demetrius loves Helena, the impasse is resolved, and all's right with the world.

Puck's response to this comedy of changing partners is the famous, "Lord, what fools these mortals be," but the feelings of the four lovers, as ridiculous as they seem to the observer, are very real and quite sublime to the participants. We the audience, who have been lovers ourselves, feel the full confusion of this paradox, on the one hand laughing with Puck in the wings and on the other caught up in the enchantment, which Demetrius tries to explain to Theseus in these words:

> . . . I wot not by what power—
> But by some power it is—my love to Hermia,
> Melted as the snow, seems to me now
> As the remembrance of an idle gaud
> Which in my childhood I did dote upon;
> And all the faith, the virtue of my heart,
> The object and the pleasure of mine eye,
> Is only Helena.
>
> [4.1.163–70]

Now we might even be tempted to laugh at this beautiful poetry as Demetrius's self-serving explanation for his own fickleness, which caused the whole mess in the first place. But whatever we think of Demetrius, Shakespeare does not allow us to dismiss his words so lightly. When he says, "I wot not by what power— / But by some power it is," he echoes an earlier line of Hermia's, "I know not by what power I am made bold" (1.1.59), her explanation to Theseus of how she can defy her father's will. The verbal echo lets us know that Shakespeare is in the wings behind Puck, laughing at him laughing at the lovers and, in the process, telling us about a sublime power that may take different, sometimes ridiculous, forms, whether Hermia's adolescent rebellion or Demetrius's falling in and out of love. Blind men battering blind men.

Certainly, the lovers have a sense of having been in the grip of such a power as they talk over their night's experience with each other:

> *Dem.*   These things seem small and undistinguishable,
>   Like far-off mountains turned into clouds.
> *Her.*   Methinks I see these things with parted eye,
>   When everything seems double.
> *Hel.*   So methinks;
>   And I have found Demetrius like a jewel,
>   Mine own, and not mine own.
> *Dem.*   Are you sure
>   That we are awake? It seems to me
>   That yet we sleep, we dream.
>
> [4.1.186–92]

They have experienced the sublime in the ridiculous, and the experience has been like a dream. We have empathically experienced this dream with them and at the same time have been sharing in Shakespeare's larger dream, *A Midsummer Night's Dream,* of a sublime power informing ridiculous events.

What is a dream after all but the embodiment of the sublime in the ridiculous. Freud discovered this when he found a royal road among the apparently aimless byways of his own dreams. In one way or another men have always been aware that dreams represent a spontaneous unwilled creativity unfolding from within us, synthesizing the sublime and the ridiculous, the truths of the Delphic oracle in the vicissitudes of indigestion. Shakespeare's dream is no exception. It is constructed entirely around the tension between, and, paradoxically, the fusion of, sublime and ridiculous. One of the central questions of this play is, "How shall we find the concord of this discord?" (5.1.60). The central metaphor of the play is the evanescent union of the fairy queen, Titania, and the ass, Bottom, a marriage of the sublime and the ridiculous if there ever was one.

To experience the play is to experience a dream. As I immersed myself in the play and then tried to describe my experience, I began to feel like Bottom, dazedly trying to make sense of his own midsummer night's dream within a dream. You may remember that Bottom is rehearsing the part of Pyramus for the play within a play, waiting for his cue, when Puck magically places an ass's head on his shoulders. Thus transformed, he inadvertently frightens off his fellow actors, but when the fairy queen Titania sees him, she falls in love with him instantly. She takes him off to her bower, where, after an enchanted evening, he falls asleep in her arms. I cannot think of better words to describe my dream of Shakespeare's play than the words Bottom uses to describe his dream when he wakes at sunrise, alone, his workaday head back in its proper place but his mind still trailing clouds of glory from his moonlit metamorphosis:

> . . . I have had a most rare vision. I have had a dream, past the
> wit of man to say what dream it was. Man is but an ass if he go
> about to expound this dream. Methought I was—there is no man
> can tell what. Methought I was—and methought I had—but man
> is but a patched fool if he will offer to say what methought I had.
> The eye of man hath not heard, the ear of man hath not seen,

man's hand is not able to taste, his tongue to conceive, nor his heart to report, what my dream was. I will get Peter Quince to write a ballad of this dream: it shall be called "Bottom's Dream", because it hath no bottom. . . . [4.1.203–215]

"Man is but an ass if he go about to expound this dream"; words are always inadequate to express the fullness of experience. They are impossible attempts to articulate the inarticulable. Commentator after commentator on the play notes the fact that Bottom's warning applies to the commentator himself and then blithely goes about to expound the dream anyway. I have been more cautious than most, intimidated by the idea of making the sublime ridiculous and making an ass of myself. But here again, the problem paradoxically becomes the solution. Bottom is the only mortal in the play who sees the fairies, but he must become an ass to do so. Bottom, the ass, eager to play every part in the play, is like Yeats's "blind man battering blind men," and Shakespeare's message is similar to Yeats's: by committing ourselves fully to the blindness of experience and the blindness of words, we can articulate the inarticulate and achieve a vision of the inarticulable. The Flesh becomes Word. Bottom becomes bottomless. "It shall be called Bottom's dream because it hath no bottom." Three centuries later, Freud (1900) came to a similar conclusion and expressed it in words that echo Bottom: "There is at least one spot in every dream at which it is unplumbable—a navel, as it were, that is its point of contact with the unknown" (p. 111). Freud made this discovery just as Bottom made his, by trying to articulate the bottom of his own dreams. Bottom's wisdom, that man is but an ass if he seeks to expound dreams, is consistent with Freud's: every exposition, every interpretive dream bottom, has a hole in it, a navel that opens onto a world beyond the dream and beyond exposition. To expound the dream, to make the unconscious conscious, to articulate the inarticulable.

Bottom's soliloquy is unquestionably the navel of Shakespeare's dream. It is the place where the sublime meets the ridiculous. Bottom's words epitomize this meeting. They are a flagrant garbling of Saint Paul's First Epistle to the Corinthians (2:9–10): "Things the eye hath not seen, and ear hath not heard, neither have entered into mans mind, which things God hath prepared for them that love Him. But God hath opened them unto us by His Spirit, for the Spirit searcheth all things, yea, the bottom of God's secrets."[3] Bottom's words may seem at first hearing to make a farce of Saint Paul, but in a way they express Saint Paul's truth more profoundly than Saint Paul's words do. Saint Paul implies that God's secrets have a bottom. Bottom comes closer to the truth, and closer to the twentieth century, when he suggests that they are bottomless. Modern physics has arrived at the same conclusion. Heisenberg (1941, p. 93), for instance, has said that "all perception must . . . be suspended over an unfathomable depth." He saw this as an implication of complementarity. We can comprehend only one level at a time, but we have an apprehension of the infinity of multileveled reality, or, as Heisenberg puts it, "Our mental approach to reality takes place, at first, on separate levels which link up, so to speak, only behind the phenomena in an abstract space." This linking up of separate, seemingly incompatible, levels of awareness in an abstract perceptual space is what gives an unfathomable depth to all experience. To apprehend all levels at once is to experience the bottomless. This is precisely what Bottom captures in his glorious garbling of incompatible modalities: "The eye of man hath not heard, the ear of man hath not seen, man's hand is not able to taste, his tongue to conceive, nor his heart to report, what my dream was." This is nonsense, but it is also poetry. It has the particular power of poetry that Bohr (1954, p. 79) described: "The power to remind us of harmonies beyond the grasp of systematic analysis . . . achieved by the juxtaposition of words related to shifting observational situations, thereby emotionally uniting manifold aspects of human knowledge." The eye hath not heard; the ear hath not seen. We hear these words at first as ridiculous and funny, but they leave behind an echo of the sublime. They capture much more poignantly than Saint Paul's "correct version" the ineffable quality of Bottom's experience and of what happens at the navel of any experience.

If it seems that Bottom's dream and his attempt to describe it fit surprisingly well with my ideas about creativity and my attempt to describe them, it is no coincidence. During the weeks when I was not writing about *A Midsummer Night's Dream*, my secondary reading consisted of *A Midsummer Night's Dream*, *A Midsummer Night's Dream*, and approximately twenty papers and two books of criticism about *A Midsummer Night's Dream*. My mind was supersaturated with thoughts and feelings about Shakespeare's play, and all my ideas about creativity crystallized out of that solution. In fact, even that last metaphor for creativity, to crystallize out of a solution, derives from *A Midsummer Night's Dream*. It was meant to combine the scientific flavor of "articulation through interaction" with the poetic flavor of Spender's "dim cloud of an idea which . . . must be condensed into a shower of words." But behind these two definitions is Shakespeare's, which, although it remained in solution, has all along been the hidden theme of my presentation:

> . . . As imagination bodies forth
> The forms of things unknown, the poet's pen
> Turns them to shapes, and gives to airy nothing
> A local habitation and a name.
>
> [5.1.14–17]

Shakespeare here defines the creative process as biphasic, first bodying forth forms of things unknown, then turning them to shapes with a local habitation and a name. I believe this is the same biphasic process that Freud described as primary and secondary process and that I have described as behavioral and verbal articulation. To be consistent with Shakespeare, we would have to extend the notion of behavioral articulation to include not only behaviors but feelings, fantasies, and dreams as well. These "forms of things unknown" are all nonverbal articulations, conscious but not yet self-conscious. Self-consciousness comes with the verbal articulation of "A local habitation and a name." The entire creative process moves from unconsciousness to consciousness to self-consciousness, from airy nothing to forms to words.

What then is "airy nothing"? It is something at many levels. It is Spender's "dim cloud of an idea"; it is my supersaturated solution; it is the inarticulate and the inarticulable, the ridiculous and the sublime. Most generally, it is the unknown. More specifically, it is the unconscious, the stuff that dreams are made on. Indeed, Shakespeare's phrase "imagination bodies forth / The forms of things unknown" could stand as a description of dreaming, in which the things unknown are the airy nothings of the unconscious and imagination is the spontaneous creative activity of the human psyche, autonomously bodying forth dreams and transferences.

If airy nothing is the stuff that is bodied forth in dreams, on another level it is the indeterminate quantum stuff that is bodied forth in the universe, the probability wave of nature. Bohr (1954, p. 77) has emphasized this tantalizing analogy between the indeterminacy of the unconscious and the indeterminacy of subatomic nature and between the impression of a thought in consciousness and the impression of an electron on a photographic plate. Whether we are dealing with a dim cloud of an idea or an electron cloud, whether we are registering a thought or a subatomic particle, we are giving to airy nothing a local habitation and a name. Another physicist, Lawrence Bragg, generalizes this analogy in a comment on the wave/particle paradox: "Everything that has already happened is particles, everything in the future is waves. . . . The advancing sieve of time coagulates waves into particles at the moment 'now.'"[4] Perhaps Bragg read Shakespeare too.

To coagulate waves into particles, to condense a dim cloud of an idea into words, to crystallize out of a supersaturated solution, these are all metaphoric children of the universal metaphor for creativity: to give to airy nothing a local habitation and a name. At this universal level, airy nothing is the ineffable, the spirit of God moving on the face of the waters. To give this airy nothing a local habitation and a name is to imitate and participate in divine creativity, making something out of nothing. Shakespeare tells us that imagination is the motive power that informs this process. Imagination must then represent man's share in the creative power of God, the spirit Saint Paul talks of that "searcheth all things, yea, the bottom of God's secrets." But we do not need to put a theological construction on it. For instance, Shakespeare clearly suggests that imagination, the power that moves the poet's pen, is the same power that moves Hermia's defiance of her father and Demetrius's labile loving. It is the power that bodies forth dreams and also bodies forth adolescent rebellions, infatuations, betrayals, love, war, and, ultimately, human history. Thought of as impersonal and collective, like Freud's It, imagination is the power that moves us from the known past through the sieve of time to the unknown future. Thought of as personal, like Freud's I, it is the power by which we actively transform the past into the future.

I have equated what Shakespeare calls imagination or an unknown power, the motive force in *A Midsummer Night's Dream*, with the energies of what Freud calls the It and the I, the motive forces in psychoanalytic theory. Actually, Shakespeare's unknown power is a broader concept than Freud's psychic forces, representing a continuum of creativity in nature ranging from inanimate to suprahuman forms. Freud's It and I are simply the human embodiments of this creative power. This idea of a larger power operating at many levels is quite consistent with Freud's (1920) concept of Eros.[5] It also resonates with

Waelder's important conceptualization of Freud's structural theory toward the end of "The Principle of Multiple Function" (1930). Waelder emphasizes the place of id, ego, and superego on a continuum of natural forces. He calls them "three phases of psychic life [that] correspond to stages of organic life," each with its own particular activity. He suggests (pp. 82–83) that the instinctual pressures of the id are common to all organic life; that the ego is a mechanism of central control that emerges "at the time of the separation of the individual from collective vegetation" or perhaps only with the appearance of the central nervous system; and, finally, that the superego, as the name implies, is the distinctive tendency of man to transcend himself, to go beyond his own id and ego interests, to take himself as an object, in the sense both of objective observation and of subjective moral valuation, and also very importantly to recognize the independent existence of a world around him apart from his own ego. Waelder's superego embodies what I have been calling self-consciousness, the awareness of self as self and, concomitantly, of other as other, of object as object. It is essential to this conception, though Waelder does not spell it out, that language is not an ego function but a superego function, that only through the self-transcending awareness of the superego can we identify a local habitation or give a name to anything. Waelder's id, ego, and superego are not three entities but three modes of psychic activity, three levels of organization of psychic energy, or, as I would extrapolate it, three levels of the broader creativity of articulation through interaction that also informs the course of evolution and the quantum course of inanimate history. This extrapolation is consistent with Waelder's adumbration of a link, on the one hand, between the id and collective vegetation and, on the other, between the superego and transcendence. It is also consistent with Shakespeare, whose fairies represent the unknown power that moves not only human interactions but the course of natural events as well, that forges the links in a Great Chain of Becoming from inanimate nature to God.

Interestingly, Waelder's view of the structural theory is very close to the Renaissance concept of the tripartite soul, which in turn has much to do with Shakespeare's poetic definition of creativity. Sixteenth-century psychology (Burton 1621; Phillips 1964) described the soul as consisting of three subsouls, the vegetative or quickening soul, the sensitive or sensible soul, and the rational or intellectual soul. Phillips (1964, p. 148) describes the functions of the lowest of these, the vegetative soul, in terms reminiscent of Waelder's id: "To this soul or power, which man has in common with vegetable and animal life, were ascribed the faculties of nourishment, growth, elimination, reproduction, and the other instinctive physiological processes." The next in order, the sensible soul, found in animals and in man, was thought to consist of a set of faculties that are identical to what we now call ego functions. The two principle faculties were those of apprehending (knowing) and of moving. Apprehending included an outward component, sense perception, and an inward component, consisting of common sense (reality testing), phantasy or imagination, and memory. Moving included the "inward and outward animal motions in the body" (Burton, p. 160), meaning affectivity and motility.[6] Finally, the rational soul, consisting of the understanding and the will, separated man from the animals. The understanding included the ability to apprehend universals as well as particulars (essential for concept formation and language), the capacity for self-reflection, and the moral sense, the capacity to judge good and evil. This conception of the rational soul is very close to Waelder's conception of the superego and much broader than the Freudian superego as it is usually construed.

Now let me try to weave together the separate threads of Renaissance psychology, Shakespeare's poetry, and my idea of creative articulation, which owes something both to Shakespeare's poetry and to Waelder's synthesis of Freud and Renaissance psychology. It must be that, when Shakespeare wrote "imagination bodies forth / The forms of things unknown," he was referring to processes of the sensitive soul, which produce what we might call the ego articulations of dreams, fantasies, feelings, and actions. Likewise, when he wrote that "the poet's pen . . . gives to airy nothing / A local habitation and a name," he must have been referring to processes of the rational soul that produce the superego articulations of language and conceptual classification. In this context, an id articulation would occur at the infrahuman, infraconscious level of physiology.

Generations of playgoers have come away from *A Midsummer Night's Dream* thinking that it was simply a deft and charming set of variations on the theme announced by Helena at the end of the first scene:

> Things base and vile, holding no quantity,
> Love can transpose to form and dignity:

> Love looks not with the eyes, but with the mind,
> And therefore is wing'd Cupid painted blind.
>
> [1.1.232–235]

This is of course an important theme, but I am claiming that Shakespeare goes far beyond it, showing the blind misapprehensions of love as closely related to dreaming and to poetry and, ultimately, as emblematic of creativity at every level of creation. Certainly there is no doubt that, in the poetic definition of creativity I have been discussing, Shakespeare was referring to something much broader than the nature of poetry. The lines themselves refer specifically to the poet, but, in the context of the speech that contains them, poetry is clearly seen as but one vicissitude of the imagination. This is the speech in which Theseus describes the lunatic, the lover, and the poet as each under the sway of imagination and each exemplifying a different articulation of it. It comes as Theseus and his bride-to-be Hippolyta stop to reflect on the confused tale they have just heard from Hermia, Lysander, Helena, and Demetrius about their magical night in the woods:

> *Hip.* 'Tis strange, my Theseus, that these lovers speak of.
> *The.* More strange than true. I never may believe
> These antique fables, nor these fairy toys.
> Lovers and madmen have such seething brains,
> Such shaping fantasies, that apprehend
> More than cool reason ever comprehends.
> The lunatic, the lover, and the poet
> Are of imagination all compact:
> One sees more devils than vast hell can hold;
> That is the madman: the lover, all as frantic,
> Sees Helen's beauty in a brow of Egypt:
> The poet's eye, in a fine frenzy rolling,
> Doth glance from heaven to earth, from earth to heaven;
> And as imagination bodies forth
> The forms of things unknown, the poet's pen
> Turns them to shapes, and gives to airy nothing
> A local habitation and a name.
> Such tricks hath strong imagination,
> That if it would but apprehend some joy,

> It comprehends some bringer of that joy:
> Or, in the night, imagining some fear,
> How easy is a bush suppos'd a bear!

[5.1.1–22]

It is of course ironic that the character who speaks these profound words does so disparagingly. The speech is itself an example of the sublime bodied forth in the ridiculous. Just as the lover finds "Helen's beauty in a brow of Egypt," so Shakespeare finds sublime poetic truth in the prosaic intellectualizations of Theseus. Theseus is a positivist. To him, airy nothing is precisely that. If he were writing this chapter instead of me, he might dismiss the insights of the lunatic, the lover, and the poet as unfalsifiable. He might give them each a different fourth-digit code number in DSM-IV under epistemologic disorders. But he would be missing the point. His insight is valid. The lunatic, the lover, and the poet, like the adolescent, the analysand, and the physicist, do have something in common. They are all dreamers. They apprehend more than cool reason ever comprehends. But Theseus, through the eye of cool reason, can see this only as ridiculous, while we, through the eyes of a dreamer, can see it also as sublime. Shakespeare gives us access to this larger perspective by making Theseus the victim of dramatic irony. He scoffs at antique fables, but the audience knows that he is himself a character out of Greek mythology. He does not believe in fairies, but the audience, like Bottom, has just seen them. In fact, the fairies represent the very something Theseus dismisses as airy nothing. They are the spirits of imagination, embodied in the mid-summer madness of the four adolescent lovers as well as in Bottom's moment of poetic inspiration, and they are the unknown power that informs the generativity of the marriage beds they bless and the emergence of concord out of discord in the natural world they inhabit.

Conclusions

To recapitulate, I have proposed that there is a creative power that takes the general form of articulation through interaction; that this power manifests itself at different levels in many forms, including adolescent rebellion, transference, science, and poetry as well as in the collective creativity of human history, the organic creativity of evolution, and the quantum creativity of the probability wave. I have tried to show that this creative power is closely related to Shakespeare's conception of creativity in *A Midsummer Night's Dream,* to give to airy nothing a local habitation and a name. As personified by the fairies and as variously articulated—by Hermia and Demetrius as an unknown power, by Bottom as the spirit of God, and by Theseus as imagination— Shakespeare's conception of a creative power spans the same range from processes of inanimate nature to processes of human interaction to processes of verbal articulation of these lower-level processes.

When we dream, love, hate, make love or war, interpret our dreams, make the unconscious conscious, measure the electron, or write a poem, we find and define a momentary bottom in the bottomless wellspring of creativity. We articulate the inarticulable, and man is but an ass if he tries to do that. But we cannot help it. Man *is* but an ass; we *are* blind men battering blind men. But as we try to articulate the inarticulable and fail, at the same time we succeed in articulating the inarticulate—in bringing light to our blind spots. The process continues dialectically over time, articulation through interaction, and slowly the inarticulate approaches the inarticulable. In the words of Hippolyta's reply to Theseus:

> But all the story of the night told over,
> And all their minds transfigur'd so together,
> More witnesseth than fancy's images,
> And grows to something of great constancy;
> But howsoever, strange and admirable.
>
> [5.1.23–27]

NOTES

This chapter was originally conceived and delivered as a presentation before a live audience and was not written in a style usual for journal articles. I have made only minor changes in preparing it for publication because the audience or reader response to the paper as originally written is central to the meaning I am trying to convey. A change in organization or style of presentation would change that audience/reader response. In the process of writing, I became aware that I had unconsciously been trying to evoke in my audience a response analogous to the response I myself had to *A Midsummer Night's Dream,* which had, in turn, been analogous to responses expressed by several characters within the play, most notably Bottom, to their dreams within the *Dream.* I hope this response can be shared by my readers as it was by my listeners. I should probably state at the outset that this is not reader-response criticism. Although I describe and analyze my own response in detail, it is as a means, not as an end in itself. My approach is predicated on the conviction that reader responses reflect, in varying ways, authors' meanings and intentions and provide a very important means of coming to know them. If a reported response of a central character within the play is the same as my response to the play and also the same as my audience's response to my discussion of the play, then I would claim with Hippolyta that all these "minds transfigur'd so together, / More witnesseth than fancy's images, / And grows to something of great constancy" (5.1.24–26). I would further claim that the source of that constancy is Shakespeare's meaning and the response he was trying to evoke in his audience.

1. All references are to the Arden edition (Brooks 1979) and are cited by act, scene, and line number.

2. The actual Strachey translation is the more familiar, "Where id was, there ego shall be." My translation is intended to highlight a connotation of the original German, "Wo Es war, da soll Ich werden," that is obscured by the Latinate "id" and "ego." The most literal translation, suggested by Bettelheim (1982, p. 89), is, "Where It was, there should become I."

3. Spelling modernized, from the 1557 Geneva New Testament, as cited in Dent (1964, p. 121).

4. Quoted in Clark (1971, p. 345).

5. Although Freud (1920) confines his discussion of Eros—the constructive, assimilatory force "which holds all living things together" (p. 50)—largely to its role across different levels of organic life, from the protista to humans, he implicitly invokes it as the force "of whose nature we can form no conception," which is embodied in "the chemical affinity of inanimate matter" (p. 58), in the evocation of life out of inanimate matter and of consciousness out of living matter (p. 38).

6. This is identical to Freud's (1915) conception of affectivity and motility as representing inner-directed and outer-directed motor discharge processes (p. 179n). The power of affectivity was also called "appetite" and included the concupiscible and the irascible powers,

precursors of the sexual and aggressive drives, operating in accordance with a pleasure/unpleasure principle (Burton 1621, pp. 160–161).

REFERENCES

Bettelheim, B. 1982. Freud and the soul. *New Yorker* (March 1), pp. 52–93.

Bloom, H. 1973. *The Anxiety of Influence*. New York: Oxford University Press.

Bohr, N. 1954. Unity of knowledge. In *Atomic Physics and Human Knowledge*. New York: Wiley, 1958.

Brooks, H. F., ed. 1979. *The Arden Shakespeare: A Midsummer Night's Dream*. London: Methuen.

Burton, R. 1621. *The Anatomy of Melancholy*. New York: Vintage, 1977.

Clark, R. W. 1971. *Einstein: The Life and Times*. New York: World.

Dent, R. W. 1964. Imagination in *A Midsummer Night's Dream*. In J. G. McManaway, ed. *Shakespeare 400*. New York: Holt, Rinehart & Winston.

Freud, S. 1900. The interpretation of dreams. *Standard Edition,* vols. 4, 5. London: Hogarth, 1953.

Freud, S. 1915. The unconscious. *Standard Edition* 14:166–215. London: Hogarth, 1957.

Freud, S. 1920. Beyond the pleasure principle. *Standard Edition* 18:7–66. London: Hogarth, 1955.

Freud, S. 1933. New introductory lectures, 31. *Standard Edition* 22:57–80. London: Hogarth, 1964.

Ghiselin, B., ed. 1952. *The Creative Process*. New York: New American Library.

Heisenberg, W. 1941. On the unity of the scientific outlook on nature. In *Philosophic Problems of Nuclear Science*. New York: Pantheon, 1952.

Kuhn, T. S. 1962. *The Structure of Scientific Revolutions*. Chicago: University of Chicago Press.

Phillips, J. E. 1964. *The Tempest* and the Renaissance idea of man. In J. G. McManaway, ed. *Shakespeare 400*. New York: Holt, Rinehart & Winston.

Waelder, R. 1930. The principle of multiple function: observations on overdetermination. In S. A. Guttman, ed. *Psychoanalysis: Obser-*

vation, Theory, Application: Selected Papers of Robert Waelder, New York: International Universities Press, 1976.

Winnicott, D. W. 1953. Transitional objects and transitional phenomena. In *Collected Papers: Through Paediatrics to Psycho-Analysis.* New York: Basic, 1958.

Yeats, W. B. 1921. The second coming. In R. J. Finneran, ed. *The Poems of W. B. Yeats.* New York: Macmillan, 1983.

Yeats, W. B. 1933a. Crazy Jane talks with the bishop. In R. J. Finneran, ed. *The Poems of W. B. Yeats.* New York: Macmillan, 1983.

Yeats, W. B. 1933b. A dialogue of self and soul. In R. J. Finneran, ed. *The Poems of W. B. Yeats.* New York: Macmillan, 1983.

14 CREATIVITY AND THE TRANSFORMATIONAL PROCESS

CARL T. ROTENBERG

The purpose of this chapter will be to discuss how the art object can function as a selfobject and how its aesthetic qualities and its selfobject functioning are interrelated. On acceptance of this construct, we have a modification of the traditional psychoanalytic theory of creativity. This enlarged theoretical perspective is broadly important in three ways. (1) It expands our capacities as clinicians to understand and therefore treat the creative artist effectively. (2) It similarly expands our clinical capacities to address the potentially evoked creative capacities in every individual. (3) It addresses our capacities to apply psychoanalytic knowledge in that challenging yet intellectually polemical cultural world at large that lies "beyond the basic rule," that is, the culturally significant area of creativity and art. Elsewhere (Rotenberg 1987), I have described the relationship between the audience at large and the art product as selfobject. Here, I will focus on the self of the creative artist and try to denote the properties of his relationship with his work as selfobject.

I have introduced a technical term, the "selfobject." It is a term that derives from Kohut's (1977) investigation of narcissism and, ultimately, his new theories about the nature of the self. A selfobject is an "object" that functions for the self so as to foster the preservation of the continuity and cohesiveness of the self. It bolsters the self's capacity both to feel and to undertake initiative. A function of selfobject relatedness is to foster the *transformation* of the self. Optimal selfobject functioning buttresses the self in its qualities of continuity as opposed to discontinuity, organization versus chaos, cohesiveness versus fragmentation, initiative and vitality versus deadness and empty boredom, and transformation versus stalemate and deadlock. Selfobject functioning refers to a set of subjective experiences rather than to a set of events that can be directly apprehended by an external observer. Selfobject functioning takes place in the realm of experiential subjectivity, and it can be directly "observed" only by someone who shares that subjectivity. Its effects can be indirectly observed; people who have functioning selfobject experiences available to them behave and function differently.

The word "object" in the psychoanalytic sense refers to a relationship with a person. Psychoanalysis has described how we relate to external objects in two fundamentally different ways and how the same object may be the bearer of two different kinds of relationships. First, we relate to people as separate autonomous entities, to whom we direct our care, concern, and love and who are the targets of our drives. Second, we relate to people as selfobjects. Their responses to us, subjectively interpreted, are the material from which we take the responses needed by the self for its functioning.

Relatedness with an artwork seems to refer to a relationship with an inanimate thing. If I view a painting, for example, my relationship seems to be to the material entities of pigment and canvas, not to a person. We recognize, however, that, in the aesthetic experience, the experiential relationship is not primarily with the material qualities of the art object. The self is influenced through its interplay with the condensed symbolic assertions of the art object, including the symbolic meaning of its material qualities, that constitute the objectification of its feeling (Langer 1953). The experiential relationship is with the aesthetic assertions of the artist who created it. Therefore, in viewing another's work or even one's own, the self is influenced by the reflected human assertions of the work. To the extent that one's own self is influenced by one's own work, the paradox is relieved by the recognition that what returns to us are primarily reflections coming from nonconscious and unconscious sources, and they are then received by the conscious self as to some extent foreign or as though from another person. In the creative act, or in the immersion of creative involvement with an artwork created by another person, the experience can be described from a psychodynamic viewpoint as a selfobject relationship with potentially transformational properties.

So, again, I am describing the process of the self's hoped-for transformation through its relationship with the emerging product as selfobject. Let us look at the interrelationship between a self and its created selfobject in closer detail. The psychological experience of the creating self has a number of different qualities.

Inner Necessity

Kandinsky (1912) has described the deep "inner necessity" of the artist in relationship to the work. Bruner (1962, p. 25) has talked about the domination of the self of the artist by the work, and he reminded us of the Zeigarnik phenomenon in psychology, which describes the necessary submission of the self to the requirement of completion of a task. Creative work seems to require the deep dedication of the artist to his cause. This concentrated focus may be phenomenologically similar to the single-mindedness of the obsessional symptom or the drivenness of compulsive behavior disorders. This is not to imply psychopathology but only to describe the feeling of urgency and exclusivity that creative activity requires. Looked at from a psychodynamic viewpoint, the selfobject in the artwork is relentlessly pursued because of the felt necessity of the artist's obtaining the particular form of feedback and sustenance he requires. In this instance, the sustenance takes the form of externalized information, which is absorbed as needed, so that the artist can then make the next step in his progression. For the visual artist, this information takes the form primarily of line, form, color, composition, surface, and so on—that is, in the form of whatever information is relevant to the experiment he is pursuing. The artist's cause and his submission to it are sacred and elicit devotion.

Enactment

Translating the inspiring force from within to without requires enactment. Enactments are central to all selfobject relations, though their operation may be invisible or intangible. How enactments proceed clinically and the relation of "enactment" to the more traditional term "acting out" is a subject beyond the limits of this chapter. In art, the materiality of the art process and the visibility of the activity encodes in externally validatable form the enacting initiatives between self and selfobject. The notion of enactment is so central to art that Kuhns (1983), in his work on the psychoanalytic theory of art, defines culture in general as "a tradition of enactments." In personal relationships, enactments may be less visible, although here, too, the self acts on the selfobject so as to inspire, recruit, seek, or compel the responses needed by the self. In art, enactments are more evident. The artist, even in conceptual and minimal art, is required to act in order to influence a material medium to create and record the externalized (material) shape or configuration of inner purpose. Writers inscribe paper, painters paint in varying ways on material such as canvas, sculptors "enact" with the material of clay, and musicians manipulate sound through their directions to instruments and players. Often the sheer monumentality of the effort required by the enactment may, intentionally or not, embellish the artistic purpose. For example, it is difficult to consider the artistic messages of man's heroic majesty portrayed on the Sistine Chapel ceilings without pausing to consider the heroic enactment of the lone aging artist painting precariously on a high scaffold in the uncontrolled climate of St. Peter's cathedral vaults. In art, the artist exerts his intentionality on a material medium, and he thereby creates an object of importance to him. The importance he perceives in his creation then operates in a feedback circuit to provide him information that influences the self-organization from which his next enactment will proceed. This feedback circuit works both microscopically in time units of instants and macroscopically over weeks, months, and years. The artistic value of the work to others may not be a direct consequence of the artist's conscious intentions. Rather, the forces that determine the artistic product probably act according to the psychoanalytic principle of overdetermination.

Materiality

The material stuff of the artistic product etches a permanent representation of the artist's hopes at that moment. In nonartistic selfobject phenomena, the record of the transactions is lost. The episode is transient, elusive, and it leaves no tangible record. The artistic product is a record of the selfobject relationship at that moment in time. The evolving artist will not, at a later date, be able to retrace his steps and paint again a painting in the same style as he did, say, a decade ago. At the instant of his self-evolution, those organizing forces in his self will select the particular hue, intensity, line, color, shape, composition, and so on that his encoded feelings require for their objectification. The information received from the placing of these will subtly transform his observing self, so that each attempt will take place from a different vantage point and perspective.

Aesthetic Elements

In the material interaction with the art object, the subjective elements important to the evolution of the artist are the artistic elements of line, form, color, composition, and the other artistic essentials that constitute each artist's technique for the development of his own brand of artistic illusion making. As psychotherapeutic clinicians, who are concerned with clinical narrative, we tend to attune most in our investigation of art to the narrative contents rather than to the formal components. This contrasts with artists' subjective preoccupation, which is often focused more on the creation of new vistas in these elemental areas, and whose creative satisfaction will derive, say, from the unique way they contrast color in an illusionary space or the way they portray yet fracture flatness, rather than, say, the particular images that are portrayed while these efforts are in progress. For the artist, line, form, color, composition, and so on have an importance that the therapist must understand rather than designate as defensive. These aesthetic elements have primary significance as expression of feeling, emotion, mood, and intellect. It is important to understand this at this juncture since the artist's conscious and nonconscious reflections, as they are reported, are often devoted to the effect on the developing artistic self of his own perceived evolution in each of these areas.

CASE ILLUSTRATION

This case illustration involves a young woman artist whose life's purpose is dedicated to advancing herself artistically. As she has affirmed, "My whole life depends on it."[1] Prior to treatment, she suffered from severe work inhibition, and only recently has she been able to give herself over to her work consistently. Her work inhibition was dependent, among other things, on a profound chasm in her self-esteem, which pervaded her personality.

251

Carole is a forty-two-year-old, single female who was referred for treatment by a social service agency. At the time of treatment, she was employed in an art-related educational field but not as an artist per se. She is a graduate of a recognized art college, where her art education emphasized illustration, engraving techniques, and graphic design. Her ambition is to be a successful illustrator of children's books, and she wants to contract for work of this nature on a free-lance basis, as opposed to being on salary. She seeks a higher level of autonomy and professional independence.

Prior to her casework with the referring agency, she had "lived like a hermit," and three years of both individual and group work with the agency helped her emerge from an interpersonal shell to an outer world of moderate social relatedness, particularly with women. Still, from her improved position, she complained that she did not feel that there was "any center" to her and that she felt a void. Her caseworker became concerned about the state of this patient's ego functioning, and she sought a consultation. The patient had formed an intense idealized relationship with the social worker that recapitulated some of the themes in her early relationship with her mother and, to some extent, actually offset massive early maternal deprivations. On referral, the patient felt "kicked out," just as she had felt kicked out by her mother abruptly at the age of four.

The patient is the eldest of three siblings born to a working-class family in a major industrial city. Her father was a sporadically employed plumber, whose occasional employment meant that the family lived "all over the city." She has two younger siblings, a sister five years and a brother seven years younger. About her early life, she said that, "When I look back, it was mostly a bankrupt childhood." She experienced both parents as failing her extensively in her developmental years. With her mother, there was a sense of early relatedness, which the patient recalls with vague memories of dressing up in her dresses and high heels. However, this relatedness ended abruptly when the patient was four because her mother developed multiple sclerosis with rapid neurological progression and physical impairment. As a result of the mother's symptoms, the high-heeled shoes were thrown out, and dressing in idealized robes, concretely and symbolically, terminated abruptly. The mother rapidly declined in her ability to look after her responsibilities to house, self, husband, and children. The patient, as the eldest sibling, was thrust prematurely into surrogate parental responsibilities as soon as she was deemed able to handle them. The father was described as an immature man who could never accept the mother's illness and the removal of her "wifely functions." He was also described as being highly arbitrary, unapproachable, insensitive, ungiving, and uncooperative. He had a hot temper, and his angry outbursts were directed mostly at the patient. The patient never felt that she could satisfy her critical and demanding father, and she often felt angry and cheated at having to give of herself so much in looking after her siblings. She longed for a life in which she "could be able to play."

One relationship with some positive yield was with an older female cousin; in this relationship, some of the longed-for need for attention and being fussed over was lived out.

It was around the age of four that the patient discovered she had a talent for art, and so the stage was set for this to form an area of potential compensatory functioning for her. At school, she was the "class artist," and teachers and students alike often selected her out for attention and encouragement on the basis of her superior artistic abilities. She attended a highly competitive high school for music and art. She remembers those years as being happy and successful ones. In spite of her successful graduation from art college and successful employment in the printing industry she continued to have serious self-doubts in the area of her artistic skills and competence. This was coextensive with major gaps in her self-esteem felt in other areas.

A dream reflects the struggles of this patient's self in the face of massive selfobject failure. "The dream was about my father, my cousins, and a lot of strangers. I was living at home. Our house was a chaotic mess. In the dream, I was me as I am now. I dreamt that I was trying to go on a date with a man. Miscellaneous things happened. An older woman came into the picture, somewhat like my older cousin. I was in her dresses and trying on her shoes. She was glamorous and going shopping, buying beautiful things, clothes, etc. My father appeared in the dream, and whatever he did upset me. I was trying to get into the bathroom. I tapped him on the shoulder, and he turned on me. He screamed and shouted. Finally, he ran out of another room and started beating me up. I remember raising my arms to protect myself and then I awoke." This dream reflects the paralysis of this woman in terms of her social and sexual relationships and in relationship to her functioning selfhood generally. It also reflects her relentless, if blocked, pursuit of "beautiful things," later perpetuated in her ambition for artistic excellence.

In her treatment with me, the patient continued to make forward strides with intervening rough periods. I saw her on a once-a-week basis for two years, after which she was much improved. The therapy ended because of my relocating in another city. When the transference was positive, I was experienced as a strong, helpful, idealized parent who helped her to deal with her problems of living. I was also the appreciative parent. Hesitantly, at first, the patient brought in her artwork to sessions, and my commenting on it was experienced by her as being affirming. Her showing her work to me was difficult because her wishes to show her work proceeded against a fundamental self-experience of shame and unyielding incapacity. When the transference was negative, I was experienced as being empty, void, unresponsive, and uncaring. The void in her self-experience showed itself to be an intersubjective void, that is, a lacuna evident in the area of "optimal responsiveness" (Bacal 1985), with the selfobject immensely needed for both mirroring and idealization. At the beginning of treatment, the patient felt trapped in obsessional paralysis, yielded to hesitant initiatives, and focused action with accompanying self-satisfaction about her achievement. At the termination of treatment, her work dominated the forefront of her consciousness. She spent the majority of her time on a succession of artistic projects in a push toward self-improvement in these areas. The success of this once-a-week psychotherapy occurred as a result of the formation of a number of different kinds of needed selfobject relationships, some of which occurred in the transference and some with the artwork itself.

In the following section, I shall discuss this patient's artwork.[2] A progression of the patient's drawings demonstrated significant evolution in the artist's expressive and creative self. The drawings were vivid in narrative display, and they lent themselves to the press of psychodynamic interpretations based on content. The foremost focus in this chapter, however, is on the formal issues already mentioned. The patient did discuss the content issues, and these were significant. What were of greater concern to her were the formal issues, and it is in the development of these that she sought significant creative evolution.

1. *Color.* This patient sought to develop her own color sense, and her technique involved the highly detailed and focused use of color

pencil, conjoined later with Magic Marker both on the surface and on the rear of her paper. In the earlier pictures, her use of color was highly variegated and unrestrained in a way that detracted from pictorial unity. In the later pictures, her color use was more restrained and therefore eloquent, as she showed evidence of developing a synthesis of her color skills. There was clearly a predominant unifying color theme, rather than several, and each element in the picture was subordinated to the dominance of that theme and related to it. Whether with emotionality or with color, synthesis, and integration, the successful achievement of harmony of expression represents significant achievements of the self.

2. *Form and composition.* Similarly, with the earlier picture, the various elements were in themselves successful, but their successful formal interrelation was haphazard, and the spaces between them, for example, lacked harmony. Each element stood more for itself than for the picture as a whole, and, as a result, the picture conveyed a sense of poor fit and even fragmentation. Contrast this with the later pictures, and we find unity of compositional theme in the latter. More playfully expressed in this picture was the interplay around the theme of the picture plane, represented by a pane of glass, which was established yet magically penetrated. Just as the color was synthesized, so was the formal arrangement of elements more harmonious and more simply yet articulately in relation to one another. Place any pictorial element in a different location, and the picture becomes less successful, a statement that was less true of the earlier picture.

3. *Line.* Line as an expressive element in art has been evident since art's inception. Think of the difference in line between, say, the cypress trees of Van Gogh and the scenery of his contemporary Seurat, and you will feel right away how emotionally expressive line can be. In the early drawings of this patient, her line may have been more realistically exact and illustratively clear, but it was far more tight and fussy and, at the same time, less expressive. To demonstrate her development in the personal expression of line, we might consider her experiment with drawing freehand, that is, not looking at the paper while she drew. This experiment was devised as a conscious attempt to loosen herself up and find her expressive bearings rather than to be expressively determined by the so-called real shape and configuration of things. Her loosening of line was also evident in her later drawings, in which her artistic attention was present and evident, without requiring the detailed fuss of earlier drawings.

These achievements represent a few microsteps in the evolution of this artist's professional self. They are accompanied by an intensification of purpose, a consolidation of initiative, a shoring up of her self-esteem and emotional excitement, and a subjective conviction of being further along her own personal road. In each formal area, she underwent a similar process, which was palpable as she talked about her artistic endeavors in the therapeutic situation. She would undertake an experiment under the sway of great feelings of risk, she would see the visible result, she would assess the outcome in terms of her goals and expectations, and then she would react emotionally to the enacted product of her efforts as one might react to another person. Her experience of a new advance—for example, in color expression—would be received by her affects as one might receive from an optimally responding selfobject in the personal realm. Along with her artistic progress, she made realistic steps in the direction of achieving professional autonomy. In short, the achievements described have occurred pari passu along with progressive achievements in her personal self and are an integral part of that self-transformation.

Conclusions

This chapter has called attention to the selfobject significance of the art object for its maker and to the role that the aesthetic elements play in the self-transformation of the creative self. One important corollary with clinical significance is that the therapist of the creative artist must understand that the aesthetic elements have at least equal emotional significance for the creator alongside illustrative content. For the therapist to force his interpretation on the patient—that is, that the content has primary meaning—is not to enter the patient's world, is not to convey understanding, and would not be a neutral act of investigative inquiry. Instead, forcing the importance of narrative content on the consciousness of the creative person would be the re-creation of a potential transference paradigm in which the therapist-caretaker forces his idiosyncratic world on the patient while ignoring the primary significance of attuning to the patient's self-expressions.

NOTES

1. It is possible to describe this individual here yet preserve her anonymity because she has not shown her work publicly and therefore has

not received general recognition. John Gedo has described the difficulties involved in reporting the clinical details of the treatment of known artists because of their public reputation. Therefore, there is some advantage in being able to discuss an artist who is not renowned.

2. This chapter was originally given as a verbal presentation. That format allowed the showing of slides of the patient's work. In this chapter, because of editorial format, the pictures will be described verbally rather than illustrated.

REFERENCES

Bacal, H. 1985. Optimal responsiveness and the therapeutic process. In A. Goldberg, ed. *Progress in Self Psychology.* Vol. 1. New York: Guilford.

Bruner, J. 1962. *On Knowing: Essays for the Left Hand.* Cambridge, Mass.: Harvard University Press.

Gedo, J. 1983. *Portraits of the Artist.* New York: Guilford.

Kandinsky, W. 1912. *Concerning the Spiritual in Art.* New York: Dover, 1977.

Kohut, H. 1977. *The Restoration of the Self.* New York: International Universities Press.

Kuhns, R. 1983. *Psychoanalytic Theory of Art.* New York: Columbia University Press.

Langer, S. 1953. *Feeling and Form.* New York: Scribners.

Rotenberg, C. 1987. Selfobject theory in the artistic process. In A. Goldberg, ed. *Progress in Self Psychology.* New York: Guilford.

15   JAMES JOYCE AND STEPHEN DEDALUS: OBJECT AND SELFOBJECT RELATIONSHIPS IN THE SUCCESSFUL AND BLOCKED CREATIVE PROCESS

HOWARD S. BAKER

Within the vast literature on James Joyce, a controversy exists concerning young Stephen Dedalus, who is generally considered to be both an autobiographical and a fictional character (Gordon 1974–1975). The question is whether Stephen, in *A Portrait of the Artist as a Young Man* (Joyce 1916) and *Ulysses* (Joyce 1922), is depicted as a genuine artist or a dilettante. Richard Ellmann (1982), in the definitive biography of Joyce, seems to believe that Joyce meant to show through Stephen the successful evolution of a young artist. Other critics (Andreach 1964; Carens 1984) feel that Joyce's intent with regard to Stephen is ironic. They maintain that Joyce portrays Stephen as having the intellect and desire to be an artist but as being, in fact, unable to create.

Stephen is very bright and shows many aspects of the creative personality. But his life lacks the essential supportive elements vital to bring his potential to fruition. In this regard, he is in sharp contrast to Joyce, his creator, whose enormous output was made possible by a network of family, mentors, friends, and associates. Their affirmation of him allowed his genius to be realized in fact, not merely remain the stuff of dreams. Given the similarities in situation and potential between this autobiographical fictional character and his creator, these supportive elements, which Joyce denied his character but which were present for himself, provide an important key to understanding creativity.

The situational similarities between Joyce and Stephen, as pointed out by Ellmann (1982) and Epstein (1984), are striking, but the differences are even more so. June 16, 1904, is Bloomsday. On this day, the action of Joyce's masterpiece, *Ulysses,* takes place. The date was not chosen randomly; it was on that very date that Joyce had what in today's parlance would be called his first date with Nora Barnacle (they went for a walk). Like her namesake and ship bottoms, the young chambermaid from Galway and Joyce attached themselves to each other. She became his longtime mistress, the mother of his children, and, eventually, his wife. The commemoration of that date is a fitting tribute to her since she was principal among several people who provided a "holding environment" (Winnicott 1965) that was vitally necessary for Joyce to produce his art. While it is obvious that the writing, often a lonely experience, was done by Joyce and Joyce alone, it is not an exaggeration to say that the process involved others and would not have occurred without their help.

Stephen Dedalus, the protagonist in *Portrait,* returns in *Ulysses.* On June 16, his new contact is Leopold Bloom, an impotent failure and cuckold, and, indirectly, his masturbating wife, Molly. The relationship between Stephen and the Blooms provides a stark contrast to the one between James and Nora Joyce.

Although there is no specific, known reference from Joyce's hand that it was his specific intention to illustrate the creative block in Stephen's character, it is difficult to understand how the differences in their lives could have been randomly developed. Stephen may even have served as a vehicle for Joyce to disown or partially resolve aspects of his personality that he knew to be destructive. In any case, these contrasts may help the clinician understand fundamental aspects of the effective and the blocked creative process.

Using biographical data from *Portrait* and *Ulysses* to understand Stephen and material from Ellmann (1982) and Epstein (1984) to know Joyce, one may draw parallels and differences between the fictional character and the real man. There are, of course, difficulties inherent in this approach. One risks missing important biographical details. The genius of the novels provides much data on Stephen's intrapsychic life. However, no such window opens directly into Joyce's mind. Nevertheless, there is such overwhelming consistency in the available evidence that one may cautiously make useful "clinical" comparisons.

A pattern repeats: parents, educators, and friends consistently fail to offer Stephen sufficiently empathic emotional responsiveness. Dreading to repeat further injury, Stephen develops a lifelong pattern of dealing with emotional turmoil and conflict by defensive withdrawal from people, becoming incapable of forming intimate relationships. This character flaw, based on both unfortunate actual interactions and on their intrapsychic consequences, results in interpersonal relationships too impoverished to sustain and support Stephen's creative process. In Winnicott's (1965) terms, Stephen presents a false self to the world. Kohut and Wolf (1978) might find him a contact-shunning personality and Balint (1968) a philobat.

In Joyce's life, by contrast, people were available with enough consistency for him to develop a basic character structure that (1) admitted intimacy in relationships with many reliable and helpful people and (2) led him actively to avoid limiting or destabilizing relationships. This does not mean that his object relationships were always stable, responsible, or even reasonable. They were not. He had, however, a pattern of involved relationships that was not available to Stephen. Thus, Joyce found the sort of holding environment that he needed to write, and Stephen did not.

Both men's childhood environments were devastated emotionally and economically by their fathers' alcoholism, which caused frequent moves to ever more impoverished neighborhoods. Their mothers valued them, but they were intrusive in some ways. Their educations were rigorous but marred by invasive and stultifying elements of Irish Catholicism. Both had visual problems severe enough to be considered mild handicaps. The backgrounds of creative individuals frequently contain such factors (Goertzel, Goertzel, and Goertzel 1978; Lytton 1971). Combined with Joyce's and Stephen's innate brilliance, the intrusiveness, marginality, and chaos that marked the childhood and adolescence of each both enabled and necessitated the sort of habitual oppositional cognitive style that is routinely found in creative people (Noy 1984–1985).

Joyce's life, however, may be differentiated from Stephen's in many significant ways. For example, (1) Joyce had a basically positive relationship with his father; (2) his mother offered valued support at crucial times; (3) his siblings were sources of strength; (4) his friends were usually emotionally available; and (5) he was able to establish and maintain an effective, loving heterosexual relationship.

James Joyce, then, provides an example of the sort of creative person who Kohut (1976, p. 814) says requires "a specific relationship with another person—a transference of creativity—which is similar to what establishes itself during the psychoanalytic treatment of . . . narcissistic personality disorders." Kohut (1977) calls that relationship a sustaining self-selfobject relationship. Stephen needed similar relationships, but, because the early intrusions and rejections were too great and were not balanced by enough empathic support, his dread to repeat those injuries forced him to reject even the minimal selfobject sustenance that was available. In Winnicott's (1965) terms, he evaded relationships by hiding his true self and presenting a false self to the world.

Winnicott (1965, p. 148) specifically states, "Only the True Self can be creative, and only the True Self can feel real." Noy (1984–1985, p. 446) understands that to mean "that only if the individual succeeds in maintaining a 'free sphere' of true selfness beside the sphere dominated by the False Self can he use his natural talent and choose the solution of creativity and originality to attain some sense of self-individuation." My thesis is that, because he had the continued availability of people who functioned as needed selfobjects, Joyce was able to achieve that free sphere of true selfness. Stephen could not because his childhood selfobject environment was excessively traumatic and (at least through age twenty-two, when *Ulysses* ends) his adult selfobject environment was not sufficiently empathic to enable belated development.

If this thesis is valid, it follows that disruptions in Joyce's selfobject milieu should result in an interruption in his creative process. Indeed, there are at least four examples.

1. When Joyce returned to Ireland in 1909, a "friend" claimed to have had a liaison with Nora while Joyce was courting her. This supposed disruption in his relationship with Nora devastated him, and he was totally incapacitated until another friend, Byrne, was able to convince him that the story was false. It appears that he was able to resume his work within hours of Byrne's intervention.

2. While Joyce was experiencing particularly difficult problems writing *Portrait*, struggling with publishers about *Dubliners,* and not on speaking terms with his previously very supportive brother, he and Nora had an argument. Joyce wished to remain in bed with Nora despite the presence of the maid in the apartment, but Nora refused. Particularly vulnerable and in need of support, this seemingly minor disruption in his relationship with Nora led him to fling the entire manuscript

of *Portrait* into the fire. His sister snatched it back, burning her hands in the process, but Joyce could not resume work for several months. He continued only after Ezra Pound wrote him, offering profuse encouragement and an offer to have the first chapters published in serial form. Pound had not seen the manuscript and extended this help on the basis of one poem and Yeats's evaluation of Joyce's work.

3. When the Joyces' daughter Lucia was in the throes of her worst mental illness (schizophrenia, for which she ultimately endured many years of chronic hospitalization), he was unable to continue work on *Finnegans Wake*.

4. "On January 17, 1932, [Joyce] . . . informed Miss [Harriet Shaw] Weaver [publisher of *Finnegans Wake*] that since his father's death he had been plunged into such 'prostration of mind' that he was considering once again abandoning [work on that novel]" (Ellmann 1982, p. 643).

An overall difference exists between the object and selfobject relationships of Stephen Dedalus and James Joyce. The healthier relationships Joyce enjoyed were vitally necessary for him to produce, and, when they were disrupted, his productivity stopped. Being unable ever to gain such support, Stephen produces little and gives scant evidence that he will become able to change in such a way as to alter this pattern and overcome his creative block.

In *Portrait,* Stephen has produced only one poem. Two years later, he has returned from Europe and is forced to work unhappily as a schoolteacher. His friend Lynch lets us know that, even at this point, Stephen has produced little more than "a capful of light odes" (Joyce 1922, p. 415). Stephen simply has not created much, whereas Joyce, by the same time in his life, had published three short stories, several poems, and a handful of literary reviews. Joyce had also written the beginning chapters of his first novel, *Stephen Hero*.

Portrait, a substantial alteration of that first novel, ends on an ominous note. Stephen writes in his journal, "I go to encounter for the millionth time the reality of experience and to forge in the smithy of my soul the uncreated conscience of my race" (Joyce 1916, pp. 252–253). Certainly, this is a noble sentiment, but, in the next and final entry, he invokes the mythic Dedalus, "Old father, old artificer, stand me now and ever in good stead" (p. 253). However, if Dedalus is his father, then he is Icarus, and Icarus refused to heed his father's advice, flew too high (detaching himself too far from the world), and met a catastrophic end. Stephen insists that he will fly high and alone, avoiding advice or support, and, by age twenty-two, he most assuredly is not successful in escaping his island prison and creating much of anything, let alone the "conscience of my race."

Finally, I cannot agree with Tashjian (1982) that Stephen has resolved his adolescent identity crisis. His insistence on being an artist is so vigorous that it makes us suspect he "doth protest too much." The quality of his object relations indicates a militant denial of dependency or even relatedness. His thinking and behavior are more indicative of identity foreclosure than identity consolidation (Erikson 1963). Unable to find confirmation of the true self, the false self gains ascendency. It is primarily Stephen's brilliance that enables him to appear to function well.

Although Stephen has the biological endowment and the determination without which no one can be an artist, his talent has remained nascent because he has not encountered people who could provide the necessary holding environment. Furthermore, if he did, his intrapsychic limitations would leave him incapable of tolerating the necessary intimacy. These same intrapsychic limitations cause pessimism for his "future." It holds little literary merit, but I would suggest that a more accurate title would be *A Portrait of a Young Man Who Wants to Be an Artist, but Hasn't Succeeded because of Limitations within the Psyches of Both Himself and Those He Has Encountered.*

Object and Self-Selfobject Relations: Joyce's Involvement versus Stephen's Isolation

Stephen has a lifelong defensive pattern of turning inward, of frank withdrawal, at times of stress. As a seven-year-old at Clongowes Wood, his boarding school, he was miserable. He would repeatedly comfort himself by flapping his hands over his ears and listening to the swirling sound. When he became the school hero for protesting unjust punishment, the other boys carried him on their shoulders, but he was relieved when the exuberance ended: "The cheers died away in the soft grey air. He was alone. He was happy and free" (Joyce 1916, p. 59). Although examples abound, Stephen's insistence on isolation is, perhaps, most clear during the following interchange with his best friend, Cranly. Stephen is twenty and about to leave Ireland for the Continent:

I will try to express myself in some mode of life or art as freely as I can and as wholly as I can, using for my defense the only

263

arms I allow myself to use—silence, exile, and cunning. . . . I do not fear to be alone or to be spurned for another or to leave whatever I have to leave. And I am not afraid to make a mistake, even a great mistake, a lifelong mistake and perhaps as long as eternity too.

Cranly, now grave again, slowed his pace and said:

—Alone, quite alone. You have no fear of that. And you know what that word means? Not only to be separate from all others but to have not even one friend.

—I will take the risk, said Stephen. [Joyce 1916, p. 247]

He will indeed, for the risk of attachment is greater than the risk of being alone. The interchange also shows us a disingenuous quality since it is very clear that Stephen was cut to the quick by the inattentiveness of Emma, a young woman he fancies and who he fears prefers Cranly—he does actually fear "to be spurned."

Immediately following the interchange with Cranly, the remainder of the novel changes to an interior monologue in the form of diary entries. Ellmann (1982, p. 358) concludes that this "had a dramatic justification there in that Stephen could no longer communicate with anyone in Ireland but himself."

At the same age, Joyce also departed for Paris, but in a different style. He had managed to get friends to arrange for possible admission to medical school there. Lady Gregory agreed to help financially, and Yeats met him in transit in London and gave him encouragement and introductions.

This pattern of gaining support, encouragement, and even thoughtful criticism persisted throughout Joyce's life. Although some of the literary giants of his day were critical of both Joyce's personal life and his works—for example, Harold Nicholson (Epstein 1984)—he had many champions. Yeats and, to a lesser extent, Lady Gregory remained constant. Ezra Pound acted as his champion, providing encouragement and arranging for the publication of Joyce's works. Sylvia Beach even expanded her Paris bookstore, Shakespeare and Company, into a publishing house in order to get *Ulysses* into print. There were many others.

Their encouragement remained in spite of Joyce's difficult personality. To know him was to enjoy his brilliant mind and wit but also to tolerate his alcoholism and to suffer his not infrequent insults and endless demands for "loans," which he rarely intended to repay. Yeats is quoted saying, "Such a colossal self-conceit . . . I never saw . . . in one person" (Ellmann 1982, p. 101). What is extraordinary, however, is that, again and again, people, including Yeats, generously helped and encouraged Joyce and that he obviously expected that they would do so. For example, at the age of twenty, Joyce decided to introduce himself to George Russell, the poet. He went to his home at ten in the evening. His knock was not answered, and he waited until after midnight, when Russell returned. "Joyce knocked at the door anyway and asked if it was too late to speak to him. 'It's never too late,' Russell courageously replied" (Ellmann 1982, p. 99), and they talked for two hours.

What evidence we have of the response of the literati to Stephen is quite different. The "Scylla and Charybdis" chapter of *Ulysses* takes place in the National Library, where he encounters the same George Russell; T. W. Lyster, the Quaker librarian; John Eglinton, assistant librarian and essayist; and Richard Best, the head librarian's assistant. Stephen presents his lengthy theory about Shakespeare and *Hamlet,* which they listen to with bemused skepticism. They do not reject him out of hand, but they also briefly discuss a party to be held that evening at the home of George Moore. They have invited Buck Mulligan, one of Stephen's friends, who is by no means as gifted as Stephen. Stephen is not invited, and not being invited hurts. Even worse, Russell discusses a volume of poems by young Irish poets. None of Stephen's modest output is to be included. Stephen is excluded from the inner circle.

That same chapter contains some of the negative interactions typical of Stephen's friendships. Mulligan repeatedly plays him for the fool, and Lynch points out how little Stephen has produced. In the first chapter of *Ulysses,* "Telemachus," Mulligan, who has moved into the Martello Tower, which Stephen is renting, is so obnoxious that Stephen leaves, vowing not to return to the place where he pays the rent. Mulligan "proceeds, in the first few pages, to destroy all the images that Stephen has created throughout *Portrait.* Mulligan usurps more than Stephen's home; he usurps Stephen's ideas, his intellectualizing process, and his rationalizations for life" (Bowen 1984, p. 435). Later, in the episode at the whorehouse ("Circe"), Stephen gets into a terrible jam. Lynch simply gives up on trying to help and abandons him, leading Stephen to refer to him as "Judas" (Joyce 1922, p. 600).

As noted, Joyce was just as difficult a person to befriend as was Stephen. Both men had many friends, but Joyce's show steadfastness and tolerance particularly when they are compared to the likes of

265

Mulligan and Lynch. Oliver Gogarty was the model for Mulligan, and his friendship with Joyce bears careful scrutiny. Gogarty was aware that Joyce was working on an autobiographical novel (there is no evidence that Stephen at the same age was so engaged). "[Joyce] was turning his life to fiction at the same time that he was living it. . . . The sense that they were characters in his drama annoyed some of his friends, especially Gogarty, who did not much care for the role of culprit in a court where Joyce was both judge and prosecuting attorney" (Ellmann 1982, p. 149). Indeed, Gogarty's trepidation was well founded. He did (probably drunkenly) comment about town that Joyce had deeply hurt his dying mother by refusing to profess the Catholic faith. Mulligan similarly insulted Stephen. It was Gogarty, however, who paid the rent at the Martello Tower. In *Ulysses,* it is Stephen. Mulligan forces Stephen out of Stephen's home; Joyce angrily leaves Gogarty's home.

Gogarty's response to Joyce's rejection is important. He continues to try to maintain the friendship. Five years later, in 1909, when Joyce returns to Dublin for a visit, Gogarty repeatedly, and almost obsequiously, tries to meet with him, but Joyce refuses. This contrasts with how Mulligan responds in the novel. Stephen complains about how Mulligan treated him after the death of his mother. Mulligan responds with little in the way of apology, offering instead an extended discourse on how the slight was unimportant. It is typical that, despite rather intense provocation, friends often try to remain loyal to Joyce; they continue to care about him. If Stephen complains, his friends may become defensive and show so little empathy as to make matters even worse.

While their friends generally responded differently, the Catholic church, as it was interpreted by many priests in Ireland at the time, was a profound, pernicious, and similar influence on both Joyce and Dedalus. Throughout their educations, the teacher-priests were overwhelmingly intrusive, reserving particular condemnation for unavoidable sexual urges. Even when the priests do seem to respond with understanding, they are later shown to be hypocrites. At age seven, at Clongowes, Joyce was whipped unjustly for something he did not do. The incident is faithfully retold in *Portrait.* Stephen and James both complained to the rector of the school, who said that he would speak to the offending priest. Later, both find out that there was no serious intent to raise the matter with the priest.

The concept of Mother Church with outstretched arms and the understanding, forgiving God are overshadowed by fear of damnation.

Most of chapter 3 of *Portrait* consists of a virulent sermon on hell, similar to one that Joyce had heard at a high school retreat. It drips with sadism. Both he and Stephen respond with terrified self-abnegation and obsessional efforts to deny their burgeoning sexuality.

This unfortunate brand of Catholicism invaded the home. An actual event, faithfully recounted in *Portrait,* is of a Christmas dinner. James and Stephen are filled with delight and relief on their first visit home from boarding school. The subject of Parnell, the Irish nationalist leader, comes up. Their governesses, both called Dante, vilify Parnell because he was a "sinner" who had committed adultery. Exploiting this scandal, those interested in maintaining the Irish-British tie destroyed Parnell's political career and delayed the advent of Irish independence. Committed to Irish nationalism, the fathers and other guests were devoted to Parnell. The men grew enraged at what they considered traitorous attacks, and the governesses grew even more enraged at the tolerance of sin. Matters grew so rancorous that the Joyces' Dante immediately left their employ, and the character disappears from the novel. One suspects that Joyce must have delighted to "murder" her so. Neither mother was able to intervene in this scene that so devastated the festivities, for they too were prisoners of the church.

In summary, the church was an intrusive force that dampened sexual feelings and required some form of intrapsychic defense from all but the deadest adolescent boys. Stephen and Joyce both responded by divorcing love from sexuality and indulged in the sensual excesses of regular visits to prostitutes. For Joyce, this was a temporary solution, giving way to both the reintegration of sex and love in his marriage and the development of sublimation in his art. By age twenty-two, Stephen achieves neither goal.

While the church may have had a similar influence on James and Stephen, their families were only superficially similar. Both were first born in large families. Their fathers were from the landed classes, but their alcoholism drove the families into severe poverty. As noted, the mothers were both prisoners of an unsophisticated form of Irish Catholicism. Joyce, nevertheless, found considerable support from his family. His relationship with his father, John Joyce, was affectionate. Ellmann (1982) notes that the poor relationship between Stephen and his father was not much like James's relationship with his father but was more reminiscent of that between James's brother Stanislaus and their father.

Ellmann's (1982) biography shows that James's mother, Mary, was devoted to him but was at times intrusive. At the time that corresponds to the hiatus between *Portrait* and *Ulysses* in Stephen's life, Joyce made his first visit to Paris, and his letters to his mother "continually prodded her for sympathy, not merely to obtain money, but to sustain his ambitions. . . . Having put himself several hundred miles away from her, he depended upon her more heavily than before. His mother was part of the stable world he was engaged in renouncing; yet he did not want her to renounce him" (Ellmann 1982, pp. 129–130). At this safer distance, he could ask, and she responded by sending wonderfully encouraging letters that also included whatever money she could spare. She was deeply religious, and Joyce put her to the supreme test by denying the Catholic faith. "She was disconcerted but did not abandon him" (Ellmann 1982, p. 294). In important, if inconsistent and unconscious, ways, both of Joyce's parents facilitated resolution of his Oedipus complex and encouraged the consolidation of sublimation as a healthy defense.

Joyce's brother Stanislaus turned his own life into a veritable shambles through his draining and generally successful efforts to salvage James's life. Stanislaus provided endless financial support, despite very limited means. He moved to Trieste to join James and Nora, there often pulling his drunken brother from the gutter and dragging him home. Two sisters, Eileen and Eva, also joined their brothers in the very difficult task of keeping James's house on an even keel. As these events in Joyce's life occurred well after the age of twenty-two, when Stephen disappears, there is no way to assess Stephen's sibling relationships adequately. Strong sibling support was certainly present, however, for Joyce.

While Joyce's family life was often troubled, Stephen's became appalling, as summarized at the beginning of the last chapter of *Portrait:*

> He drained his third cup of watery tea to the dregs and set to chewing the crusts of fried bread that were scattered near him, staring into the dark pool of the jar. The yellow dripping had been scooped out like a boghole and the pool under it brought back to his memory the dark turfcolloured water of the bath in Clongowes. . . . [His mother then scrubs his neck and ears as if he were still a child.]

—Well, it's a poor case, she said, when a university student is so dirty that his mother has to wash him.

—But it gives you pleasure, said Stephen calmly.

An earsplitting whistle was heard from upstairs and his mother thrust a damp overall into his hands, saying:

—Dry yourself and hurry out for the love of goodness.

A second shrill whistle, prolonged angrily, brought one of the girls to the foot of the staircase.

—Yes, father?

—Is your lazy bitch of a brother gone out yet?

—Yes, father. . . .

—Ah, it's a scandalous shame for you, Stephen, said his mother, and you'll live to rue the day you set your foot in that place [the university]. I know how it has changed you. [Joyce 1916, 174–175]

This dismal picture of family life joins other episodes to reveal an assaultive father and a mother who is both seductive and critical. This combination is, of course, a prescription for failure to resolve the Oedipus complex. Stephen's failure in this sphere helps to account for his backing away from competition, a possible latent homosexual aspect to his personality, and his troubled heterosexual relationships.

John Joyce was far from a perfect father to James, but they maintained a basically loving and positive relationship. John made James his sole heir, and James wanted to have *Finnegans Wake* published on July 4, his father's birthday. Joyce stated in a letter to Harriet Shaw Weaver, "My father had an extraordinary affection for me" (quoted in Ellmann 1982, p. 643).

Even if it was present, which is doubtful, Stephen never internally experienced such love from his father, Simon. A telling episode occurs at age fifteen or sixteen, when Stephen accompanies his father to Simon's hometown of Cork. They are going to sell the last family property to reduce the escalating debts created by Simon's alcoholism. Stephen is so overwhelmed while walking next to his father that his internal experience becomes fragmented. Desperately, he tries to comfort himself with these thoughts: "I am Stephen Dedalus. I am walking beside my father whose name is Simon Dedalus. We are in Cork, in Ireland. Cork is a city. Our room is in the Victoria Hotel. Victoria and Stephen and Simon. Simon and Stephen and Victoria. Names" (Joyce 1916, p. 92).

Shortly thereafter, the property is sold, and Simon gets drunk and says, "There's that son of mine there not half my age and I'm a better man than he is any day of the week" (Joyce 1916, p. 95). By themselves, these incidents need not have a traumatic effect, but they are typical of this father-son relationship, one marked by so much competitiveness and distance that little in the way of a sustaining relationship can form between father and son. In the "Circe" episode of *Ulysses,* Stephen summarizes his relationship to his father in a hallucinated vision. Simon swoops down through the air, leading huntsmen after a fox that is running to escape after burying its grandmother. Here we see both Stephen's vision of his father as an avenger and one of Stephen's habitual defenses of running into isolation to escape.

Immediately following Stephen's return from Cork to Dublin, he begins what is to become another habitual defense, loveless sexual stimulation. He goes to Nighttown for the first time and encounters a prostitute: "He would not bend to kiss her. He wanted to be held firmly in her arms, to be caressed slowly, slowly, slowly. In her arms he felt that he had suddenly become strong and fearless and sure of himself. But his lips would not bend to kiss her" (Joyce 1916, p. 101). The timing of this behavior leads us to suspect that it is at least partly motivated by an effort to seek comfort from the assaults of his father.

Stephen's sensual defenses are, of course, also derived from his relationship with his mother. Carens (1984, p. 305) notes Brivic's argument "that Stephen is ambivalent toward all women, because he even sees his mother as 'betrayer and whore.' " Important intrapsychic fundamentals of this relationship appear in the "Circe" chapter, when Stephen hallucinates her as chiding him for his ingratitude and trying to claw at his heart. He shouts back, "*Non Serviam!*" (Joyce 1922, p. 582). Taking his walking stick, he screams, "*Nothung!*" (p. 583), and flails about with it. This is a direct reference to Siegfried's sword, which is broken to end the old order and establish the dominance of the new. But Stephen breaks a chandelier, and the stick remains intact, just as his guilt toward, oedipal attachment to, and impotent rage at his mother remain intact. It is not surprising, then, that Stephen has been unable to establish a loving heterosexual relationship by age twenty-two, instead remaining addicted to the sensual stimulation of prostitutes.

While Joyce knew his share of prostitutes, he did maintain a profound relationship with Nora from Bloomsday until his death in 1941. Their relationship was not without tumult, but, "if her allegiance would always be a little mocking, it would be nevertheless thoroughgoing'' (Ellmann 1982, p. 157). She was not anything like an intellectual companion, even referring to *Finnegans Wake* as "chop suey" (Epstein 1984). "In spite of her deficits in education, [she] was independent, unself-conscious, instinctively right" (Ellmann 1982, p. 249). She remained constant and tolerant through James's alcoholism, early poverty, and even an affair. Joyce, however, tested her love in even more profound ways. Not only did she have to accept the worst in him, but she also had to "recognize all his impulses, even the strangest, and match his candor by confiding in him every thought she has found in herself, especially the most embarrassing. She must allow him to know her inmost life, to learn with odd exactitude what it is to be a woman. This test, the last, Nora passed successfully" (Ellmann 1982, p. 294). She seemed secure enough in herself that she did not need to feast on being Mrs. James Joyce. While providing him essential human insights, she had little need to exploit her husband's stature.

When Stephen meets the Blooms, they are not similarly free of wishes to use him to gratify their own, often unhelpful, needs. Molly hopes that she will be able to end the boredom of her existence by forming a sexual liaison with him. She indulges the unlikely fantasy that this will inspire him to new heights of creativity, and she will then delight in having inspired genius. Bloom often has his own designs for Stephen. Toward the end of the "Eumaeus" chapter, Stephen begins to sing beautifully, leading Bloom to think of commercial vocal successes, concert tours, and aristocratic audiences, all under his artistic management. As he thinks this, Joyce comments by having a horse deposit "three smoking globes of turds" (Joyce 1922, p. 665).

It would be grossly unfair and inaccurate to say that Bloom is not also motivated by positive emotions. After Stephen gets into terrible trouble at the whorehouse, Bloom looks down at him and is overcome with paternal longing. Bloom has lost a son in infancy and has also lost his father to suicide. He has great reason to long for the opportunity to function as a father surrogate for Stephen. But this is not to be. Through the beginning of *Ulysses,* we wonder "what would happen when Bloom and Stephen finally get together. In [the] 'Eumaeus' [chapter] the answer [is] nothing, or very little" (Bowen 1984, p. 533). Bowen is convinced that Bloom and Stephen will never effect a permanent relationship, and their parting at the end of the "Ithaca" chapter promises little hope of further meetings.

The pattern is consistent. Joyce finds and is able to accept intimacy and support from many sources. Perhaps because of his genius and extraordinary sense of humor, people are willing to tolerate him to such an extent that Joyce can establish relationships that are clearly capable of performing what Kohut (1977) calls selfobject functions. Stephen finds no such people, and it is likely that his conflicts and inadequate defenses will force him to maintain distance even if he does wander into a relationship that holds genuine promise.

Literary-Structural Evidence for Joyce's Involvement with Others

In addition to the biographical data already presented, the literary structure of Joyce's writing offers evidence of his strongly held belief that the artist can and must rely on others. Most obvious is the fact that the title and form of *Ulysses* parallel Homer's epic. Although often with tongue in cheek, Joyce arranged each of the chapters to follow a similar episode in the classic work. Bowen (1984, p. 516) notes that the "Circe" chapter also borrows "heavily from Goethe's *Faust*." The "Oxen of the Sun" chapter, which takes place in the delivery suite of the Holles Street Hospital, deals with the concept of birth. Playing against the delivery of a child, Joyce considers the gestation and birth of writing. The chapter begins in Latin and quotes from or imitates most of the historic languages and literary styles "from Old English through the contemporary argot" (Bowen 1984, p. 510). The chapter builds to the birth of "the word," but, in typical Joycean fashion, when the word finally arrives, it is "Burke's," a local bar.

The aesthetic theory that Stephen espouses in *Portrait* reflects his detachment. He believes that the artist remains behind the work, detached, like the god who pares his nails while the events of the world take place. In *Ulysses,* Stephen presents some views about Shakespeare. As he is talking, it is clear that he does not believe what he is saying despite his intoxication with the complexity of his ideas. The theory, which he does not believe, suggests that, in writing *Hamlet,* Shakespeare was working through his anguish about affairs that Anne Hathaway was having. These affairs were supposedly what drove Shakespeare to London. While Stephen does not believe a word of what he is saying, Joyce told friends that he thought there was great merit in the concept (Ellmann 1982, p. 364). Stephen, then, holds an aesthetic theory of the creator being detached from his work. Joyce believes otherwise. He is certainly not detached from what he is writing. As is clearly evidenced by the extensive parallels between his own life and those of his characters, Joyce relies heavily on his world for material, and he uses the creative process to work through his disappointments, delights, and sorrows.

Summary and Conclusions

Explanations for creative blocks based on problems in resolving the Oedipus complex have been well explored. For example, Freud (1916) noted how such a failure of resolution may force a person to avoid success since it may bring some people too close to oedipal victory (see also Brown 1971; and Krueger 1984). Others are lost in compromise formations or symbolic gratification of libidinal drive conflicts. For them, the sublimation necessary for creativity is impossible. These and related explanations may be sufficient to explain creative block and to guide successful treatment. However, Kohut (1976) and Winnicott (1965) have added a new dimension to understanding creativity.

In order to create, Joyce needed sustaining, empathic relationships, in which the other person often functioned as a selfobject. This need appears to be present in many, perhaps even most, creative people. Kohut (1976) notes the relationships between Freud and Fleiss and between Picasso and Braque. He contends that these relationships offered vital support at the time that these men made some of their most daring progress. Ellmann (1948) states that Yeats would have been a relatively minor poet if judged by his works prior to the point at which he married. Careful study might reveal similar relationships between Leonard and Virginia Woolf; Leopold, Constanze, and Wolfgang Mozart; Eugene and Carlotta O'Neill; Frédéric Chopin and Georges Sand.

Groups as well as individuals may fulfill the selfobject function. In a recent videotape about Franz Kline, Elaine de Kooning talked fondly about the environment in Greenwich Village during the 1940s and 1950s. These artists created a group process that provided each other with an environment that invigorated the whole of American abstract expressionism. The composers known as the Russian Five and the French Six functioned similarly. In an entirely different area, the development of the Apple Macintosh computer occurred among a group of highly creative people. Through their interactions, they also provided each other extensive, affectionate support and help that facilitated this technological advancement.

Noy (1984–1985) believes that genuinely creative people like Joyce, Woolf, Picasso, and the rest think in an original way *habitually*. For them, "originality . . . must be regarded not as an isolated mental act . . . but as a habitual response based on the permanent ability to use a much greater repertoire of organizing programs than does the non-original [person]" (p. 425). He demonstrates that this pattern is necessitated by childhoods that are usually marked by being highly valued children who were encouraged to be original but who were intruded on by their families and cultures. As many also felt themselves to be childhood "outsiders," they often have developed a pattern of seeing themselves as different or marginal. Facilitated by a marginal status and a certain heightened omnipotence, originality, then, may function as a healthy and necessary defense against intrusiveness. This pattern was present in the lives of both James Joyce and Stephen Dedalus, necessitating and enabling creative thought patterns.

Creative thought patterns are not, however, enough to produce meaningful artistic products. More is required. Along with Kohut (1984) and Winnicott (1965), Noy (1984–1985, p. 439) is "convinced that the struggle to maintain a cohesive and well-integrated [true] self . . . is a never-ending struggle, occupying the healthy [and the creative] mind as well as the pathological one for its entire life." Although they do not use the same terms, Kohut and Winnicott both understand that the goal of a firm sense of a true self requires a satisfactory holding or selfobject environment.

This requirement is greater for the creative person since the creative process can be frightening and debilitating. Deliberately concealing his identity, Noy (1984–1985, p. 435) quotes "one of the most creative and original minds in our field. . . . 'When I begin to work on developing my own ideas, I become more and more anxious. I know that the more I depart from the common opinion, the more I will be attacked, excommunicated, and rejected by many of my best friends.' " Kohut (1976, p. 818) puts it like this:

> During creative periods, the self is at the mercy of powerful forces it cannot control; and its sense of enfeeblement is increased because it feels itself helplessly exposed to extreme mood swings which range from severe precreative depression to dangerous hy-

pomanic overstimulation, the later occurring at the moment when the creative mind stands at the threshold of creative activity. . . . And when his discoveries lead the creative mind into lonely areas that had not previously been explored by others, then a situation is brought about in which the genius feels a deep sense of isolation.

For most, this simply requires a sustaining relationship, or the creativity cannot be risked.

It is a fundamental and, I believe, accurate tenet of self psychological theory that the ability to regulate self-esteem and to calm and soothe the self is never achieved *entirely* by intrapsychic means. The selfobject is someone or something external to the self that assists in accomplishing those goals. To some varying degree, then, everyone turns outside the self to those who can and will function as selfobjects. The extent to which one is compelled to do so is dependent on both (1) the internal, structural ability to accomplish these tasks and (2) the amount of stress to which the self is exposed. The creative process is often accompanied by nearly hypomanic overstimulation, pre- and postcreative depression, and catastrophic loss of self-esteem when the product is not well received. Even if the capability to calm and soothe the self and to regulate self-esteem is sufficient under usual circumstances, for those who experience such affects when they create, there will be an intensified need to turn outside the self for calming and encouragement. If no one is there, as was the case with Stephen but not with Joyce, the creative process poses an intolerable threat to the integrity of the self. It cannot be risked. The concept of the creative loner is, therefore, often little more than a romantic myth.

Like others, but perhaps more so, the artist must choose who will function as central selfobjects with considerable care. Not only will they be needed frequently, but they will also count on the artist to function as a selfobject. The other has selfobject needs too. Nora was a good choice. Her selfobject needs apparently were not excessive, so she was able to tolerate very emotionally threatening behavior on Joyce's part. He had at least one affair, which many women would find intolerable. But he also had a far more demanding mistress, his art. Had Nora needed constant attention from her husband, she might have interfered with Joyce's creative efforts.

One may choose a spouse, but no such option is possible with parental selfobjects. Here again we see a difference between Joyce and Stephen. John and Mary Joyce did not interfere with their son's in-

275

terests. They generally encouraged him. This contrasts with Mrs. Dedalus, who complained bitterly about Stephen's involvement at the university. The person who functions as a selfobject cannot be dismissed, and, if he or she is unwilling to tolerate the artist's creative work, a conflict arises. Shall the artist be true to his work, which also may function as a selfobject (Kohut 1976), or shall he be true to his spouse or parent? For Stephen to choose his parents, he would have interfered with his work, but to choose the work would have placed him in a position of losing any shred of selfobject support that he could have got from his parents. He could not win.

With respect to creativity, failure to resolve the Oedipus complex is particularly pernicious. Persistence of these intense libidinal conflicts results in reduced ability to establish intimate relationships. This reduction, in turn, precludes adequately meeting selfobject needs. People like Stephen Dedalus withdraw from self-selfobject relationships because they dread to repeat the pain of nonempathic responses. They also withdraw because intolerable drive conflicts surface. For people like Stephen who are unable to establish intimacy, further growth is impossible, and creative productivity may be blocked because they are unable to form satisfactory self-selfobject relationships rather than merely because they are trapped in libidinal conflicts.

It is beyond the scope of this chapter to discuss extensively the therapeutic implications of these findings. However, the therapist who encounters a patient with a creative block may more fully appreciate the needs these patients have for a supportive "holding" or selfobject environment. While exercising careful control not to act out of countertransference pressures, therapists may also find it useful judiciously to break the barriers of abstinence to create elements of such a facilitating environment within the therapeutic relationship. For example, while working with one blocked, creative visual artist, I visited his studio and extensively discussed compositional and other technical aspects of his work. Through mutual acquaintances in the artistic community, he knew that I have studied art seriously and am committed to expressing myself in this area. This breaking of the barrier facilitated his conviction that I genuinely understood his creative efforts and had a salutory effect on the therapeutic relationship. He became far more productive. He carries a diagnosis of bipolar affective disorder but has shown an evenness of mood unknown in years of previous therapy with highly respected and competent analysts.

By intensifying the self-selfobject relationship, the psychiatrist provides a self-consolidating holding environment for the patient. This environment alone may facilitate creative output. More important, it gives an opportunity, within the therapeutic relationship, to examine the consequences of disruptions in self-selfobject relationships directly. A magnifying glass is then held to the creative process, highlighting its thrilling successes and bitter inhibitions. Within the context of the therapeutic alliance, interpretations may then be offered to help the patient see what firms and disrupts his experience of self-cohesion and how these moments of solidity and disruption directly effect his ability to work.

It is true to the peculiarities and perversities of the Joycean tradition to conclude a consideration of his creative process by quoting someone else. Eugene O'Neill (1956, p. 7) begins *Long Day's Journey into Night* with this dedication:

For Carlotta, on our 12th Wedding Anniversary
Dearest: I give you the original script of this play of old sorrow, written in tears and blood. A sadly inappropriate gift, it would seem, for a day celebrating happiness. But you will understand. I mean it as a tribute to your love and tenderness which gave me the faith in love that enabled me to face my dead at last and write this play—write it with deep pity and understanding and forgiveness for *all* the four haunted Tyrones. These twelve years, Beloved One, have been a Journey into Light—into love. You know my gratitude. And my love!

REFERENCES

Andreach, R. J. 1964. *Studies in Structure: The Stages of the Spiritual Life in Four Modern Authors*. New York: Fordham University Press.
Balint, M. 1968. *The Basic Fault*. London: Tavistock.
Bowen, Z. 1984. Ulysses. In Z. Bowen and J. Carens, eds. *A Companion to Joyce Studies*. Westport, Conn.: Greenwood.
Brown, W. A. 1971. The meaning of success in a person with a "success phobia." *Psychiatry* 34:425–430.
Carens, J. F. 1984. A portrait of the artist as a young man. In Z. Bowen and J. Carens, eds. *A Companion to Joyce Studies*. Westport, Conn.: Greenwood.

Ellmann, R. 1948. *Yeats, the Man and the Mask.* New York: Macmillan.

Ellmann, R. 1982. *James Joyce.* Oxford: Oxford University Press.

Epstein, E. L. 1984. James Augustine Aloysius Joyce. In Z. Bowen and J. Carens, eds. *A Companion to Joyce Studies.* Westport, Conn.: Greenwood.

Erickson, E. H. 1963. *Childhood and Society.* New York: Norton.

Freud, S. 1916. Some character-types met within psycho-analytic work. *Standard Edition* 14:309–355. London: Hogarth, 1957.

Goertzel, M. G.; Goertzel, V.; and Goertzel, T. D. 1978. *Three Hundred Eminent Personalities.* San Francisco: Jossey-Bass.

Gordon, W. A. 1974–1975. Submission and autonomy: identity patterns in Joyce's *Portrait. Psychoanalytic Review* 64:535–555.

Joyce, J. 1916. *A Portrait of the Artist as a Young Man.* New York: Viking, 1968.

Joyce, J. 1922. *Ulysses.* New York: Vintage, 1961.

Kohut, H. 1976. Creativeness, charisma, group psychology: reflections on the self-analysis of Freud. In P. H. Ornstein, ed. *The Search for the Self.* New York: International Universities Press.

Kohut, H. 1977. *The Restoration of the Self.* New York: International Universities Press.

Kohut, H. 1984. *How Does Analysis Cure?* Chicago: University of Chicago Press.

Kohut, H., and Wolf, E. 1978. The disorders of the self and their treatment: an outline. *International Journal of Psycho-Analysis* 59:413–424.

Krueger, D. W. 1984. *Success and Fear of Success in Women.* New York: Free Press.

Lytton, H. 1971. *Creativity and Education.* London: Routledge & Kegan Paul.

Noy, P. 1984–1985. Originality and creativity. *Annual of Psychoanalysis* 12–13:421–448.

O'Neill, E. 1955. *Long Day's Journey into Night.* New Haven, Conn.: Yale University Press.

Tashjian, L. D. 1982. Aspects of internalization and individuation: James Joyce's *Portrait of the Artist as a Young Man. Adolescent Psychiatry* 10:75–84.

Winnicott, D. W. 1965. *The Maturational Process and the Facilitating Environment.* New York: International Universities Press.

16 MASTER AND APPRENTICE: THE MENTORING RELATIONSHIP IN THE DEVELOPMENT OF ADOLESCENT CREATIVITY

DAVID A. HALPERIN

There is an increasing appreciation of the role played by the mentoring process in the development of artistic creativity. No longer is the creative process examined in exclusively intrapsychic terms. Rather, there has been an increasing recognition that, as Bloom (1982) writes,

> the origins and aims of poetry together constitute its powers, and the powers of poetry, however they relate to or affect the world, rise out of a loving conflict with previous poetry, rather than out of conflict with the world. There is, despite much contemporary criticism, a referential aspect to a poem, which keeps it from coming into being only as a text, or rather keeps a text from being merely a text. But this referential aspect is both masked and mediated, and the agent of concealment and of relationship always is another poem. There is no unmediated vision, whether in poetry or in any other mode, but only mediated revision, for which another name is anxiety, in the Freudian sense of "anxious expectations." [P. viii]

Thus, the focus of critical scrutiny has been transferred from an investigation of the individual artist acting in isolation to an examination of the creative process as being part of a continuing dialectic between the artist and his progenitors—between the mentor/master and the apprentice.

The transition from adolescence to maturity and the vicissitudes experienced by the adolescent artist as he achieves maturity are the focus of three entertaining and provocative films starring Peter O'Toole. These films—*The Stunt Man, My Favorite Year,* and *The Creator*—constitute a cinematic trilogy that examines the processes of mirroring and idealization as aspects of the development of the adolescent artist. This chapter examines these aspects of the creative process as it is presented in a popular medium but with a rare degree of sophistication.

The Stunt Man highlights the issues that these films raise. Cameron, a Viet Nam veteran, is fleeing from the police, who are pursuing him for an unnamed misdemeanor (in actuality, a crime à la "Alice's Restaurant"). He blunders onto the production site of a film by running across a bridge. As he crosses the bridge, he sees a car racing toward him. He jumps aside and throws a rock at the driver. The car crashes into the water, and the driver drowns. Unknown to Cameron, the crash was a film stunt (although the driver's drowning was not in the script). The drowning may have been caused by the driver's having panicked while in the water, or it may have resulted from Cameron's having injured the driver with the rock. After the car and the driver are retrieved from the water, Eli, the film director, offers Cameron refuge from the pursuing policemen if he will take over the dead man's task and become a stuntman. Cameron accepts this offer. During the course of the production, Cameron forms a relationship with Eli's mistress and seduces her. Together, they plan to leave the production site after Cameron performs the stunt in which his predecessor died. Ultimately, Cameron does perform the stunt and crashes into the bay, but, unlike his unfortunate predecessor, he succeeds in freeing himself from the sinking car. However, his girlfriend decides to return to the director. The film ends with Cameron arguing with Eli over the fee he should be paid for successfully performing the stunt.

Summary of a film tends toward reductionism because visual metaphor and nuance, central to an appreciation of the underlying structure of the film, are excluded. Despite this limitation, an exploration of the underlying structure of this film is rewarding particularly for the light it sheds on the creative process as examined through the lens of the psychology of the self.

The setting of the film is the Del Coronado Hotel in southern California. The Del Coronado is a unique High Victorian landmark whose profusion of gables, towers, and pinnacles makes it a destination for the tourist and an exciting backdrop for an otherwise depressingly mundane suburb of San Diego. It is an oasis, a Xanadu surrounded by Miami Beach. The juxtaposition of the Del Coronado and its surroundings forces the viewer to confront the magical nature of the American dream with its contradictory and paradoxical amalgam of pragmatism and idealism, aesthetics and cinderblock. The very creation of the Del Coronado belongs to a period when California was regarded as a yet unsullied Garden of Eden—an Eden before the Fall, with all the biblical connotations of innocence and asexuality (not surprisingly, its greatest claim to fame is that the duke of Windsor met Wallis Simpson in its dining room). While the main building survives, the price of its survival is the construction of exceptionally tacky and unimaginative concrete towers on its grounds. In short, it is a place where the fantasy of omnipotence is confronted with the reality of compromise.

Cameron is to participate in the creation of a film about World War I. The film is to be an antiwar film, but one that is not ostentatiously pacifist. In his first day on the set, Cameron confronts the enigmatic nature of cinematic reality as the soldiers (bit players and stuntmen) die and miraculously revive. In an extraordinary scene, the dead disinter themselves, shake off their mud, and stand erect. Their disinterment and resurrection parallel the manner in which Eli, the director, will, ultimately, provide for Cameron's miraculous resurrection. In a comparable fashion, the apprentice approaches the mentor as an agent of his birth as a creative artist (as the patient approaches the psychoanalyst as the agent of his rebirth). In the film, the dead painlessly revive, a metaphor for the process of initiation in which the apprentice approaches the mentor with the fantasy that apprenticeship is a painless process (as the patient enters psychoanalysis with the expectation that it will provide for the rapid resolution of his conflicts). The rage that Cameron ultimately expresses at Eli for not fulfilling his part of the bargain is like the rage that the young artist expresses as he experiences the anxiety of isolation and asserts his artistic autonomy. It parallels the anger and disillusion that is often present at the termination of an analysis when the patient discovers that the process of psychoanalysis has not provided for rebirth but only, in Freud's (1937) memorable words, "replaced neurotic anxiety with everyday discontent."

In choosing as its subject World War I, the film examines the manner in which our perceptions of our leaders reflect our use of idealization and our denial of reality. The world entered into World War I on a wave of popular hysteria and idealistic patriotism. Both sides anticipated a rapid romp on the road to victory and national fulfillment. A crude Darwinianism portrayed war as a glorious arena in which the fittest would prove their right to empire and domination. The bitter films of the 1920s and 1930s are products of a generation whose idealizing fantasies of military glory and making the world "safe for democracy" were realized in the ceaseless, senseless, and dehumanizing war of the trenches. Viet Nam was the product of a comparable national idealism (and grandiosity). The United States has found it difficult to return to its conception of itself as the last, best hope of mankind. It has had to express its rage at its formerly idealized leaders and explore the grandiosity that was expressed in the self-confidence that led them to distort the purpose and scope of our military intervention, and it has now begun to recreate a sense of national cohesiveness and, by erecting a memorial, to put the war behind it.

The Stunt Man and Cameron's cynicism and alienation reflect the perceptions of a generation whose belief that a war was simply an exercise in futile destruction was disregarded by authorities whose grandiosity had replaced their sense of reality. The film finds its current relevance in its reflection of the enduring nature of the "generation gap," for example, the enduring reality that the adolescent artist inevitably stakes out his artistic position through shattering the vessels of adult authority. This dialectic extends even to benign and creative relationships such as that of the psychoanalyst and the analysand (hence, the frequent portrayal of the psychoanalyst as aloof, disengaged, avaricious, and detached).

The most strikingly realized character of *The Stunt Man* is Eli, the director. Portrayed by Peter O'Toole, his very name evokes the biblical story of Creation ("Eli" is "my God" in Hebrew). As in Genesis, Eli does separate light out of darkness and create form. His words have a deified cast, for example, "Come near to me." He wears a black turtleneck sweater that resembles a clerical collar. As with divine beings, his gender identification is ambiguous (he has consummated his relationship with his girlfriend only once). He presents an androgynous facade throughout the film. To reemphasize the ambivalent role he plays, Eli is photographed silhouetted against a hakenkreuz—the bent cross or swastika, an ancient sun symbol that represents to modern man the most potent symbol of demonism. His ambiguity is reflective of his split agenda: (1) the completion of the film as the creative expression of a task-oriented group whose leader he is and whose efforts he bends in the solution of artistic dilemmas and (2) the completion of the film as an expression of his own narcissism. Cameron, like all adolescents, responds to Eli's expressions of concern by rejecting them. He justifies his rejection by focusing on the narcissistic agenda without considering his role as a responsible group leader.

Eli is the pivot around whom Cameron, the film crew, and the creation of the film revolve. However, his is not an unchallenged divinity, as Cameron discovers when he forms relationships with other members of the crew. For example, an older stuntman befriends Cameron and provides him with a more realistic picture of the actual relationships within this ambiguous world. A screenwriter (read psychoanalyst) provides Cameron with factual details that flesh out Cameron's understanding of Eli's relationship with the other actors. He helps Cameron understand his use of splitting as a means of defense within the unreal world of the film.

Initially, Cameron strongly identifies with the film world. He idealizes Eli and the other actors as his mentors and protectors against a hostile outside world. Gradually, he becomes increasingly disillusioned with the world of film and art. His increasingly intimate relationship with the lead actress (Eli's former girlfriend) provides an oedipal and competitive basis for his disillusionment. Yet, Cameron rationalizes his changing attitudes toward Eli as reflecting his increasing disdain for Eli's narcissism and his coming to view Eli's direction of the film primarily as a product of his narcissism. When the actress points out to Cameron that there are other aspects to her relationship with Eli than the purely sensual/sexual, Cameron is forced to confront Eli in his role as a task-oriented group leader facilitating the creative progress of the film crew. Cameron begins to appreciate that the creativity of the artist lies in the ability to transcend competitive struggles with mentoring figures and to cathect the energies previously utilized, primarily in competitive strivings, onto new objects, which are then endowed with this new vitality. The actress enables Cameron to place his idealized (now devalued) object, Eli, in perspective when she points out to him that, while the creative process is inherently competitive, it becomes meaningful only when placed within a public and accessible context. In short, she enables Cameron to realize that meaningful creative activity is possible only within the context created by other artists. Finally, she reminds Cameron that the artist is essentially separate from his creation and that, whatever shortcoming Eli's androgyny may create in terms of their individual relationship, his very passivity may even help her gain access to her own artistic potential and strength. Her very presence raises another and more complex question. What is the role of the adult female muse in the development of the adolescent artist? Perhaps the relationship between Thomas Wolfe, the preeminent American adolescent artist, and Aline Bernstein, his older female mentor, is more prototypical than previously imagined?

Cameron's initiation into adulthood occurs when he allows himself to separate from Eli and assume equality with his once-idealized mentor. The initiation occurs when he returns to the scene of his birth into the cinematic world—the site of the accident on the bridge. This time, he reenacts the crash scene, but, unlike his predecessor, he is able to crawl out of his vehicular tomb and surface. The film concludes with a "comic" coda to his immersion into the dangerous element. He surfaces, lands, and immediately starts to argue with Eli about his fee for the stunt. Like many analyses, the individual's growth into maturity is signaled by his willingness to argue over the banalities of life—the fees and schedules. In these arguments, there is a recognition that only in the acceptance of the mundane is the artist (or the individual) able to advance beyond infantilization and a childlike idealization of his craft.

These issues are approached more directly in the film *My Favorite Year*, where Benjamin Stone reminisces about his mentoring relationship with Allan Swann (a fading film idol who is part Barrymore and all ham). The initial focus of the film is on the idealizing transference that pervades the relationship between the youthful Stone and a fading Swann—exemplified in Stone's statement, "We need our heroes." The film portrays the process of maturation in which Stone finds a dignity in his having been born Benjamin Steinberg of Brooklyn, and Allan Swann is able to accept the humanity of having been born Clarence Duffy of Liverpool. Both protagonists grow into an acceptance of their past and into being able to face the future without denying their past.

My Favorite Year derives much of its dramatic tension from its portrayal of Stone's coming to grips with his idealizing transference and his having to choose among a variety of models for identification. In its exploration of alternate models for mentoring, it highlights the dilemmas faced by the adolescent artist in the process of growth. One individual presented to Stone as a model is Kyser, the "King of Comedy." Kyser is an aggressively provocative, albeit honest, artist who survives through dominating and emasculating his subordinates (one of them is rendered speechless by him until the very end of the film). His denial of his vulnerability makes him into a hero (in a particularly funny scene, he caricatures a Mafia don and refuses to water down his caricature despite the don's threats), but his inability to accept his own vulnerability, which makes him into a hero, also makes him ultimately unavailable to Stone as a viable object for identification. On the other hand, Allan Swann's charm is compounded primarily out of his vulnerability. He revels in his passivity and explains his numerous marriages to Stone as the product of his acquiescence—"They wanted me." Their commonality of weakness and their ability to accept their vulnerabilities enable Swann and Stone to form a mutually productive relationship. Stone and Swann change as a result of their interaction with each other. Unlike Eli of *The Stunt Man*, who remains locked in his helicopter, omnisciently directing the actors who scurry beneath the propellor blades, Swann accepts Stone's challenge to accept his vulnerability and rises to the level of the cinematic facade (the hero) that he portrays. *My Favorite Year* illustrates that the gifted teacher is gifted precisely because of his ability to learn from his students.

The dyadic and interactive nature of the mentoring relationship is underlined once more in Peter O'Toole's most recent fable, *The Creator*. While this film has not received as positive a critical reception as either *The Stunt Man* or *My Favorite Year*, it illustrates the issues raised in the other films in a succinct (and entertaining) manner. In *The Creator*, O'Toole is an aging, archetypically eccentric, absent-minded scientist. His affectual life has been profoundly blunted since the death of his wife in childbirth. However, he has chosen a novel mode of solving his depression—he plans to recreate his wife by cloning her tissue. His experiment is entitled "The Big Picture." While setting up his experiment, O'Toole adopts Boris as a laboratory assistant. During the early stages of their relationship, Boris idealizes O'Toole. He mirrors him and succinctly states, "I want to be just like you." Boris accepts O'Toole's mentoring in the social, sexual, and academic arenas. With O'Toole's guidance, Boris forms a relationship with a nubile fellow student, Amy. Boris's development of a relationship with Amy parallels

O'Toole's beginning to form a relationship with a free-spirited nymph who wanders into his life. Ironically, Boris's relationship with Amy provides O'Toole with a role model that allows him to bury his relationship with his dead wife. Ultimately, O'Toole's new relationship allows him to replace the asexual fantasy of reproduction through cloning with the more complex relationship of fatherhood. At film's end, both Boris and O'Toole are anticipating fatherhood.

In *The Creator* and *My Favorite Year*, a model of the mentoring relationship is presented. In both films, the importance of individuation within the dyadic relationship is highlighted. They emphasize the importance of mutuality within the mentoring relationship and the fact that, if a mentor is so locked into his position of authority that he is unable to grow, then mentoring becomes a species of cloning. These films underline the fact that true education must respect the individual's need to grow in all areas—that, without this respect for every aspect of the individual's life, education becomes a form of indoctrination. In this regard, the recent movement toward limiting the work hours of residents and interns is significant because it recognizes that the postdoctoral student requires the opportunity to grow in many areas—that creating physicians who are so numbed that they barely possess a technical competence is self-defeating in both educational and emotional terms.

O'Toole is a spokesman for an older, superficially archaic conception of the process of scientific education. He represents, with all his fey charm, the conception of the scientist as an educated man, not simply a well-trained technician. Lewis (1967) has spoken about the need for discourse between the sciences and the humanities. With the film's wry manner, the importance of this discourse is emphasized by the difference between O'Toole and the other scientist, Dr. S, who is also presented to Boris as an object for identification. Dr. S's primary expertise is in the area of grantsmanship—he views his academic activities primarily as vehicles for personal advancement or for control. Ultimately, his toadying and manipulation receive their appropriate reward—he becomes O'Toole's assistant.

My Favorite Year and *The Creator* substitute whimsy and humor for an exacting examination of the nuts and bolts of the educational process. Nonetheless, these films underline a truth about mentoring that is too often forgotten in these narrowly task-oriented days—that education is a two-way street and that, without mutuality, it degenerates into rigidity, maneuver, and indoctrination. Kohut's (1971) caution about the uncritical acceptance of idealization and mistaking mirroring for genuine growth during the course of the mentoring process is still relevant. Its relevance was illustrated during the 1960s—and it is hoped that they will point toward less divisive modes of change during the final years of this century.

Conclusions

Three recent films starring Peter O'Toole are provocative commentaries on the process of mentoring and the role it plays in the development of creativity in the adolescent artist. The vicissitudes of the mentoring relationship, with its progression from idealization and mirroring to deidealization, are examined. Particular emphasis is placed on the importance of a mutually interactive relationship between mentor and apprentice in which real personal growth as well as technical education occur. In the absence of mutuality, the mentoring relationship degenerates into the relationship of a master to an apprentice/servant. In this latter relationship, the mentor's efforts reflect a primarily narcissistic orientation in which he attempts to control the subordinate.

While the appearance in adolescent artists, such as Rimbaud, of profound creative genius is ultimately inexplicable, their departure, as in the more recent and mundane examples of the adolescent stars that flame brightly, briefly, and out, illustrates again the importance of the mentoring relationship in creating and preserving the adolescent artist's creative potential. The history of such individual tragedies is often one of young artists who established close relationships with mentoring figures who defined their role in exclusively academic or business terms without considering the individual needs of the adolescent artist (Halperin 1987).

REFERENCES

Bloom, H. 1982. *Agon*. New York: Oxford University Press.

Freud, S. 1937. Analysis terminable and interminable. *Standard Edition* 23:211–253. London: Hogarth, 1964.

Halperin, D. A. 1987. Arthur Rimbaud: the poet as an adolescent. *Adolescent Psychiatry* 14:63–81.

Kohut, H. 1971. *The Analysis of the Self*. New York: International Universities Press.

Lewis, A. 1967. *The State of Psychiatry*. New York: Science House.

17 PORTRAIT OF THE ARTIST AS ADOLESCENT PRODIGY: MOZART AND THE MAGIC FLUTE

JOHN E. GEDO

In 1931, the biographer Stefan Zweig sent Sigmund Freud copies of a series of letters from Wolfgang Amadeus Mozart to his cousin Maria Anna Thekla Mozart. Zweig added, "I hope that you, as one who understands the heights and depths, will find the enclosed . . . not entirely irrelevant: these nine letters of the 21-year-old Mozart . . . throw a psychologically very remarkable light on his erotic nature, which, more so than that of any other important man, has elements of infantilism and coprophilia. It would actually be an interesting study for one of your pupils, for all the letters revolve consistently around the same theme" (Hildesheimer 1982, p. 109).

With the exception of a brief paper by Esman (1951), psychoanalysts have failed to respond to Zweig's challenge: the nature of Mozart's provocative letters to his seductive cousin, almost certainly his first sexual partner, has given rise, instead, to the scatological portrait of this supreme musical genius recently popularized on stage and screen. The authors of these fictions cannot be blamed, of course, for the widespread tendency to confuse their efforts with history or biography; at any rate, their compelling dramatic presentations threaten to elevate a very particular response by the composer to the circumstances of his late adolescence to the dignity of a character diagnosis. At the age of twenty-one, this prodigious creator was just passing the midpoint

Reprinted with permission from *Medical Problems of Performing Artists*, vol. 1, no. 3, September 1986. Published by Hanley & Belfus, Inc., 210 South 13th St., Philadelphia, PA 19107.

of his three decades as a composer: the public may therefore be forgiven for its inability to remember that, in ordinary human terms, he had not as yet left the family nest.

The correspondence with Maria Anna Thekla followed Mozart's visit to Augsburg, ancestral home of his paternal family, in the course of a sixteen-month journey to Munich, Mannheim, Paris, and intermediate points that marked the youthful virtuoso's first separation from his hitherto ever-present father. Not only did this initial effort to seek his own fortune lead this previously submissive youth into rebellion against the sexual prohibitions of his conservative upbringing. In rapid succession, it stimulated Mozart into the only romantic passion he was to experience in the course of his brief life of less than thirty-six years— his love for the aspiring operatic soprano Aloysia Weber. It then forced him to attend his fifty-eight-year-old mother, who accompanied him to Paris, during her sudden terminal illness. Finally, it eventuated in his decisive rejection by Aloysia Weber and the dispiriting decision to accept a minor musical post from his father's unsympathetic patron, Hieronymus Colloredo, prince-archbishop of Salzburg.

From a present-day vantage point, Mozart's sad retreat to Salzburg in January 1779, just before his twenty-third birthday, may be seen as the end of his adolescence. From the perspective of musicology, there seems to be little disagreement with the judgment that the works of supreme merit that elevate Mozart above his contemporaries are ushered in by the Symphony in C (K. 338) and the Sinfonia Concertante for violin and viola in E-flat (K. 364), composed in the year that followed the climactic events of his adolescence.[1] Work on his first operatic masterpiece, *Idomeneo* (K. 366), and the great Serenade for Thirteen Winds (K. 361) started in the fall of 1780.

Mozart's biographers of recent years tend to downplay the personal significance of the coprophilia demonstrated in the letters of the young composer.[2] These scholars rightly point out that the German burgher of the late eighteenth century is not to be credited with the civilized refinements of our day. Similar crudities, in smaller doses, to be sure, are found in letters of both Mozart's father and mother; according to Wolfgang, they were the stuff of common discourse in the drawing room of his Mannheim hostess, the wife of the kapellmeister Cannabich. More interesting from our viewpoint is the fact that none of Mozart's surviving letters from later periods are scatological: the relationship with Maria Anna Thekla seems to have released inhibitions of the phallic and the anal components of Wolfgang's psychosexuality at the same time.

We might note in passing that on rare occasions similar, if briefer, anal outbursts punctuated Mozart's cursory letters to his older sister, Nannerl, during the three journeys he made to Italy with his father between December 1769 and March 1773, from the ages of fourteen to seventeen. If we accept Wolfgang's first independent venture, the trip to Paris without his father, as the end of his adolescence, it may be equally cogent to look on his initial separation from his mother, a month before his fourteenth birthday, as the starting point of this era of his life.

These were heady times, even for a boy already used to giving triumphant recitals for the kings of France and England and the Holy Roman Emperors. To put the matter somewhat differently, he was now old enough to grasp the magnitude of his accomplishments. In July 1770, when Pope Clement XIV awarded him the Order of the Golden Spur, Wolfgang wrote his sister, "Mademoiselle, j'ai l'honneur d'être votre très humble serviteur et frère. Chevalier de Mozart." An English rendering might be, "Young lady, I have the honor of being your very humble servant and brother. Sir Wolfgang Mozart." He then added, in Italian, "Addio. Keep well, and shit in your bed make a mess of it."[3] Clearly, the switch from a formal French, the language of the courts, into vulgarities in a foreign vernacular conveys the boy's sense of incongruity about attaining the highest honors available to an artist even though he had scarcely left childhood behind him. We may assume that similar tensions between the stature of his art and his personal immaturity produced the scatological self-mockery of Mozart's letters to his cousin.

The most perceptive of Mozart's recent biographers, Wolfgang Hildesheimer (1982), reports an incident that took place sometime during the last four years of Mozart's life, which I believe had similar significance. A Viennese hostess once recalled that, when she played music from *Figaro* at a soiree, Mozart "sat down, told me to keep playing the bass and began to improvise variations so beautifully that everyone present held his breath, listening to the music of the German Orpheus. But all at once he had had enough, he jumped up and, as he often did in his foolish moods, began to leap over table and chairs, miaowing like a cat, and turning somersaults like an unruly boy" (p. 271). The child who was forced into becoming the German Orpheus by the age of five never learned to tolerate that his acceptance forever depended on his enchanting us through his lyre. His outrage about this took the form of reverting to the antics of an unruly boy—or a tomcat. In a society tolerant of scatology, coprolalia does not make the point with similar clarity.

As an adolescent, Wolfgang was still unconscious of his mounting grievance about the universal exploitation of his unique talents; on the contrary, he was still overtly delighted about the privileges their exercise brought him. Witness the joyful and flirtatious fantasy he elaborated about the queen of Naples at the age of fourteen (in a letter of May or June 1770 to his sister Nannerl): "The King has had a rough Neapolitan upbringing and in the opera he always stands on a stool so as to look a little taller than the Queen. She is beautiful and gracious, and on the Molo . . . she bowed to me in a most friendly manner at least six times." The later testimony of Mozart's father, Leopold, that the child virtuoso used to burst into tears if he sensed that his audience was not serious about music—that is, if he was made to feel that he was being viewed as a curiosity or an act in a sideshow—suggests that Wolfgang's increasing disenchantment with the role of performing artist stemmed from his distaste for the faddish enthusiasm of an undiscriminating public for the entertainments he provided.

It is widely known that the most significant recognition Mozart received in his lifetime was the statement Joseph Haydn made to the young composer's father in 1785. As Leopold Mozart reported it, Haydn declared, "Before God and as an honest man I tell you that your son is the greatest composer known to me either in person or by name" (Hildesheimer 1982, p. 297). Of course, by that time Mozart was in the process of composing his matchless series of piano concerti, string quartets, and piano sonatas.[4] He was on the threshold of work on *The Marriage of Figaro* (K. 492). In other words, he was no longer in need of external confirmation of his genius. It was precisely during the adolescent journeys to Italy that he did receive such vital affirmation of his worth as a composer.

In the summer of 1770, Wolfgang and Leopold Mozart stayed in Bologna, where the fourteen-year-old boy began work on his first opera seria, *Mitridate, Ré di Ponto* (K. 87), to be premiered in Milan at the end of the year. At the same time, Wolfgang took lessons in composition from the outstanding contrapuntist of the era, Padre Martini, and was awarded the diploma of the Academia Filarmonica after a bare fortnight of work. The success of Mozart's first opera for Milan obtained for him several commissions to compose major pieces for the stages of that musical capital. These honors, which permitted him to collaborate as an equal with some of the outstanding singers of the century, culminated in December 1772 with the production of the opera *Lucio Silla* (K. 135). Thenceforth, the seventeen-year-old knew himself to be without peer as an operatic composer; like Tamino, the protagonist of his ultimate work for the stage (K. 620), he was in possession of a magic flute.

As the increasing success of the adolescent Mozart suggests, his career was carefully, not to say shrewdly, managed by his father, Leopold. Wolfgang always acknowledged his father's savoir faire and experience in all practical matters, but he was impatient to throw off the intrusive control through which Leopold accomplished his prudent ends. It is unclear whether the son was consciously aware of his desire for autonomy; his letters to Leopold from Mannheim and Paris explain his hope not to have to return to Salzburg on the ground that Archbishop Colloredo was an insufferable tyrant. The present-day reader of these letters cannot overlook the displacement of Wolfgang's hostility from Leopold to his authoritarian patron. What we cannot discern from these texts is whether the adolescent was being intentionally disingenuous.

We are here face to face with the most difficult extramusical problem in Mozart studies: there is no scarcity of authentic documents, but there is every reason to mistrust the veracity of those who produced them. Leopold Mozart was convinced that it was foolhardy and unsafe to write letters containing information someone might use against him. Some autographs have survived that end with postscripts intended for his wife alone, which she was supposed to detach and destroy; these reveal that the body of the letter consists of disinformation meant to mislead potential enemies. Wolfgang was undoubtedly aware of these tactics, and their usefulness was clearly not lost on him. It is unclear when he began deliberately to mislead his father, but his letters after the spring of 1781, when he moved to Vienna, obviously never reveal the unvarnished truth to anyone.

Soon after he was summoned to Vienna by Archbishop Colloredo, following the successful production of *Idomeneo* for Munich, Mozart provoked a quarrel with his hated employer. This naturally led to a breach that procured the composer's freedom as well as the additional "benefit" of never again being able to earn a living from music in his hometown. The resultant separation from Leopold was then secured in August 1782 by Wolfgang's marriage to Constanze Weber, the younger sister of his previous inamorata, Aloysia. Despite the romantic beauty of the love music of Mozart's contemporaneous opera *The Abduction from the Seraglio* (K. 384), the heroine of which is another Constanze, most biographers agree that his marriage was lacking in romantic passion. Many sources contend that Mozart was flagrantly unfaithful to his wife, and some believe that, toward the end of his life, she reciprocated in kind. All in all, this marriage of convenience seems mostly to have served the purpose of permanently alienating Leopold Mozart, whose unforgiving rancor about this betrayal permeates all his subsequent letters.

Leopold Mozart's reaction to his son's emancipation and Wolfgang's Machiavellian manipulativeness in procuring his freedom from parental meddling suggest that their previous relationship may not have been as untroubled as the unfailingly positive tone of their comments about each other in all their correspondence might lead one to believe. Wolfgang invariably portrayed his father as a fount of wisdom and benevolence, not unlike the character of the wise Masonic leader, Sarastro, in *The Magic Flute*. Leopold, on the other hand, wrote all and sundry about his son, "the miracle" bestowed on Salzburg by a loving God. Leopold carefully compiled notes on his travels and made provision for the preservation of the letters written to a business associate from these concert tours starring Wolfgang. These measures were intended to form an archive to document a biography of his son he planned to write.

A dozen years of triumphs through his child prodigy, from the time the six-year-old pianist climbed into the lap of the empress Maria Theresa to receive her kiss until the production of *La Finta Giardiniera* (K. 196) for the elector of Bavaria just before Wolfgang's nineteenth birthday, erased the distinction in Leopold's mind between his own achievements and the great musician he had nurtured. After a successful concert, he was capable of writing to the same business associate, "I made" so much money. No doubt, over the years, this illegitimate appropriation of his accomplishments became unacceptable to Wolfgang, necessitating the complex maneuvers that led him to stay in Vienna while Leopold was forced to stick to his mediocre position in Salzburg. It would seem that, in *The Magic Flute*, Leopold was a model not only for Sarastro but also for the stifling Queen of Night—it is she, after all, who provides the opera's protagonist with the magic flute.[5]

In my judgment, the decisive turning point in Mozart's feelings about his father occurred when Wolfgang met Aloysia in Mannheim, shortly after he began his sexual liaison with his cousin. It has often been noted that the relationship with Aloysia began on the highest plane of romantic idealism and that the scatological letters to Maria Anna Thekla were written at the very time when Mozart's passion for his musical protégée, Aloysia, blossomed. Perhaps we may compare the manner in which Wolfgang emotionally split these realms of experience to the contrast between the two pairs of lovers in *The Magic Flute:* his aspiration to marry Aloysia, whose actual character he was completely unable to see, resembled Tamino's chaste love for the princess Pamina; Mozart's simultaneous affair with his boisterous cousin is echoed in the earthy relations between the bird catcher Papageno and his Papagena. The duet that marks their successful mating, in the course of which they alternate in calling out each other's names, like a pair of lovebirds, is prefigured in passages from Wolfgang's letters to his newfound sexual partner: "Why not?—Strange! I don't know why I shouldn't—Well then—you will do me this favor.—Why not?—Why should you not do it?—Why not?—Strange! I shall do the same for you, when you want me to. Why not? Why should I not do it for you? Strange! Why not!—I can't think why not?"

Mozart's all-but-conscious awareness that Papageno represents a vital aspect of his own being may be confirmed by an incident he related in a letter to his wife, early in October 1791: "During Papageno's aria with the glockenspiel I went behind the scenes, as I felt a sort of impulse today to play it myself. Well, just for fun, at the point where Schikaneder [who sang Papageno] has a pause, I played an arpeggio. He was startled, looked behind the wings and saw me. When he had his next pause, I played no arpeggio. This time he stopped and refused to go on. I guessed what he was thinking and again played a chord. He then struck the glockenspiel and said '*Shut up.*' Whereupon everyone laughed." We could get no clearer indication that Mozart was asserting that *he* was Papageno and that only he could play the magical instruments of the Queen of Night.

Mozart's coaching catapulted the sixteen-year-old Aloysia Weber into instant operatic stardom—a brilliant singing career that included the roles of Donna Anna in *Don Giovanni* (K. 527) and of Constanze in *The Abduction* and that, in uncanny fashion, came to an end shortly after Mozart's death, a dozen years later.[6] Mozart spelled out his fantasy about a future joined to that of Aloysia in a letter of 1778 to his father: he wanted to be her accompanist and to take her on a concert tour of Italy! In other words, he wished to turn the passive experience of being an adolescent prodigy under the tutelage of a benign dictator into its active counterpart.

In psychoanalytic terms, we may conclude that Wolfgang loved Aloysia on a narcissistic basis. In his unconscious, she represented his infantile self, to be protected and promoted by a loving tutor—without exploitation! We can hardly fault Aloysia for sidestepping such a suffocating embrace, however greatly we may wish to support the claims of a genius for the emotional sustenance he would claim from those around him. We may note in this connection that, in *The Magic Flute,* Pamina does accept Sarastro's tutelage, abandoning that of her stifling mother, the Queen of Night; but her personal life is tied to that of someone other than this tutor, the hero Tamino. Perhaps at age thirty-five, facing imminent death, Mozart was finally able to reconcile himself to the impossibility of his desire for Aloysia. Or did he still wish that a Sarastro had been available to him so that he might have preserved his idealism about women?

In either case, it cannot be a coincidence that the music he wrote for *The Magic Flute* had a unique personal significance for Mozart. In July 1791, in the most emotionally revealing passage in his entire correspondence, he wrote his wife: "I can't describe what I have been feeling—a kind of emptiness, which hurts me dreadfully—a kind of longing, which is never satisfied, which never ceases, and which persists, nay, rather increases daily. . . . If I go to the piano and sing something out of my opera, I have to stop at once, for this stirs my emotions too deeply. Basta! [enough]." I assume that this unparalleled breakthrough of uncontrolled affect was stimulated by memories of the crucial adolescent experiences stirred by working on *The Magic Flute.*

These experiences ended in the worst manner possible, for Aloysia Weber's decisive rejection of his offer of marriage, in Munich, early in January 1779, took Mozart entirely by surprise. He had last seen the girl ten months earlier, in Mannheim, and in the interval she had obtained a superb position at the court of the elector of Bavaria and no longer needed Mozart's assistance. In Mannheim, she had done nothing to discourage Wolfgang's interest in her, so that he understood the apparent change in her attitude as proof of her duplicity. *Così fan tutte,* as Mozart and his Italian librettist, da Ponte, cynically put it a decade later—"women are like that."

I think we may assume that Wolfgang's initial reaction consisted of the painful emptiness, the ceaseless frustrated longing that recurred when he was composing *The Magic Flute*. His bitterness sometimes found a voice in his letters in brief references to Aloysia's treachery. Unconsciously, he seems to have hungered for revenge in the form of Don Juanism: even if we cannot be certain that Mozart actually led the life of a successful libertine, his understanding of the implacable determination of a Don Giovanni to persist in his mistreatment of women bears witness to the depth of his outrage. In *The Magic Flute*, this attitude is represented by the evil figure of the would-be rapist Monostatos—a personification of sadistic lust.

Of course, in waking life Mozart did not play the role of a stage villain, but he did give Aloysia's sister Constanze a hard time after their marriage through his unreliability, in both financial and sexual matters.[7] His actual adult persona came closer to that "amorous butterfly," the adolescent page Cherubino, than to any of his other operatic characters, and he generally veiled his emotions through the rococo cynicism prevalent in his da Ponte libretti. Having been exploited by his father through his adolescence and by the only woman he could ever idealize at the threshold of adulthood, he became the exploiter in turn, abusing all his friends and relations through attitudes of entitlement and a ruthless manipulativeness.

The story of Mozart's escalating delinquencies after the death of his father in the spring of 1787 is widely familiar. What needs to be emphasized here is the significance of the fact that, despite the actual distance between father and son, both literal and metaphoric, Leopold's very existence seems to have restrained Wolfgang from the wild improvidence that characterized the last four years of his life. The historian Uwe Krämer believes that Mozart became an inveterate gambler (Hildesheimer 1982, p. 184). Whatever the truth may be in this regard, there is no doubt that Wolfgang wasted astonishing amounts of money and ran up enormous debts, mostly by borrowing from indulgent friends. Recent biographers have agreed that his behavior during these difficult years was unacceptable by any standard; from a psychiatric perspective, it can only be called psychopathic. Yet, Mozart the composer went from strength to strength at the same time.[8]

To put the matter differently, vicissitudes in his personal life generally did not seem to influence Mozart's productivity or the quality of his music. If he went through one period of relative apathy, this occurred immediately after Aloysia jilted him. In 1779 and much of 1780, he produced only a half dozen works—but, as I have already mentioned, some of these for the first time achieved the supreme quality of his greatest music. Mozart's adolescence was filled with creative activity; his best works of those years would do honor to any other composer and are put in the shade only by the miracles of his maturity.[9] In other words, the never-to-be-healed disappointments Wolfgang suffered at the conclusion of his adolescence affected his music only in terms of its content: the composer's hidden melancholy, always cloaked under a seamless facade of elegance, jesting, courtly *galanterie,* or cynicism, lent its ambiguous character to much of his music. W. B. Yeats asked, "Can you separate the dancer from the dance?" I do not believe we can separate Wolfgang from his music.

Nowhere does the duality of Mozart's personality—the poignant depths screened by a surface smooth as silk—show itself more clearly than in his works for the stage. After all, his music is always completely appropriate for the text; the latter, therefore, provides us clues to the composer's message that are lacking in his instrumental compositions. The lack of moral commitment in Mozart's operas, particularly those on da Ponte libretti, was explicitly repudiated by his Romantic successors, such as Beethoven and Wagner. Indeed, it is difficult to grasp that Mozart does not wholeheartedly endorse the psychopathy of Don Giovanni, that "soul of ice" (*anima di bronzo*), as Leporello calls him, or the corrosive cynicism of that evil spirit, the Don Alfonso of *Così Fan Tutte*—that his complex philosophy was forged in response to the wounds of his adolescence. In *The Marriage of Figaro,* the other side of his nature found its voice in Cherubino's virginal apostrophe to Love, "Voi chi sapete," or the Countess Almaviva's laments about disappointed expectations, "Dove sono" and "Porgi amor." The tragic aura of Mozart's G minor masterpieces, the Quintet (K. 516) and the Symphony no. 40 (K. 550), to mention only the most celebrated examples, seems to convey a similar message.

Conclusions

From a psychoanalytic standpoint, we feel uneasy about attributing the crystallization of an unfortunate character structure to emotional vicissitudes at the threshold of adulthood. If the exploitation of Mozart's genius by his father or his first beloved proved to be crucial events that curdled his personality, we are tempted to postulate the occurrence of early childhood traumata that foreshadowed these adolescent troubles. Indeed, such predisposing transactions may well have taken place, but we have no specific information about the first six years of Wolfgang's life, those preceding the family concert tours that impelled Leopold Mozart to compile a written record about his prodigious son. Reports of Wolfgang's docility and sunny disposition as a boy virtuoso may very well be the stuff of legend—we simply do not know.

We do have reliable accounts of Mozart's cool reaction to the death of his mother—his expression of conventional clichés barely masking total indifference. Perhaps he had merely grown away from her through the long years of absence and the intrusive tutelage of his father. Perhaps his affability hid the resentment of a child exposed for financial gain to the hazards of the life of a vagabond. Perhaps his earliest years were marked by other injuries to his self-esteem. It is difficult to imagine the stolid Frau Mozart as the prototype of the brilliant coloratura of the Queen of Night, but she may have been capable of unsuspected emotional intensity when she gave birth to Wolfgang after five of her previous children had died. Mozart's ultimate representation of an elemental matriarch may, after all, allude to a terrifying maternal image from a past he could recapture only at the threshold of his own death.

NOTES

1. Mozart's works have been assigned numbers in a catalog originally prepared by Ludwig von Köchel; hence, they are conventionally referred to by "K." numbers.

2. In addition to Hildesheimer's (1982) superb, psychoanalytically sophisticated book, it is worth noting Blom (1972) and Sadie (1983).

3. Quotations from the correspondence of Mozart and his father are taken from Anderson (1966), with the exception of Mozart's letter to his cousin, which was published in Hildesheimer (1982).

4. To be precise, in 1785 Mozart produced the Piano Concerti in D Minor (K. 466) and in C (K. 467), the String Quartets in A (K. 464) and in C (K. 465), and the Piano Sonatas in B-flat Major (K. 454) and in C Minor (K. 457).

5. It has long been doubted that E. Schikaneder deserves sole credit for the libretto of the opera. After the demise of the others concerned, a member of Schikaneder's troupe named Giesecke claimed to have

written much of it. I am suggesting that Mozart may have had more to do with the book than has ever been generally believed; we do know that he always took an unusually active part in devising the final text of his operas.

6. We have witnessed a similar phenomenon in our time, that of the strange career of the great dramatic soprano Maria Callas, whose unparalleled power on the stage began and ended with her relationship to her husband, the Italian industrialist Meneghini.

7. Mozart's hostility to his wife was also manifested through his inability to finish any of the numerous compositions he undertook at her behest. Although most of these pieces were of no great significance, they include that magnificent torso, the Mass in C Minor (K. 427), which was performed in Salzburg with Constanze as a soloist on the occasion of the Mozarts' only visit to his family and birthplace, in October 1783.

8. In this period, Mozart created his last three symphonies (K. 543, 550, 551), *Eine Kleine Nachtmusik* (K. 525), the last piano concerto, in B-flat Major (K. 595), the Clarinet Concerto (K. 622), the Clarinet Quintet (K. 581), the String Quintets (K. 575, 589), the Sonatas in F Major (K. 533) and in D Major (K. 576), the Requiem Mass (K. 626), *Don Giovanni* (K. 527), *Così Fan Tutte* (K. 588), *La Clemenza di Tito* (K. 621), and *The Magic Flute* (K. 620).

9. Especially notable are the Symphonies in G Minor (K. 183) and in A Major (K. 201), the Violin Concerti, particularly the one in A Major (K. 219), the Bassoon Concerto (K. 191), the Piano Sonatas for the electress Palatine (K. 301–306), the Piano Sonata in C Major (K. 296), and the Piano Concerti in B-flat Major (K. 238) and in E-flat Major (K. 271).

REFERENCES

Anderson, E., ed. and trans. 1966. *The Letters of Mozart and His Family.* New York: St. Martin's.
Blom, E. 1974. *Mozart.* London: Dent.
Esman, A. 1951. Mozart: a study in genius. *Psychoanalytic Quarterly* 20:603–612.
Hildesheimer, W. 1982. *Mozart.* New York: Farrar, Straus, Giroux.
Sadie, S. 1983. *The New Grove Mozart.* New York: Norton.

MASKED I GO FORWARD—PLAY RESEARCH
AND CREATIVITY: OVERVIEW

ROBERT HORAN

The title of this section is drawn from an essay by Paul Rabinow (1982) concerning Descartes. As Rabinow tells us, "Masked I Go Forward" was Descartes's motto. I find that it is as descriptive of recent play research as it is of reflexive anthropology. Indeed, Rabinow's discussion of the impossibility of a positivist anthropology draws on Descartes's life as an actor and a player. A playful motto seems appropriate both to the man we tend to think of as a consummate rationalist and to the ideas suggested in these chapters. "Mask" suggests doubleness, fictive selves, semblance as well as dissemblance—and such a concern echoes throughout these papers. "Forward" picks up the argument used by Brian Sutton-Smith (1966) in his exchange with Piaget—namely, that play is constitutive as well as assimilatory. Both the masking and the going forward shape and, if you will, disfigure the "I"—an "I" who is perhaps more of a player than a cogitator.

The first paper in this section, Brian Sutton-Smith's "Creativity and the Vicissitudes of Play," provides a history of ideas about play and adolescence. Sutton-Smith, the prolific and well-known student of children's play and folklore, has made many contributions to these fields, but one of his most stubborn points is that the idea of play in the West has been constructed of various layers of idealization. It certainly is not new to suggest that ideas have histories, but, perhaps because of the idealization that Sutton-Smith has drawn our attention to, the idea of play as ahistorical and even atemporal persistently survives in both popular and elite lore. One of Sutton-Smith's central contributions, then, has been to deconstruct ideas about play and to describe how we often discuss our own motives and desires when we allegedly discuss play. Sutton-Smith explores three associations of play and adolescence and identifies each association with a writer. He finds in Erik Erikson an elaboration of the notion that play projects and reflects an inner reality; in G. Stanley Hall he discovers the conception of play as a process of organizing primitive intrapsychic and evolutionary elements; and in Margaret Mead he locates an association of play with sexuality. Sutton-Smith explicitly relates each of these associations with Romanticism—a philosophical position that not only encourages such associations but also encourages the author's efforts to claim "epistemological priority" for play. He is concerned with several of the Romantic metaphors for play, which have been used to explain adolescence. Underlying his analyses is an argument for the "epistemological priority" of play, for what he describes in one passage as "the vision of a world in which the members are consumed with the internal and passionate truths of games." Here, the author draws our attention to "the play of the streets," the texture of actual lives, as what gets left out of idealized conceptions of play. His implication is that the actual lives of adolescence are similarly obscured by idealization. Sutton-Smith's paper concludes with a sobering assessment of our chances for comprehending either adolescence or play as they are actually lived, given our history of attraction to Romantic ideas. This chapter brings the approach of the history of ideas to a topic that for many of us has ceased to be a problem. To paraphrase Bertrand Russell's remark to Whitehead, Sutton-Smith is to be commended for not attempting to deceive us about the "great obscurity" of this problem.

John L. Caughey's chapter is based on the author's research on "imaginary social worlds" (Caughey 1984). His essay offers us a remarkable way to consider one genre of fantasy. While the symbolic interactionists in sociology, following George Herbert Mead, have made us aware of the power of our social relations in forming our beliefs, attitudes, and conduct, Caughey has turned from the world of external social others to internal ones. While it is a commonplace that our identities are shaped—all arguments seem to be about the degree to which this occurs—by our relations with family, friends, strangers, coworkers, and so forth, Caughey suggests that we also have social relations with people we not only do not know but who may be entirely fictional. In his chapter we meet individuals to whom Laverne and Shirley, Baretta, and Alan Alda are "significant others." Although Caughey does not diminish the possibilities for frame breakdown, for "going too far" with these relations, one of his most important con-

302

tributions is to show that this is a social phenomenon and that it cannot be wholly accounted for as individual pathology. Caughey's argument is essentially a humanistic one—his chapter is an attempt to persuade the reader of the power of fictions and of art in our real-life efforts "to play with the possibilities of self." As clinicians, teachers, and all who regularly deal with adolescents know, "the range of possibilities of self" for adolescents seem at times to be overwhelming. Caughey's essay presents us with information about a significant way in which adolescents try on and try out possibilities.

Diana Kelly-Byrne enters territory that will be familiar to those who use play in treatment settings. Kelly-Byrne describes an intensive research project with Helen, a seven-year-old girl. The author reminds us that, while research has suggested that children's play is different on their own territory than it is in school, laboratory, or clinic and, further, that play is different when it is engaged in than when it is merely observed, modeled, or diagnosed, there really are no studies that are based on these ideas. Therefore, the research that Kelly-Byrne reports on is unique. The chapter at hand recounts the phases of the play that Kelly-Byrne engaged in with Helen, and it attends to the shifting dynamics of their personal relationship as well. Kelly-Byrne argues that Helen uses the sanctioned, literary medium of play to mask her exploration of personal and relational issues. Here, play—as story—is shown not merely to reflect the child's already crystallized concerns but as a means by which the child learns of and contends with those concerns. This chapter will surely be of interest to those who still believe that play is merely a projection of desire and dread.

Jay Mechling presents his chapter as a thought experiment about the nature of cheating and its relation to play and creativity, especially in adolescents. Mechling's investigation begins with the understanding that cheating is wholly contextual. In this way, he joins cheating to the class of context-dependent activities, which includes play and creativity. As in the other papers in this section, Mechling is less concerned with producing creativity from play than he is with understanding both as transformational processes that permeate social life. Mechling offers us eight ways to look at cheating that range from the conventional "cheating is a sin" to the Batesonian notion that "cheating is a member of the class of actions called 'transcontextual syndromes,' which also includes play and creativity." His interdisciplinary approach to this problem includes a number of examples from his extensive research.

Mechling's readings of cheating effectively destabilize cheating. The variety of possibilities for interpreting cheating direct us toward the active, processive, and possibly creative dimensions of cheating. Certainly, he opens this problem in a way that our normative judgments infrequently do.

Robert Horan discusses the relationship between the playfighting of adolescent boys in a residential treatment center and the adult staff who care for and attempt to treat them. As a combined result of our cultural idealization of play and the staff's perception that social order is their most important job function, playfighting was regarded as a nuisance behavior until it was brought front and center in the form of a crisis. Horan looks at the invisibility of this play form, the process of learning to see it, and its structure. Horan concludes that the play of these emotionally disturbed young men is an important piece of their social life—and not as a rehearsal for adult functions or as a reflection of social or intrapsychic reality.

These chapters discuss several varieties of actual play. In the process we meet a number of players and get some idea of what it might mean to engage in such play. The idealization of play considered in Sutton-Smith's paper is so pervasive that it would be unwise to suggest that these essays have altogether avoided it. Nonetheless, the variety of subjects permits us to surround the problem, if not to penetrate it. Sutton-Smith interprets the history of the ideas associating play and adolescence; the papers by Caughey and Kelly-Byrne concern solitary and dyadic imaginative play; whereas the papers by Mechling and Horan have to do with more social and antistructural play forms. Throughout, there is argument against the notion of play as epiphenomenal and for the notion that play is constitutive as well as reflective of social life. As those who work with them are well aware, adolescents often argue against those who would confine them to a "stage," to a developmental step. While what he or she actually is may be inchoate, most adolescents are passionately aware that they are something. Acknowledgment of this is invariably the first step in helping those who are in some way troubled.

REFERENCES

Caughey, J. 1984. *Imaginary Social Worlds: A Cultural Approach.* Lincoln: University of Nebraska Press.

Rabinow, P. 1982. Masked I go forward: reflections on the modern subject. In J. Ruby and B. Myerhoff, eds. *A Crack in the Mirror: Reflexive Perspectives in Anthropology.* Philadelphia: University of Pennsylvania Press.

Sutton-Smith, B. 1966. Piaget on play: a critique. *Psychological Review* 73:104–110.

18   CREATIVITY AND THE
VICISSITUDES OF PLAY

BRIAN SUTTON-SMITH

My task is to illuminate the role of play in the confluence of creativity
and adolescence. As adolescence can be argued to begin and perhaps
continue with nineteenth-century Romanticism, my first play concept
at that historical point is that of the young and passionate John Keats
(1795–1821), for whom, along with many others of his time, a central
term, the imagination, incorporated the notions of free play and artistic
creativity. Furthermore, according to his colleague, Samuel Taylor
Coleridge, these states of mind were to be found most prominently in
the minds of youths. Play, creativity, imagination, and youthfulness
were, therefore, overlapping concepts all very much idealized within
the discourse of that time and all having to do with the way in which
poets could capture, through the free play of their imagination, states
of being from earlier historical periods. We have the paradox that the
Romantics used history in order to define themselves against the changes
of the industrial, urban, and political revolutions, just as it may be
contended that we use our own adolescence today, in part, to define
ourselves. They idealized prior history in their reach for cultural stability, just as we may, perhaps, idealize or seek to control phases of
human growth within our own reach for personal stability.

The first concept of play, then, to be disentangled for our understanding of adolescence stresses that play is a kind of imagination or
creativity. But first, just in case you find nothing unusual in this identification, I must remind you that the dominant kind of play that was
actually available at the time and place that these philosophers and

poets were engaged in their philosophical discourse was festival play, which consisted largely of rough and crude forms of aggression, sociability, and sexuality. There was bear baiting, bull baiting, football, country dances, jugglers, minstrels, tumbling, wrestling, dancing dogs, mummings and masquerades, bowling, skittles, cockfighting, dice and chess, racing, and hunting, to give a few lusty examples. As one authority has put it, it is not hard to believe that the people of the times enjoyed witnessing the pain of others, inflicting pain on others, and experiencing pain themselves in the name of play. Clearly, this was not the kind of play that the philosopher Kant had in mind when he identified free play as that essential intermediary between sensory experience and formal reasoning through which the imaginative grasp of reality was formed (Warnock 1978). Nor was it the kind of play that Friedrich Schiller (1795) could have had in mind in his quote about a man being a man in the full sense of the word only when he plays. Kant, Schiller, Coleridge, and Keats were talking only of some kinds of philosophical or poetic "play" of the imagination. They were ignoring the play of the streets, which appears to get no reference at all in their writings, except, perhaps, in the occasional mention of "mere play" as compared with "good play."

How, then, has the association of play, imagination, and the arts fared in our own times? We know that they were identified as the same activity by Spencer, who introduced this association into English-speaking social scientific discourse. As he said, "Play and art are the same activity because neither subserves in any direct way the processes conducive to life and neither refers to ulterior benefits. The proximate ends are their only ends" (Spariosu 1982, p. 29). It is still commonplace among modern popular books on child care to find the authors treating all children's forms of free expression, including their art activity, as play. In his classic *Education through Art,* Read (1943) defends the proposition that play is a form of art, in contradistinction to Margaret Lowenfeld's (1935) earlier statements that art is a form of play. Either way, the association continued.

Despite the popularity of this association over 200 years, it has not received much support from those few philosophers and psychologists who have dealt with it at all rigorously. Philosophers in the "expressive" traditions of art—for example, Bosanquet, Croce, and Collingwood—who might be most expected to identify the two do not do so. Nor is the association maintained by the post-Kantian philosophers

Cassirer, Langer, and Goodman, who have considered the relation. As Cassirer (1944) says, "In play as in art we leave behind us our immediate practical needs in order to give our world new shape. But this analogy is not sufficient to prove a real identity" (p. 163). Berlyne (1960), Gardner (1982), and Groos (1901), among the few psychologists who have carefully considered the matter, also avoid the identification.

On the other hand, if we attempt to unite play with creativity rather than with art, there has been considerable consensus that the two should be associated. Since the 1960s, there have been correlational (Lieberman 1979) and experimental (Pepler and Rubin 1982) studies in which linkages appear to have been established. Furthermore, play literature from the evolutionary tradition, which suggests that animals needing more flexible adaptations are likely to play more, have been used in support of these associations (Bruner 1972). Unfortunately, more recent and careful experimental work seems to suggest that many of the results in these studies may have occurred as a result of experimenter bias or tutorial effects (Simon and Smith 1985). So, despite the inherent good sense that the variability that characterizes play and the variability that characterizes creativity might well be related, current evidence is not very supportive. In sum, play and art and play and creativity, for all their historical conflation, have not so far been very profitable empirical couplings.

The remaining association, between play and imaginative activity, is the only one of the Romantic conflations that appears to be in good health. The studies of Jerome and Dorothy Singer (1981) show that playful children who are also imaginative have decided advantages over children who are not imaginative. They are indeed the superior beings that Schiller had in mind. The children are less aggressive, more capable of concentration in schoolwork, less troubled, and happier; they have better self-control and better reality discrimination; and their verbalizations are richer in metaphoric creativity. Their focus on play as a form of imaginativeness finds agreement among the play researchers of early childhood who have also centered most of their play analysis on pretense, finding that easier to observe reliably than other kinds of play. I need mention only the work of the two leading play researchers, Greta Fein (1986) and Katherine Garvey (1977), by way of illustration.

So, we may ask, why has the association between play and art, or play and creativity, fared poorly and that between play and the imagination fared relatively well? My best intuition here is that the Romantic tradition is alive and well in modern play theory and that it is this tradition that has kept alive the basic synthesis of play and the imagination. The synthesis of play and art or play and creativity has been more troubled in those few minor spots where it has been thought about or investigated with any thoroughness. The immediate practical reason why imagination has had this advantage, I believe, has been its connection with play therapy and the depth psychological disciplines that have governed that practical therapeutic form. For, in play therapy, the basic concern is with mediating the child's fantasy life through outward symbols and, if possible, making a transfer from the play symbols of inward life to the verbal symbols of inward life and, therefore, to the normal processes of psychotherapy. The message of the greatest of play theorists of this kind, Erik Erikson (1963), is that the inner life is retrievable through play and, furthermore, that the inner life as trust, autonomy, industry, identity, and so on is what human growth is all about. For Erikson, the greatest challenge for the adolescent is in his or her internal synthesis of personal and social processes. As he has said, "Maybe the fact that I am an immigrant to this country made me feel that the problem of identity holds a central position in the disturbances we encounter today. . . . I had changed nationalities. . . . I faced one of those important redefinitions that a man has to make who has lost his landscape and his language and with it all the 'references' on which his first sensory and sensual impressions and thus some of his conceptual images were based. Migration can do that" (quoted in Evans 1967, p. 41).

What I am leading to is that perhaps the relation between imagination and play established by the Romantics was itself underlain by something more fundamental in the Western world—the increased concern first with individuality, later with alienation, and then with inward life. For Romanticism, in contrast to the Enlightenment, is an insistence that the world be subjectively and personally considered, not just objectively and rationally considered. In these terms, the modern preoccupation in psychology with solitary play (as in most play therapy, in most play experiments, and in toys for children who watch television by themselves) is a continuance of this larger traditional interest in alienation and inwardness. In these terms, we are all migrants and adolescents.

The recent definition of play by Rubin, Fein, and Vandenberg (1983) as being intrinsically motivated, being an area of freedom from externally imposed rules, being guided by organism-dominated questions, and being active not passive is couched in terms that might appeal to Keats and at the same time shows the subsumption of modern play theory by the larger Romantic, Western tradition. Those kinds of social play that are cruel and barbarous but that as a child you would rather be a part of than left out, that are hardly voluntary or autonomous even when they are most exciting, that both Rabelais and Bakhtin (Bakhtin 1984) have spoken of with some fervor, and that people like the Opies (1985) continue to record in modern life, all those are entirely ignored by this modern definition just as they were by Keats and Schiller, Kant and Coleridge. So I must conclude this first section by suggesting that the interpretation of play as imaginative provides a romantic or idealistic gloss, serving probably to support that trend toward the solitary imaginative life that is increasingly functional to the kind of civilization we have constructed. Adolescents with their supposedly enhanced inwardness and potentially playful imaginativeness become, themselves, symbolic of the kinds of mental life that will be functional for those who run our electronic futures. Adolescents and imaginative players are a fiction that we think we desperately need. In sum, I have reduced the search for play in adolescence and the continuing conflation of play with imaginativeness to the more general pursuit of the nature of "inwardness" in modern civilization, an inwardness we can recognize in the character of our novels from *Tom Jones* to *Portrait of the Artist as a Young Man*. Our state of affairs is often poignantly symbolized by such novelists, who would rather have the last word than the last friendship. When inwardness or alienation are thus both our power and our disease, it is perhaps not surprising that our cultural definitions of play, creativity, and adolescence reflect those passions. The marginal adolescent embodies for us this inner dilemma of our desire for private creativity as a response to systemic cultural alienation.

Play as Power (or as Order or as Disorder)

What is omitted from this discussion, as from that of Keats to this point, is the play of the streets. This more powerful kind of play was not encountered within modern intellectual traditions until Darwin's theory of evolution and Spencer's, who attempts the fusion of Darwin and Keats. What he and others after him had to deal with were largely the rough games and cruel forms of play that characterized the activity of children and adolescents, particularly in the nineteenth century, when so many of these youths, in America often immigrants, congregated in urban streets and carried on their feisty ethnic activities. There were various ways of doing this. For Stanley Hall, the theory of recapitulation provided a way to think of forms of folk play as an inheritance of more primitive times, which, if permitted their exercise, would lead in due course to their desuetude and to the emergence by adolescence of the potentially rational being. Hall was a progressive in supporting movements for childhood play, playgrounds and apparatuses, swings and roundabouts, that would rid the child of primitive simian urges. For others, the metaphor for controlling savages at play was not so much this evolutionary manipulation as it was the colonial manipulation of bringing them into playgrounds where they could be under mainstream American control and learn the benefits of character and cooperation that could be brought to them through organized exercises and through baseball and football (Goodman 1979). In each case, play was seen as a dangerous kind of child and adolescent power that, if brought under organized control, could serve the larger purposes of society for the development of leadership or for the domestication of the unruly. For Hall the conservative, however, those children who had been rid of their atavisms could become a superior race (*sic*), leading the rest of mankind to a higher level of civilization (Grinder and Strickland 1963). Hall's notion of the manipulation of the play of adolescents to create leaders and followers was central to the various forms of what we now know as the Boy Scouts, the YMCA, and the European "Youth" movements that flourished early in the century and to the various more explicitly fascist and elitist youth organizations that succeeded them in postwar European countries. It is not far wrong, in fact, to suggest that the organization of sports has become a major effort at political control in all modern nations, whether conducted with adolescents in their high schools or with adult persons through professional and international as well as Olympic forms of sport.

What this has lead to in the past twenty years is a clear bifurcation of play as imagination from play as games and sports. Those who deal with children in the contained worlds of nursery schools and laboratories can think of their play largely in terms of pretense and fantasy, while those who deal with them in high schools can seldom think of their play in that way. Instead, they must deal with the constant insurgence of obscene play, humor, pranks, graffiti, verbal dueling, insults, slang, mooning, cruising, necking, drinking, mocking laughter, and sexual exploits, which are a very few of the innumerable unrecognized folk play forms found at that age level. Remember, for example, that adolescents delight in humor that parodies childhood but then try to say that it is not play and that teachers should not try to control it:

Little Miss Muffet, sat on her tuffet, eating her curds and whey.
Along came a spider, and sat down beside her, and said, What's in the bowl bitch?

or,

Mary had a little lamb, the Doctor was surprised.
But when Macdonald had a farm, the Doctor nearly died.

No wonder, then, that the major mass meaning of play in this century to most adults is sports. The major function of sports or other forms of play for adolescents has been to bring them under some kind of social control. The alternative is graffiti and obscenity. It is not surprising, also, that many of us, in order to retain our idealization of play, prefer to think that organized adolescent leisure activities are not play at all, that they are something else. We reject sports, we reject gambling and games of chance, and we reject war games in our efforts to stay with the idealizations of Kant, Schiller, Coleridge, and Keats. But clearly, as far as the study of adolescence is concerned, such ivory tower views of play are of limited use. Play is a form of power as well as of imagination (see Berne 1964; Goffman 1959; Maccoby 1976). Play has to do with power, and it is used all the time by a variety of social, political, and commercial agencies to manipulate others who are made vulnerable by their need for it. Indeed, it is, perhaps, the very alienating characteristics of such organized play that make us so desperate to find that the more idealized and imaginative mind is still alive in the adolescent heart.

Play as Passion

There is one more kind of play to bring into association with adolescence, and that is sex play. As already indicated, adolescent obscenities and jokes are largely about sex, and so is much of their ordinary conversation and verbal play. Their folklore is rife with sex, whether in terms of panty raids, snapping bras, mooning, dances, necking, automobile antics, cruising, or more symbolic activities. Spacks (1981) speaks of sex as "nobody's power," that is, as dealt with by constant denial. She says, "Sex focuses the true issue, defines the crucial power—a fact denied, avoided, transformed; the central fact of adolescence" (p. 19). For his part, Keats's clearly imaginative and reputedly culturally archetypal poems are themselves replete with the passion of implicit sexuality. There is the Indian maid who has been cheated by a shadowy wooer from the clouds but forgets him as fornicating Bacchus and his merry crew, their faces all aflame, come dancing madly through the pleasant valley, rushing into the folly to join them. Or there is the "Ode to Psyche," in which the two fair creatures (who do indeed represent the philosophical principles of poetry and philosophy) "lay calm-breathing on the bedded grass; / Their arms embraced, and their pinions too." Throughout his poems, there is a constant alternation between melancholy and inebriation, with beauty described mostly in terms of natural phenomena but partly also in hints of youthful bodies, mouths, tongues, and so on. The storm and stress is under way.

Just as I have chosen Erikson to symbolize our interest in play as a kind of inwardness in our pursuit of the nature of adolescence and Hall to represent play as a kind of organization and socialization of adolescence, it is not unfitting to choose Mead (1928) as the keystone for considering play as a kind of sexuality. She brought back from Samoa the idyll that it was possible to escape storm and stress in adolescence—that sexual activity was played at by the very young and that liaisons of all kinds were typical of adolescence. She said that there was a laid back, easy-going attitude toward sexuality and that sexual permissiveness was the norm. Furthermore, she maintained, it was the role of the anthropologist to bring such examples back to the mainland as models of behavioral alternatives. Her accomplishment in doing so was lauded at the time as a discovery that the free union of the sexes was the fundamental sexual reality by such intellectual giants as Russell and Ellis. One hundred years after Keats, the long struggle to change attitudes toward adolescent sexuality reached its fruition in her work and paralleled the actual changes in American sexuality, the greatest shift in which occurred after World War I, according to Kinsey. Since Freeman's (1983) critique and various rebuttals, we are no longer sure whether Mead's female adolescent informants were giving her only a portion of the truth, as her daughter asserts (Bateson 1984), were teasing her cruelly, as Freeman (1983) claims, or were led into giving her what she really wanted to hear. Given that so much of our cultural intellectual space is spent with attempts to preclude adolescent sexuality, drug use, abortion, and delinquency, it is perhaps not surprising that we actually know very little about adolescent sexual play except for the multicolored hints occasionally yielded by folklorists and novelists. Nevertheless, along with play as fantasy and as power, it is clearly one of the major ways in which adolescence is characterized. Yet, along with play as power, play as passion is kept in the background of our consciousness of adolescence, by our "Panglossian" fever over play as creativity and imagination.

Conclusions

I have attempted to show a few of the ways in which thoughts about play and about adolescence have intersected in our cultural history and have chosen the names of Erikson, Hall, and Mead as central figures in illustrating these conflations. I think the focus of each of these theorists—on imagination or inwardness in Erikson's case, on power and its control in Hall's case, or on sex and its freedom in Mead's case—is as much a general cultural concern, an adult concern, as it is a description of adolescence. One could make a case from all this, as many have, that our adolescent psychologies, as illustrated here, are in a large part a projection of our own adult ambivalences about these phenomena. It would certainly be legitimate to respond with the assertion that, although that might well be so, it is because the adolescents are the marginal people that Hall said they are that they are particularly susceptible to manifestations in some extreme of fantasy (which is what we call it when they use it), power, and sex and, therefore, to increasing our adult anxiety about matters that already cause us such ambivalence.

Underlying these relations of play and adolescence, however, there is the perhaps more fundamental epistemological point that historical Romanticism also introduces the cultural transformation that permits play to be even considered in the serious way that I am doing here. As Spariosu (1982) has suggested, what most characterizes that time is the shift from the 2,000-year hegemony of philosophy, logic, and science as describers of the real world and art, literature, and play as only their epiphenomena. Now, the latter instead become sought as roads to real human truth, or at least to spiritual human truth, which in Keats, as we have seen, is sought through poetry. Though later in the century others will seek it through the music and the visual arts, play is at first carried along in a kind of ancillary status by these other art forms and, as we have seen, is still today identified with them in some quarters. With the theory of evolution, it gains something of its own "scientific" status, not so much for its playfulness as a kind of epistemological truth, but for its supposed preparedness as a kind of adaptive and, therefore, scientifically established function. Hence, we have so much effort to show that play can be educational, that it can help solve problems. It must, however, be admitted that this ambivalence about play long precedes the theory of evolution characterizing the recommendations of Locke and his alphabet blocks as much as it does Papert and his computer. Playfulness as a kind of truth has probably gained as much from the symbolic anthropologists as from any other source. Geertz and his Balinese cockfighters, Turner and his liminal and liminoid zones of reality, Babcock and her rites of reversal, Azoy and his Afghanistan Busakshi on horseback, MacAloon and his Olympics, all have contributed mightily to the vision of a world in which the members are consumed with the internal and passionate truths of games—though, admittedly, even in some of this discourse, there is still the attempt to deny play its epistemological priority by showing that it is being examined largely as some kind of interpretive or cognitive scheme of things in the philosophical head of the investigator.

For most of us, what Romanticism did was permit play to become a metaphor for some of our deepest concerns, and I show how it has sometimes been used in relation to adolescence. I rather suspect that, with concepts that are as fuzzy as play and adolescence and in a world that is as systematically Cartesian as ours is, we may do little more than this. Given that we mostly automatically distrust the humanities (art, literature, and play) as bearers of true knowledge, then we must also automatically be unable to fathom the nature of adolescence. In conclusion, I hope that I may have made clear my general position that our frenzy over Keats and his kind is just one more way of screening out our apprehension about, and our deep involvement in, the dilemmas of alienation, power, and passion. These are the vicissitudes of interpretation when you attempt to use play to tell you something about creativity and adolescence. There is no science here, only immense cultural fiction.

REFERENCES

Bakhtin, M. 1984. *Rabelais and His World*. Bloomington: University of Indiana Press.

Bateson, M. C. 1984. *With a Daughter's Eye*. New York: Morrow.

Berlyne, D. C. 1960. *Conflict, Arousal and Curiosity*. New York: McGraw-Hill.

Berne, E. 1964. *Games People Play*. New York: Grove.

Bruner, J. 1972. Nature and uses of immaturity. *American Psychologist* 27(8): 1–22.

Cassirer, E. 1944. *Essay on Man*. New Haven, Conn.: Yale University Press.

Erikson, E. H. 1963. *Childhood and Society*. New York: Norton.

Evans, R. I. 1967. *Dialogue with Erik Erikson*. New York: Harper & Row.

Fein, G. 1986. The affective psychology of play. In A. W. Gottfried and C. C. Brown, eds. *Play Interactions*. Lexington, Mass.: Heath.

Freeman, D. 1983. *Margaret Mead and Samoa*. Cambridge, Mass.: Harvard University Press.

Gardner, H. 1982. *Developmental Psychology*. Boston: Little, Brown.

Garvey, K. 1977. *Play*. Cambridge, Mass.: Harvard University Press.

Goffman, E. 1959. *The Presentation of Self in Everyday Life*. New York: Doubleday.

Goodman, G. 1979. *Choosing Sides*. New York: Schocken.

Grinder, R. E., and Strickland, C. E. 1963. G. Stanley Hall and the social significance of adolescence. *Teachers College Record* 64:390–399.

Groos, K. 1901. *The Play of Man*. New York: Appleton, 1913.

Lieberman, N. 1979. *Playfulness: Its Relationship to Imagination and Creativity*. New York: Academic Press.

Lowenfeld, M. 1935. *Play in Childhood*. London: Gollancz.

Maccoby, M. 1976. *The Gamesman*. New York: Bantam.

Mead, M. 1928. *Coming of Age in Samoa*. London: Penguin.

Opie, I., and Opie, P. 1986. *The Singing Game*. London: Oxford University Press.

Pepler, D. J., and Rubin, K. H. 1982. The play of children: current theory and research. In *Contributions to Human Development,* vol. 6. New York: Karger.

Read, H. 1943. *Education through Art.* London: Faber.

Rubin, K.; Fein, G.; and Vandenberg, B. 1983. Children's play. In E. M. Hetherington, ed. *The Carmichael Handbook of Child Psychology.* New York: Wiley.

Schiller, F. 1795. *On the Aesthetic Education of Man.* New York: Ungar, 1965.

Simon, T., and Smith, P. K. 1985. Play and problem solving: a paradigm questioned. *Merill-Palmer Quarterly* 31(3): 265–277.

Singer, J. L., and Singer, D. G. 1981. *Television, Imagination and Aggression.* Hillsdale, N.J.: Erlbaum.

Spacks, P. 1981. *The Adolescent Idea.* New York: Basic.

Spariosu, M. 1982. *Literature, Mimesis, Play.* Tubingen: Gunter Narr.

Warnock, M. 1978. *Imagination.* Berkeley: University of California Press.

19 MASKING THE SELF: FICTIONAL IDENTITIES AND THE CONSTRUCTION OF SELF IN ADOLESCENCE

JOHN L. CAUGHEY

In "Masked I Go Forward," Rabinow (1982) expresses an idea that has considerable currency in contemporary social science, namely, that the self or identity is "fictive." This view is implied, of course, by the very title of his essay, which reminds us that our term "personality" is derived from the Latin word for "mask." Usually, the social science view of self as fictive is connected to the problem of cultural relativity. Different cultures, subcultures, and psychological theories contain different and often contradictory assumptions about the nature of the self. Enculturated into any one such system, the individual internalizes and thinks about himself or herself in terms of a conception of personality that is partial and relative, one interpretation among many—fictive (cf. Caughey 1980; Shweder and LeVine 1984).

In this chapter, I want to develop a different, although complementary, perspective on the process by which we construct fictive identities or masks for ourselves in adolescence. I will suggest, first, that the creative process of adolescent identity construction is directly analogous to and overlaps with the process by which novelists and scriptwriters create the fictional characters of novels and screenplays. I want to suggest, second, that there is another link here, that the imaginary characters of fictional worlds constitute a significant source from which adolescents—not to mention children and adults—create their so-called actual identities.

In our culture, with its strong emphasis on "individualism," one romantic image presents the creative writer as an isolated, totally original genius who magically conjures up fictive worlds through the unique power of his or her personal imagination. The persistence of this image is evident in literary criticism that may put down a particular fiction as "imitative" or "derivative." For example, W. P. Kinsella's new novel was recently criticized in a review by Eliot Aisnof (1986), who repeatedly used the phrase "shades of" to suggest that Kinsella had borrowed this or that character or theme from previous literature. "Imitative" is one devalued opposite to our image of the artist as creative.

In fact, of course, this individualistic image is a myth. Writers in our society—like those everywhere—can create only because of their thorough enculturation in the fictional worlds of their predecessors. As the mystery writer Raymond Chandler remarked, when asked about learning to write, "Analyze and *imitate;* no other school is necessary" (Gardiner and Walker 1962, p. 92; emphasis added). One important source for the creative work of any novelist is his or her familiarity with the fictional characters and situations of the field within which he or she works. In the most original writing, these fictional antecedents remain in the background. But even here their presence can be dimly felt. In more formulaic genres—such as detective or romance fiction—previous exemplars are obviously influential. One successful romance writer offers the following advice: "A budding author should read at least 100 romances in three weeks before she writes her first novel. Otherwise, she is wasting her time" (Mathias and Richey 1986). Thus, the characters of any "new" novel are likely to be quite recognizable versions of previous fictional beings. The extreme cases here are those in which the writer works directly with characters from earlier fiction. James Bond and Sherlock Holmes, for example, have "lived on," after their authors died, when later writers brought these characters back to life in their own fictions. One of my children is currently reading a *Star Wars* novel that openly presents itself as being "based on the characters and situations created by George Lucas," who in turn borrowed these stock characters from the fiction of his predecessors. Hollywood scriptwriters, too, often work out adventures for the characters of a series that was originated by someone else.

Whether the writer works with stock characters or not, how does the creative process actually work, how does the drama get written?

There is a good deal of mystification about how creative artists get their material; supernatural analogies—the mysterious muse, "inspiration," and so on—are unsatisfactory explanations. While the process is complex, some dimensions are clear enough. Along with a certain amount of analytic thinking, the creative process significantly depends on the imaging power of intuitive, right-brain thinking. In short, as Freud (1927) long ago observed, the novelist obtains much of his material through daydreaming or fantasizing, that is, through imaginatively experiencing it. External reality dims, and the novelist's mind is taken over by a world of inner imagery, sounds, sensations, and dialogue. The novelist needs to be able to tune into this capacity and may resort to a variety of external strategies in order to facilitate daydreaming. One scriptwriter I interviewed likes to write in a warm tub since this helps him "daydream" his characters through their paces. Another novelist and short-story writer says that the mindless routine of long automobile drives, necessary in his paying job, facilitates hours of useful daydreaming. In some cases, the artist feels like a spectator watching the characters perform, but, in other cases, he transforms his own being and, merging his own emotions with those of an imagined other, adopts the point of view of the character. As the mystery writer Elmore Leonard observes, "I become the characters. I immerse myself in them. I spend so much time thinking about my characters and developing my characters in my mind so that when I put 'em into action, and when I do their point of view, I know the person, I become the person" (Jolidon 1986, p. 5). Like an actor in a play, the writer temporarily drops his own identity and assumes that of a fictional character.[1]

At first glance, such creative processes might seem unique to the world of the artist. In fact, they are common to everyone—perhaps especially to adolescents. Like the creative novelist, the adolescent is busily fashioning identity through combining personal qualities with exemplars from the cultural environment. Often, as with the novelist, the models are fictional. My data here are drawn from my general study of imaginary experience (Caughey 1984). I will focus on thirty-nine young people, most of whom were college students in the early 1980s, who described to me their relationships with fictional beings.

As in the world of art, the American value of individualism sometimes leads to misconceptions about the uniqueness of the individual personality. As Phillip Slater (1976, p. 26) observes, a young person who "calls too obvious attention to the fact that learning is based almost entirely on imitation is ridiculed by being called a copycat or a monkey." Hence, the process of role modeling is often concealed, and people may be hesitant to admit its importance. However, if the area is approached carefully, a great deal of interesting information emerges.

It is well known, of course, that role modeling often involves imitation of real people in the individual's actual social world, such as parents, peers, and friends. But it is also apparent that adolescent identity is often significantly influenced by unmet figures outside the individual's actual social acquaintances. Asked to list people important to them that they had never met, the young people in my study readily listed hundreds of different figures. These included many real people, especially celebrities they were indirectly familiar with, such as rock stars, actors, talk show hosts, sports figures, politicians, and the like. Yet, mixed in with such real people, adolescents regularly listed purely fictional beings—television characters such as Magnum P.I., Pamela Ewing, Hawkeye Pierce, and Laura of "General Hospital"; characters from novels such as Scarlett O'Hara, Gandalf, and James Bond; movie characters such as those portrayed by Woody Allen, Clint Eastwood, and John Wayne; comic strip and cartoon figures such as Batman, Snoopy, Cathy, and Astroboy. A very large stock of imaginary characters inhabits the mind of the American adolescent. One might think that such fictive beings would be less significant than such real unmet figures as sports stars. This is not always the case. Two days after the space shuttle *Challenger* blew up, one of my colleagues at the University of Maryland asked his science fiction class to compare their reactions to this tragedy with the fictional events portrayed in the film they had just seen, *Star Trek II*. One young man noted that he "felt much worse" when the fictional character Spock died, that he cried when Spock died. "I didn't know the astronauts," he said, "but I *knew* Spock, I grew up with him."

The pseudointimacy of fictional portrayals often allows us to "know" a fictional being more deeply than we know real people—after all, we can observe them in their private and intimate moments, and we can know what they "really" feel and think. Furthermore, fictional figures are larger than life, untrammeled by human limitations, wants, and contradictions. They represent qualities and ways of being in a more clear-cut and dramatic way than do real people, known or unknown. The level of emotional orientation toward such unreal figures is often surprising. One informant spoke of a soap opera character as follows:

"He is one of the most self-centered, arrogant, selfish, uncaring persons I have ever come across. . . . I watch him with feelings of hatred. . . . I am overjoyed to see other characters beat him at his own game."

Adolescents know about and feel strongly toward fictional beings—they also become intimately involved with them through imaginary social interactions. This comes about in two major ways, both of which are analogous to the creative work of novelists and both of which are important to the construction of adolescent identities.

One major means of involvement is through the consumption of fictional productions, that is, through reading, attending plays, and watching electronic media such as television and movies. Suspension of disbelief allows the individual to enter an illusory, but vivid, imaginary world populated by swarms of fictive beings. If we analyze the psychological process involved, we find that the individual connects to these fictive beings by assuming a social role that links him or her to the beings of the drama. In the least intimate case, the individual retains his or her own identity and watches in the passive role of observer or voyeur. More commonly, he or she is drawn directly into the fictive world by assuming a participatory role. For example, one young woman spoke of her involvement with the male lead in the television series "Hart to Hart," as played by Robert Wagner. Jonathan, she says, "taps many of my needs. . . ." During the show, "[I] would place myself in his wife's role," thereby experiencing Jonathan's "rapport with his wife, affection, sharing of thoughts and experiences, total respect and admiration for her." In short, she imaginatively weds herself to a fictive being.

An even more common form of connection involves identification. The process closely parallels that in which the novelist assumes an imaginary identity during creative work as well as the method by which an actor temporarily puts on a fictive identity in order to act in a play. As one woman observed, "Reading the novels of Henry James at fifteen I experienced a miracle. . . . I was transformed into someone older, more beautiful and graceful" (Brownstein 1982, p. 5). In identification, the individual drops his or her actual identity, enjoys temporary amnesia, and becomes the hero or heroine of a fictive world.[2] By projecting his or her consciousness onto the fictive being, the individual feels the figure's fictitious emotions, endures his or her pseudotragedies, and enjoys his or her imaginary triumphs. This is how fictional media engage us—by transforming us into someone else. In this sense, we all experience multiple personalities—and delusionary ones at that. It should be emphasized that this is not just an occasional process in American socialization. By the age of sixteen, the average American has spent more time watching television than attending school.

Those who would downplay the importance of media effects sometimes argue that such "escapist" experiences are insignificant because they somehow "evaporate" from consciousness after the production is over. In fact, most research suggests that media experiences have important aftereffects (Roberts and Bachen 1981). For my purposes, the most interesting are those in which fictive beings leave the page of the book or the television or movie screen and enter the individual's consciousness after the fictional production is over. The most significant way this happens is through daydreaming. Creative writers daydream fictive characters through imaginary dramas; so, too, do adolescents. As various studies have shown, Americans in general, and adolescents in particular, spend a great deal of time in the imaginary worlds of daydreaming, that is, in the drifting semiconscious experience of memories, anticipations, and fantasies. In fact, any time the individual's attention is *not* taken up with demanding tasks, engrossing actual relationships, or absorbing media productions, attention is likely to drift away into the playlike worlds of daydreaming (cf. Caughey 1984). External reality dims, and the individual enters a private, playlike world characterized by inner imagery, emotions, imaginary action, and dialogue. All such worlds are fictive because they are imaginary experiences. Even a vivid memory, that is, a pseudoexperiencing of the actual past, is an imaginary and, probably, distorted version of what actually transpired. With anticipation and fantasy, we are in an even more obviously fictive territory. The beings one meets there are, of course, not one's actual friends and acquaintances but imaginary replicas of them. Often, however, these worlds are doubly fictive because the beings one meets in daydreams are imaginary versions of fictive beings.

In some instances, the individual recalls a fictional drama witnessed earlier through a novel or a movie. Occasionally, as in childhood, this may involve simultaneous inner recall and external acting out of the fictional experience. One informant was particulary moved by *White Line Fever,* a sadistic movie in which villains do in a good-guy trucker and his noble pregnant wife. For "months" after seeing the movie, she would fantasize various scenes in her room, particularly the one in which the bad guys punched the wife in the stomach. "I would actually fall back on the bed, doubling up with pain. The things I was imagining Jan [the fictional hero] saying always made me cry. Somehow he was hurting for me more than I was hurting for myself."

Often, however, the individual goes beyond replay and, like a novelist, uses the fictive characters and situations creatively as a basis for constructing fantasies, as it were, "based on" fictional characters and situations. By working modifications in identity and action, the individual can exquisitely tune the fictive dramas to his or her personal needs and conflicts. In some cases, the individual imagines herself more or less in her own identity, typically somewhat improved, meeting with a fictional ideal being as a friend or lover. One informant liked to imagine herself "smoking and talking with" Gandalf of *The Lord of the Rings* or riding behind him on his horse. Another young woman, like many in my sample—both male and female—was particularly taken with Hawkeye Pierce, as played by Alan Alda in the television version of "M*A*S*H." "I not only view him [Hawkeye] as a friend and close companion, but I also imagined his creativity and sensitivity translated into a bedroom scene." She adds, "I still consult with him when I'm feeling particularly low and isolated. . . ." She pictures the character and herself "walking along a deserted New England beach on an early summer morning. . . . We're walking near the water, our pants rolled up from the cuff, kicking at the waves, talking, laughing. . . . This imagined scene relaxes me. . . ."

In still other cases, the individual does not just imagine meeting the fictive being. He or she imagines leaving himself or herself behind and *becoming* or turning into the fictive being. Of course, it is the individual who orchestrates these fantasies of being someone else, and there is, typically, a kind of merging of aspects of oneself with the fictive being. Sometimes this is symbolized by a kind of mixed appearance and personality. Like many of her peers, one young woman particularly admired Scarlett O'Hara of *Gone with the Wind:*

> In my fantasies I see myself dressed in one of those beautiful hoop skirt dresses complete with parasol, hat, and fan—making me your typical Southern belle. I would speak in a sweet Southern accent. I would belong to a very wealthy Southern family with a large plantation stretching out for miles. . . . In my fantasies I look like myself, and I still have some of my own peculiar habits and per-

sonality traits, but I do take on most of Scarlett's charming attributes—her vivaciousness and way of dealing with people, the way
she carries herself, and so forth.

These imaginary involvements with fictive beings are absorbing, vivid,
and pervasive. But how significant are they for the formation of adolescent identity? One model would suggest that fictive identities are
important for their vicarious, cathartic, and compensatory functions.
An adolescent without a real boyfriend can achieve emotional satisfaction through a fictive love relationship. An adolescent lacking in
self-confidence can temporarily merge with the masterful competence
of a James Bond. This is one significant function, but such a form of
explanation is incomplete when it implies that the significance of fictive
beings remains entirely apart from the actual world. My data show
how fictive beings may make their appearance directly on the stage of
everyday life.

One special occasion—Halloween—nicely introduces this process.
Invited to Halloween parties, adolescents—like children and adults—
often choose to "go as" a fictional character. Here, the individual
literally puts on the mask of the fictional being and enters the world
of the party in that guise. While the Halloween experience is usually
rather pallid, it symbolizes a much more powerful and widespread
process. Adolescents draw on fictive characters not just for fantasy
escape but as masks for real life role playing. Let us consider a few
examples.

In certain rare but illustrative cases, the process of impersonation
is sufficiently overt, and Halloween-like, that it is socially recognized
both by the individual and by his or her acquaintances. The individual
plays a fictive self socially, and others acknowledge and respond to the
individual as that character. Here, the merger of self-qualities and fictive identity is socially cemented. As a high school student at an over-
seas international American school, this informant did not have access
to the most current American television fare:

I became familiar with the character Tony Baretta of the television
series when newly arrived friends from the United States started
to call me "Baretta." I learned that I look a good deal like him—
short, stocky, and black hair. The fact that I was from New York
and had a tough-guy reputation also helped. Eventually, the series

came to Belgium, and I saw who this character was. I was not displeased at our apparent similarity. He portrayed a hard but sensitive character, a heavily muscled tough guy who at the same time could be counted on to help people through thick and thin. I also enjoyed his speech, attitudes toward smoking, and life in general.

Once I started looking at the series, my behavior, largely because of peer expectation, started to resemble that of Baretta's more closely. . . . The next day—after the series had been on—friends and fellow students would say things like, "Man, I caught you on TV last night." Soon most people called me "Baretta" or "Tony" and I was sort of expected to play this character. . . . Often I would dress like him . . . and soon I had assimilated many of his mannerisms. Although I never sounded like him, I do say many of his phrases: "You can take that to the bank," "Don't roll the dice if you can't pay the price," and so on. . . . The TV character probably helped cement my character into the mold that is now me.

In a similar but even more intimate and intricate case, two junior high school adolescents who were "best friends" began simultaneously to identify with and to be publicly typed as the fictional companions of the television comedy series "Laverne and Shirley." As in folie à deux, they played their complementary roles to each other and to their social worlds at large.

Laverne and Shirley were TV characters in a situation comedy supposed to be taking place during the 1950s. I related to both of these fictitious characters because I was given the nickname "Laverne" and Jane [her best friend] was called "Shirley." Our physical appearances and personalities, though by no means identical to these characters, were similar. . . .

Our peers as well as our teachers and family would call us these names, and this was a constant reinforcement of our roles. Our language, dress style, and our mannerisms had become like Laverne and Shirley's. We learned a lot about cars because cars were "neat." . . . Like Laverne and Shirley, we would also date guys who were friends. It was proper for us to do just about everything together, like Laverne and Shirley did. . . . Every time I watched the show I would not see TV characters, but instead I would see Jane and

I. The show also gave the impression that it was Laverne and Shirley against the world, and that is how it was with Jane and I. I really disliked seeing Laverne and Shirley in real life situations such as talk shows or in magazines. They became serious and had a grown-up quality of the 1970s that was disastrous to the carefree imaginary characters of the 1950s. It destroyed the fantasy.

To me, my relationship with Laverne and Shirley was one of the best things that ever happened in my life. First of all, it made Jane and I very close. Second of all, we were loners, and being Laverne and Shirley gave us an identity. . . . Thirdly, being Laverne and Shirley took out much of the pain that comes with growing up. We did not have to worry about being accepted or doing the right thing. . . . We lived in a carefree world where problems were comical. Problems were viewed by us as typical Laverne and Shirley skits.

Like stage actors, the adolescents who played Baretta, Laverne, and Shirley were selected for their roles because they were similar, in superficial ways, to these characters. But, in accepting these parts, they took on fictional identities; they became figments of someone else's imagination. Unlike actors, for these three adolescents, the play never stopped. Role and actor, mask and identity, became one.

These unusual cases point directly to the much more common process by which the adolescent covertly draws on fictional beings as role models, heroes, and mentors. While never acknowledging this publicly, one young man spent years of his adolescence heavily influenced by the protagonist of Ralph Ellison's novel *Invisible Man:* "True, this novel is a work of art, is fiction, but in some ways it is more than that to me. It is a piece of art that contains knowledge on how to live. This novel is a how-to-do-it book containing countless mental recipes for a healthy existence, all of which comes from Ellison's head and is passed on through the persona of the 'invisible man.' "

In a number of interesting cases, adolescent informants openly state that the fictional figure was "better" than available real people such as friends or parents. The following account shows how a fictional character changes from mother figure to role model. This case also vividly shows how deeply a fictional being can affect adolescent identity.

It all began when I used to watch "The Dick Van Dyke Show" about eleven years ago, so I was ten years old at that time. The first thing I can remember is how much I admired Laura; after all, she was slender, feminine, funny, talented, intelligent, cute, attractive, a kind mother, a loving wife, a caring friend, a good cook, a clean housekeeper, and more. . . . Laura became the person that I wanted my mother to be. . . . I would watch my mother cooking, for example, and I would imagine that my mother was just like Laura.

Things really took a turn when I got into junior high school about eight years ago. "The Mary Tyler Moore Show" had been on TV for about three years by that time, but I didn't pay much attention until I realized that I wanted to learn how to become a woman for myself . . . , and I had the perfect person to model myself after: Mary. On her show she was a career woman and still as perfect as before; she dressed well, she was slender, she knew how to cook, she was independent, she had a nice car, she had a beautiful apartment, she never seemed lonely, she had a good job, she was intelligent, she had friends, and so on. There was *still* nothing wrong with her.

She goes on to show how this process can involve deeper forms of self-transformation:

I used her personality in my . . . anticipations about myself, especially when I had a problem I would find myself thinking, "What would Mary do?" . . . I would imagine myself in the situation that I wanted to be in . . . and also that I was exactly like Mary, that I had her sense of humor, her easygoing manner, and so on. . . . This was a daily occurrence for me until about five years ago. . . . It was a way to solve my problems or to guide my behavior according to a model of perfection; a natural result was that I was pleased about how I conducted myself, especially with other people. I ended up regretting my behavior a lot less when I behaved as I thought Mary would behave. As a teenager I was very concerned about meeting role expectations, but with Mary inside my mind, it was much easier to meet those expectations.

Two other informants independently drew on characters Woody Allen portrays in his earlier movies. Both realize that their own relationship to the Woody Allen figure is directly analogous to Woody's relationship to the Humphrey Bogart character in Allen's film *Play It*

Again, Sam. Here, life imitates a fictional portrait of life imitating fiction.

Conclusions

In this chapter, I have suggested that the construction of adolescent identity parallels the processes by which novelists create fictive worlds. Like novelists, adolescents draw on fictive beings in vicarious, fantasy experience. Like novelists, adolescents take on fictive identity; they become fictional beings. Furthermore, adolescents may also use fictive beings as masks for real world role playing. For many adolescents, everyday life is a kind of Halloween.

As noted earlier, aspects of this theme have been used by screen-writers and novelists in their own fictionalizing, perhaps because their own experience makes them sensitive to the process. However, this theme is also available to draw on because of its long history in the canon of Western fiction. For example, Miguel de Cervantes's *Don Quixote,* sometimes called the first novel, depicts the negative effects of reading fictions about the doings of heroic knights centuries before. Inspired by immersion in these works, the character Don Quixote sloughs off his own identity and, imposing fantasy on reality, takes on the fictive role of a knight-errant. Masking himself in costume armor, he sets off to try and live out similar adventures. By turning us into fictional beings, art gives us new perspectives on life, helps us work through problems and conflicts, and allows us to play with the possibilities of self. Yet Don Quixote casts a disturbing shadow over the subsequent fictions of Western culture. Don Quixote aspires to an idealized, fictional way of being, but this very effort causes him to lose touch with others and with any socially shared understanding of who he really is. He is de-luded by fiction. The invasion of fictional beings into modern psychic life—aided and abetted by the extraordinary power of the electronic mass media—also has complex negative as well as positive effects.[3] In some cases, it creates rather than resolves adolescent identity confusion.

NOTES

This is a longer version of a paper presented at the American Society for Adolescent Psychiatry conference on "Creativity and Adoles-cence," Philadelphia, September 28, 1986. Some of the material presented here was originally published in Caughey (1984). This material is used with the permission of the University of Nebraska Press.

1. For a psychological exploration of an author's relationship to his characters, using the Minnesota Multiphasic Personality Inventory, see Fowler (1986).

2. For a discussion of psychological transformation during readings of fiction by adolescent girls, see Brownstein (1982). For a general discussion of romance reading, see Radway (1984).

3. For a classic account of disturbed adolescent fictional identification, see Lindner (1958).

REFERENCES

Aisnof, E. 1986. Did Leonardo invent the home run? Review of *The Iowa Baseball Confederacy. New York Times Book Review* (April 20), p. 15.

Brownstein, R. 1982. *Becoming a Heroine: Reading about Women in Novels.* New York: Viking.

Caughey, J. 1980. Personal identity and social organization. *Ethos* 8(3): 173–203.

Caughey, J. 1984. *Imaginary Social Worlds: A Cultural Approach.* Lincoln: University of Nebraska Press.

Fowler, R. 1986. The case of the multicolored personality. *Psychology Today* 20(11): 38–49.

Freud, S. 1927. The relationship of the poet to daydreaming. In B. Nelson, ed. *On Creativity and the Unconscious.* New York: Harper & Row, 1958.

Gardiner, D., and Walker, K. 1962. *Raymond Chandler Speaking.* Freeport, N.Y.: Books for Libraries.

Jolidon, L. A. 1986. Murder, he wrote. *USA Weekend* (October 31–November 2), p. 5.

Lindner, R. 1958. The jet-propelled couch. In *Fifty-Minute Hour.* New York: Bantam.

Mathias, B., and Richey, C. 1986. Romancing the prose: confessions of a Harlequin writer. *Prince Georges County Journal* (November 25), p. B-1.

Rabinow, P. 1982. Masked I go forward: reflections on the modern subject. In J. Ruby, ed. *A Crack in the Mirror: Reflexive Perspectives in Anthropology.* Philadelphia: University of Pennsylvania Press.

Radway, J. 1984. *Reading the Romance*. Chapel Hill: University of North Carolina Press.

Roberts, D., and Bachen, C. 1981. Mass communication effects. *Annual Review of Psychology* 32:310–317.

Shweder, R., and LeVine, R. 1984. *Culture Theory: Essays on Mind, Self and Society*. New York: Cambridge University Press.

Slater, P. 1976. *The Pursuit of Loneliness*. Boston: Beacon.

20 WORD CHILD:

TRANSFORMATIONS IN PLAY STORY

DIANA KELLY-BYRNE

Story is an ancient, fundamental, and invincible part of the lives of many. It takes many shapes but is always concerned with exploring and illuminating life. For centuries, mankind has used this system of thought to explore values and imponderables, to try out new visions, to debate questions, to explore the darkness of self, to stand on the verge of worlds seen but as yet unknown, and to abandon the restrictions of life.

Fantasy is story; it shares the object of story, and it is a genre to which children in Western cultures are often introduced at an early age. Many children are actively socialized to the belief that story, and fantasy in particular, is a means by which alternate worlds are created and in which the ordinary can be transformed to the extraordinary for a while. They are "taught" by various sources of socialization, including parent-child interactions of a playful nature and television shows, how to "make believe," how to "play " at being somebody else or at doing something, like flying, or how to "pretend" in activities framed as play. By such experiences, children learn that this verbal mode of acting "as if" is a powerful means by which all manner of alternatives to their everyday situations may be created. In short, these children understand the benefits that accrue from using words to spin desired webs of meaning. This chapter will describe some of the ways in which a seven-year-old white girl created several stories in her play world that enabled her to try out new visions, live in longed-for worlds, and explore some of the mystery and difficulty in everyday life. Her fictive creations allowed her control of her worlds, provided her with fun and festivity and with moments of vision and truth, and in the process may also have soothed some of the difficulty she experienced in her daily life. It can be suggested that she used this ancient form of storying to make some of the realities of her daily life more bearable. Such a response to life and the storehouse of myths with which the world provides us is a thoroughly creative one.

Creativity

The association of verbal fashioning, whether it be story, drama, or some other form of fiction, with creativity has a history of some hundred years. Originally, the word "create" was intended to establish an emphasis on human making and innovation as opposed to divine creation. The humanism of the Renaissance, linking human creation to the poet, associated the process to worlds of the imagination and, it has been argued, is the decisive source of the modern meaning of the word (Williams 1976). The word "creativity" was coined in the eighteenth century with conscious overtones of its association with art and with verbal art in particular. Such etymological details are ancestral and, therefore, relevant to the location of creativity in this discussion. Indeed, this is no accident, given that it is the eighteenth-century usage that is prioritized today in considerations of childhood creativity by such mainstream institutions as the school, the family, and the many mandarins of childhood associated with them.

In such a valuing of creativity, emphasis is on the ability to create verbal fantasies using literary, mythic, heroic, and other symbolic materials and systems for a variety of purposes. Use of such elements to generate verbal artifacts is based on the ability to operate within a subjunctivized mood in which the laws of fiction hold sway. It calls for the building of "paradigms" (cf. Kuhn 1966) whereby alternative worlds that are at once "real" and "not real" are envisaged.

Play

In play, too, the laws of fiction hold sway. In addition, play may be conceptualized as a paradoxical system of expression and communication used by humans and animals. Such a conceptualization is useful

334

because, for one thing, "paradox" is a literary term that draws attention to the "as if" quality that the behavior carries. In addition, it also focuses on the apparent contradiction carried by the behavior whereby actions are at one and the same time real and not real, thus uniting contraries. In referring explicitly to the statement, "This is play," Bateson (1955, p. 41) said that, in an expanded form, the message reads something like this: "These actions in which we now engage do not denote what these actions for which they stand would denote. . . . The playful nip denotes the bite but it does not denote what would be denoted by the bite." Thus, people engage in socially situated acts called play by the production of paradoxical statements about persons, objects, activities, and situations for various expressive and communicative purposes.

In such acts, the paradoxical alteration of real and unreal creates a structure that makes play a fitting and appealing medium for negotiating a variety of purposes and communicating multiple meanings of a symbolic and often private nature. The inherent paradox allows the behavior to be taken back by the players if they fail to engage with their audience and execute their purposes. Because the players are not held accountable for their actions in terms of the everyday world, this form of communication may be safely used to venture, test, and dream. The same terms hold for story. Such characteristics of the structure of play enable symbolic selves and worlds to be created and shared with safety, thereby giving rise to levels of involvement and relatedness, as is evident in the case at hand (cf. Haley 1955; Herne 1967; Milner 1952; Winnicott 1974).

In reference to childhood behaviors, it is still often the case that both notions, creativity and play, continue to be located within a literary paradigm within the culture, despite the fact that all human creation is not play and that the face of imagination is not monoparadigmatic. Nevertheless, as noted earlier, it is often the literary model of creativity that is valued and promoted by mainstream mandarins of childhood, whether they be teachers, parents, or others invested in the stock of childhood (Kelly-Byrne 1986a, 1986b). Once socialized to the form, some children operate it with great success, transforming and recreating their worlds and life situations in a myriad of ways.

I now wish to discuss a study of a child that illustrates the influence of the literary model of creativity, demonstrating its power and the ways in which this mode, based as it is on the ability to create fictions, was used by the child in her play with an adult to fulfill a variety of purposes of her own choosing.

The Study

Details of the case presented in this chapter are based on a study that investigated a seven-year-old girl's play and story in a relationship with an adult who was the researcher (Kelly-Byrne 1982). In this intensive case study, the stance assumed is a phenomenological one in that the event is described from the viewpoint of the participants and is itself taken to be contingent on the meaning-making performance of its members. Thus, meaning is not taken to be static or a priori but is seen rather as emergent and constituted in interaction.

The study took place over one year, during which there were fourteen visits to the home, each lasting three to four hours. The recording procedures were those used in ethnographic study (see Spradley 1980). For several reasons, it was argued that it would be advantageous to have the researcher be an active participant if the child sought such a relationship. First, it was believed that, since play is a relational matter, there is no play outside a relationship. The same may be claimed for psychotherapy; that is to say, there is no psychotherapy outside a human relationship between therapist and patient (see Gardner 1986). It was also argued that the child's play might be remarkably extended by play with a facilitative adult (cf. Vygotsky 1978). Further, as Cassirer (1961) argued in relation to speech and art, individuals are interdependent in dialogue; they do not simply share what they already possess, but rather, by virtue of the sharing process, they attain what they possess (see also Volosinov 1973).

The study is unique in having the investigator stay with the child in her own territory for longer periods of time and participate actively with her. The closest examples of such lengthy involvement come from the fields of psychoanalysis and psychotherapy, although, in such instances, the child is taken to the therapist, plays in a strange place, and does so within external time constraints of usually about an hour. Further, some psychiatrists and classical analysts, subscribing to a model of maintaining neutrality and the attendant view of scientific control, do not usually play with their patients. In short, play is usually simply observed (Piaget, 1951), diagnosed (Axline 1967), manipulated

(Bruner, Jolly, and Sylva 1976), or modeled (Smilansky 1968) but not participated in except quite incidentally (Erikson 1977).

The home was chosen because it was felt that such public settings as laboratories or nursery schools militate against observing very significant developments taking place in play. In public settings, usually, the transformations observed are those momentary accommodations that must be undergone to get things going. In such situations, relationships tend to be relatively public. Therefore, it was assumed that a very different order of relationship would emerge in a more private setting between participants who related to each other on a more established and ongoing basis. For example, in such settings as schools, the players are often hindered by continuous interruptions from teachers, time schedules, and other children. Also, it is often the case that, in public settings, the lack of close friendship among the players, as is generally the case, effectively focuses their behavior on processes of negotiation in getting a relationship going to a much greater extent than would otherwise be the case. Therefore, from studies in such settings, not only do we get little sense of what occurs after these negotiations have been accomplished, but there is also little sense of any real development and innovation in a majority of these cases (cf. Mueller and DeStefano 1973).

Although play theorists have suggested that the creative and transformational qualities of children's play have reached higher levels of competence in solitary play (Fein and Apfel 1979; Rubin and Pepler 1977; Vandenberg 1978) or when playing with friends and familiar people (Doyle, Connolly, and Rivest 1980; Matthews 1978), to date they have paid scant attention to the quality of children's play in private settings and in liaison with regular facilitative play partners other than a parent. This is a significant oversight since there is reason to believe that play is often a private and somewhat secretive phenomenon that erupts in spaces away from the watchful eyes of the mandarins of the culture.

In short, the study sought to document a single child's play in a private setting, away from the observation of unfamiliar and censoring adults. What resulted may be described as a play biography that used the procedures of active participant observation (cf. Bühler 1928). It was never intended to be diagnostic or therapeutic. Rather, it was a response to the need for several rich accounts of a number of instances of play in "naturalistic" settings (cf. Mead 1972) that concentrate on the creation of texts and contexts for play by players for various purposes of their own volition (see Kelly-Byrne 1984; Schwartzman 1978).

The Child

In this case example, the child, Helen, a seven-year-old girl, was at the time of the study an only child of extremely verbal, literacy-valuing academic parents, who lead busy professional lives. Consequently, Helen often spent time by herself. The family placed a high value on language use, literature, independence, intellectualization, and control of others by asserting verbal intellectual superiority.[1]

Synopsis of the Relationship between Child and Adult

The play relationship had an initial, a middle, and a final phase. The initial phase comprised the first five sessions, which were crucial to laying the groundwork for what was to come.

SESSION 1

The first session (discussed in detail in Kelly-Byrne [1983]) was characterized by a great deal of negotiation, as is often the case in early play encounters (cf. Corsaro 1980; Garvey 1977; Schwartzman 1976). On the first occasion, the investigator came to the child as a baby-sitter whom she had not previously met. Helen entered the relationship wearing her public face, which in this case was aloof, competent, and controlling. Helen's goal was to make a relationship with the adult and, in particular, to do so by luring her into her private world. The currency Helen used to operate her world was fantasy, and it was crucial to her purposes that she should negotiate a play frame for this relationship. When she abruptly refused the adult's offer to read her a story in the first session and instead reminded her that "perhaps they had better get to know each other first," she also included two important conditions for doing so. On the one hand, she said, "You have to come to my room." Then, as child and adult proceeded upstairs to the bedroom, Helen stopped short on the landing and said, "I tell no one my dreams, secrets, secret languages, or about my superheroes, so don't ask me about them." This complex interdiction signaled a negation of behavior that deals directly with those things close to the personal self.

However, by implication, this interdiction asserted the very opposite. What Helen implied was that her adult partner and she would share a ludic relationship in her bedroom, a partnership that by its very playful and thus paradoxical nature would deal with a play on these phenomena of her fantasy life, her secrets and dreams, but that would not deal with them in everyday, "realistic" terms (Bateson 1956, 1972). For the sharing and exploring of such matters, it is metaphor that is far more potent than secondary reality. This first session was characterized by numerous negotiations for this play frame, which suggests that play was not only the currency or means by which the adult and the child got to know each other better but also a mask for the child's most personal concerns.

After the preliminary politics of these negotiations, which dominated most of this first session, there was some play enactment that occurred, although during that playful interaction the adult was mainly an on-looker or follower of the child's instructions. However, this play of child and adult led Helen to share her fantasy autobiography with the adult, which, although indirectly expressed since it was framed as play, was nevertheless part of her personal self. This storied autobiography contained many themes that were later evinced in more or less elab-orated form throughout the fourteen sessions. The story was of an orphaned and thus deprived heroine who grew into a powerful princess with magical powers and then had a task to perform—to avenge her father's death by killing his enemy murderers. After that, her missions were to restore peace to a war-torn country and to be nice and caring to people. The story has many elements of the hero tales (cf. Raglan 1936) with their basic struggle between good and evil. Further, as in fairy tales, a premium is placed on beauty and the virtues of kindness and courage. Moreover, there is a clear cause to which the princess must attend, and her agency for accomplishing all this, in addition to her own personal virtues, is magic.

What is remarkable about this story and all others that Helen created and enacted is not only that they draw on and transform the many sources of myth, folktale, and fantasy in the culture but that, in ad-dition, they are mapped onto her own experience of her family and peer life and used to change these everyday realities momentarily. The child used make-believe to conjoin and transform all these separate materials from her life, thereby creating alternative realities and ways of exploring and knowing the self.

SESSIONS 2–5

In these sessions, only a minimum of negotiations of the social relationship occurred. It was clear that this had been established by the successful outcome of the first session. Henceforth, negotiations were more in the nature of stage managements and were directed to the roles and content of the play itself. The length of the enacted dramas increased enormously in each succeeding session, and, although Helen had become much less haughty and more flexible in everyday relationships, she still insisted on being the boss to the adult in the enacted frames. Indeed, in this relationship, the play world was the last bastion of Helen's inflexible dominance. Her need for power and control, which she had given up everywhere else in the relationship, continued to be manifested in the play area. In the play world of the first phase, evil was repeatedly perpetrated by various anthropomorphic characters—for example, Super Squirrel and Evil Dynosaurs. These characters were then confronted and punished by Super Girl or Wonder Woman, played by Helen. Afterward, the evil characters were allowed a chance for remorse and conversion, which then led to their transformation into wholesome characters. The evil characters were usually assigned to the adult for enactment.

Having enacted these long cathartic-like dramas, Helen would then often engage in regressed activity like rolling on the floor, singing in a babyish voice, lying in the adult's lap, singing, twirling about, and dancing in a caricatured fashion to the accompaniment of peals of laughter. An air of celebration and festival pervaded this phase of the play activity.

What is remarkable about the sessions of this first phase is the range of cultural material that was transformed and spun into dramatic stories. Helen generated stories that drew on biblical myths of good and evil, Greek and Norse myths, fables, and superhero tales.

SESSIONS 6–9

These sessions may be taken to represent a middle phase. During this phase, Helen's stories dealt exclusively with everyday human or mythic characters in human form rather than with animal characters. In these stories, she clearly established the "super" and "special" identity of the characters she played, but she also allowed the adult to play characters that shared these qualities. In addition, the adult was

340

allowed a more active role in the dramas, and the play was more open ended. There was increasing uncertainty of outcome for Helen as the adult began to make her own independent input. Helen was unwilling to tolerate this during the first phase of the play relationship, but during the middle phase she even welcomed the adult's impromptu contributions.

Planning stages tended to precede the enactments in which Helen talked about possible scenarios for dramatization. She was often unwilling to have these planning periods tape-recorded, from which it may be surmised that it was only in the disguises of play that she felt that her inner secrets had their paradoxical safety. The planning itself was still in the everyday world and likely to lead to some "exposure" of the inner self, which she did not wish in so direct a form.

Within the stories of this phase, there was decreasing attention to good and bad mother figures and forces of good and evil, and, increasingly, there was veiled attention to the relationships of men and women and of adults. A familiar theme was that of powerful infant daughters rescuing weak and perishing fathers from cold, foodless planets in the absence of mothers and wives. In addition, there was a preoccupation with men and women dating, falling in love, and having babies. The parts the adult and child played now mirrored, as well as reversed, the relationship between Helen and her parents.

A further development of interest is that, during the latter stories of this phase, Helen took the adult's real life name as her own and assigned the adult to the role of a child. In addition, these roles were reversed, and Helen also took the role of the baby in relation to the good mother played by the adult. Clearly, the child and adult now played the roles of desired parent and child figures. Such developments show increasing identification with the adult within the play itself and a continuation of role flexibility within the play, which was not the case in the first phase. As Helen envisaged other worlds and roles for herself, she talked in a narrative way about what would be done and then played out these scenes in highly dramatic ways. One might describe the planning narratives that preceded the play as schematic and drawn from past enactments or from literature or television. The planning narratives were more like stage sets than were the places where the alternative reality occurred. The storied plans set the place where the alternative reality occurred. The storied plans set the context but never confined the enactments, which were livelier and more open ended than the storied scenario might have implied.

SESSIONS 10–14

By the last three months of the year, what was interdicted in the first session now preoccupied hours and hours of time. There were endless discussions of the narrative or planning of the play without even getting to its enactment. It seemed that narrative and direct conversation could now deal more easily with matters close to the self. In addition, Helen now asked for some intimate details from the adult's personal life. Thus, stories about play took the place of play just prior to emergence of stories about "reality" and the details of her everyday world. Thus, Helen's own creative response to her life situation generated a system whereby she could play with the various elements in her life in a manner she enjoyed. Through this process, by the end of a year conversation and intimacy took the place of play and indirection.

Discussion

In summary, I can suggest that Helen's story and play creations worked to her advantage in transforming her implicit vision of her life situation, which she found much less than satisfactory. In real life Helen saw herself as powerless, dumb, and ugly, but in the story plays her leading character became the opposite of these—powerful, wise, and beautiful. In addition, during the latter storying phase, the principal character was also given a mother who was not only powerful but beautiful, wise, and intent on showing her beloved daughter the ways of powerful gods. It should be said that, in the everyday world, Helen's parents were both powerful, bossy figures. The mother presented herself as dominating the household and as often being absent in the cause of furthering her career ambitions. The father and daughter were often left to fend for themselves. In the play scripts, the mother figures were often faulty and usually absent, while the lacking father was rescued by the wise, powerful, and beautiful female children.

The case also suggests that, in the play relationship, as distinct from the play content, the investigator became the positive model for a mother transference. In consequence, as the story plays proceeded, the child reintroduced mother figures who were good and with whom the child identified. On occasions, she introduced bad mother figures in the roles of stepmothers or grandmothers and duly had them executed or burned to a crisp.

But these first two phases of play in which the child canceled the

342

mother and then replaced her were a prerequisite for what was to emerge in the third phase. Having canceled the negative forces of evil with which she struggled and identified with more positive ones, especially a good mother, Helen was able to deal with her underlying concerns with sexuality, both her parents' as well as her own. This is borne out by the fact that, in the end, the child wished to explore her parents' relationship, her own relationship to each of them and to them as a unit, and the details of the adult researcher's relationship with a man who was soon to become her husband. In addition, when Helen was observed in her peer play, she was preoccupied with her friends' as well as her own emerging secondary sexual characteristics.

Conclusions

We may infer that the child's creativity moved on two levels. The first level is the sanctioned historical and literary level of verbal construction, which was in itself sufficiently healing to allow the second. At the second level, the child was able, through her extraordinary play creations coupled with a supportive adult, to deal directly with her everyday relationships with her parents and with the investigator. We may argue that she took the outer and public literary medium that is sanctioned in Western society as her medium and mask and subverted these to her private ends, through which she emerged with a new kind of knowledge about herself and her worlds.

In this seven-year-old's life story, that ancient, fundamental, invincible part of the lives of many played a fundamental role. Her endless, legendary, but culture systemic–like creativity provided her with a profusion of permutations of her own life concerns that were "writ large" within the play story frames she made up during her relationship with the adult partner.

1. A more complete account is available in Kelly-Byrne (1982).

REFERENCES

Axline, V. 1967. *Dibs in Search of Self.* New York: Ballantine.
Bateson, G. 1955. A theory of play and fantasy. *Psychiatric Research Reports* 2:39–51.

Bateson, G. 1956. The message "This is play?" In B. Schaffne, ed. *Group Processes: Transactions of the Second Conference.* New York: Josiah Macy Foundation.

Bateson, G. 1972. *Steps to an Ecology of Mind.* New York: Ballantine.

Bruner, J.; Jolly, C. M.; and Sylva, L., eds. 1976. *Play: Its Role in Development and Evolution.* New York: Penguin.

Bühler, C. 1928. *Kindheit und Jugend: Genese des Bewusstseins.* Psychological Monographien, vol. 3. Leipsig: Hirzel.

Cassirer, E. 1961. *The Logic of the Humanities.* New Haven, Conn.: Yale University Press.

Corsaro, W. 1980. Role-play and peer culture. *Anthropological Association for the Study of Play Newsletter* 6(4): 9–13.

Doyle, A.; Connolly, J.; and Rivest, L. P. 1980. The effect of playmate familiarity on the social interaction of young children. *Child Development* 51:217–223.

Erikson, G. H. 1977. *Toys and Reason.* New York: Norton.

Fein, G., and Apfel, N. 1979. The development of play: style, structure and situation. *Genetic Psychology Monographs* 99:231–250.

Gardner, R. 1986. Central elements in the psychotherapeutic process. Paper presented at Swarthmore College, Swarthmore, Pa., September 19.

Garvey, C. 1977. *Play.* Cambridge, Mass.: Harvard University Press.

Haley, J. 1955. Paradoxes in play and fantasy and psychotherapy. *Psychiatric Research Reports* 2:52.

Herne, H. 1967. Play as an aesthetic concept. *Humanitas* 5:21–28.

Kelly-Byrne, D. 1982. A narrative of play and intimacy: a seven-year-old's play and story relationship with an adult. Ph.D. dissertation, University of Pennsylvania.

Kelly-Byrne, D. 1983. A narrative of play and intimacy. In F. Manning, ed. *The World of Play.* New York: Leisure.

Kelly-Byrne, D. 1984. Making a relationship: a context for fabling. In F. Kessle and Artin Goncii, eds. *Dialogue and Imaginative Play.* San Francisco: Jossey-Bass.

Kelly-Byrne, D. 1986a. The childhood stockmarket: hidden and ambivalent investments. Philadelphia: University of Pennsylvania, Graduate School of Education, typescript.

Kelly-Byrne, D. 1986b. Community literacy: infant story hours. Philadelphia: University of Pennsylvania, Graduate School of Education, typescript.

Kuhn, T. S. 1966. *The Structure of Scientific Revolutions*. Chicago: University of Chicago Press.

Matthews, W. S. 1978. Interruptions of fantasy play: a manner of breaking frame. Paper presented at the annual meeting of the Eastern Psychological Association, Washington, D.C., March.

Mead, M. 1972. *Blackberry Winter*. New York: Pocket.

Milner, M. 1952. Aspects of symbolism in comprehension of the not self. *International Journal of Psycho-Analysis* 33:181–195.

Mueller, E., and DeStefano, C. 1973. Sources of toddlers' peer interaction in a playgroup setting. Boston: Boston University, Education Department, typescript.

Piaget, J. 1951. *Play, Dreams and Imitation in Childhood*. 2d ed. New York: Norton, 1962.

Raglan, L. 1936. *The Hero*. London: Watts.

Rubin, K. H., and Pepler, D. J. 1977. The relationship of child's play to social-cognitive growth and development. In T. Foot, T. Chapman, and J. Smith, eds. *Friendship and Childhood Relationships*. New York: Wiley.

Schwartzman, H. 1976. Children's play: a sideways glance at make-believe. In D. F. Lancy and B. A. Tindale, eds. *The Anthropological Study of Play: Problems and Prospects*. New York: Leisure.

Schwartzman, H. 1978. *Transformations: The Anthropology of Children's Play*. New York: Plenum.

Smilansky, S. 1968. *The Effects of Sociodramatic Play on Disadvantaged Pre-school Children*. New York: Wiley.

Spradley, J. 1980. *Participant Observation*. New York: Holt, Rinehart & Winston.

Vandenberg, B. 1978. Play and development: an ethological perspective. *American Psychologist* 88:724–738.

Volosinov, V. N. 1973. *Marxism and the Philosophy of Language*. Translated by L. Matejka and I. R. Titunik. New York: Seminar.

Vygotsky, L. S. 1978. *Mind in Society*. Cambridge, Mass.: Harvard University Press.

Williams, R. 1976. *Keywords: A Vocabulary of Culture and Society*. New York: Fontana.

Winnicott, D. W. 1974. *Playing and Reality*. Harmondsworth: Penguin.

345

21   ON THE RELATION BETWEEN CREATIVITY
AND CUTTING CORNERS

JAY MECHLING

Every schoolchild knows that "cheaters never win" and that "cheaters only hurt themselves." These are the folk slogans children learn from adult caretakers and playmates. But every schoolchild knows, too, that cheaters sometimes do very well, hurting others along the way, and that one might wait long for evidence that a cheater has hurt himself or herself. Therein lies one of the inconvenient discoveries of childhood, the realization that playing by the rules must be its own reward.

This essay is a thought experiment, as the philosopher might say, about the nature of cheating and its relation to play and to creativity, especially in adolescents. I first became interested in this question while doing fieldwork with a troop of Boy Scouts in California at their annual summer encampment high in the Sierra Nevada. In studying their play as well as their "serious" work—that is, their advancement work toward earning badges and ranks within the organization—I began to notice how cheating operated structurally and symbolically in these activities, all this within an adolescent organization with an extraordinarily explicit commitment to trustworthiness and duty.[1]

These data drove me to the scholarly literature on cheating, only to find some surprises in the premises of that work. I returned to my initial view that Bateson's (1969) ideas about play and creativity provide the best perspective for understanding the nature of cheating. Dictionary and legal definitions of cheating pretty well match our intuitive understandings. Cheating is wholly contextual. It is action (a "text") that derives its meaning from the "frame" defining the larger context of the action. Bateson (1955) called the frame "metacommunication," by which he meant that the participants in a framed activity must communicate with each other about the frame and that the frame provides the set of rules for interpreting communication within the frame. Thus, a game's frame includes the rules within which the competitors must operate, just as the frame of an academic examination event defines what is permissible action toward succeeding in the "test."

In fact, it makes sense to take the "game" as the paradigmatic frame for understanding cheating. In games and gamelike frames, there is organized play, competition, two or more sides, criteria for determining the winner, and agreed-on rules (Roberts, Arth, and Bush 1959). This definition needs some adjustment when we want to consider solitary cheating, as in a game of solitaire at cards, but it serves well for understanding a broad range of gamelike framed activities in which one commonly cheats. Thus, a school examination is framed by examiner and examinee alike, very much like a game.

To cheat is to violate the social contract that is the frame; it is to break the rules, to "cut corners" toward achieving the goal, and to deceive the other players as well as the game actors whose charge it is to enforce the rules. Note two things about this understanding of cheating. First, cheating is wholly contextual. Using one's notes during an open-book examination is not cheating. "Looking up" answers in the library is permissible; looking them up on one's thigh during an exam is cheating. Second, cheating violates the rules of the frame but *not* the legitimacy of the frame itself, a point made by Huizinga's (1950) distinction between the "cheat" and the "spoilsport." The cheater acknowledges the reality and legitimacy of the rules while breaking them. The spoilsport denies the reality and the legitimacy of the frame and its rules, rudely drawing attention to their fragile social construction.

With this much of a general understanding of cheating and its relation to a framed context, let us examine each of eight ways of looking at cheating. I have ordered these perspectives from the most conventional to the least, moving eventually toward a consideration of the relation between cheating and creativity, the subject most central to this inquiry. The eight ways are not mutually exclusive; that is, an individual's view of cheating might combine a number of these views and not necessarily consistently.

Cheating Is a Sin

I begin with the religious, moral view because it is the one implied by the folk slogans quoted at the outset of this chapter. This is the superego speaking. One does not obey the rules of the game just because there is a social contract with penalties for violating the frame. One does not cheat because cheating is wrong. Cheating may not strictly be one of the seven deadly sins, but cheating is an action in context that may be motivated by avarice, envy, sloth, pride, or anger.

Cheating Is a Crime

Lawyers tend not to use the word "cheating," preferring instead such locutions as "fraud," "deceit," "theft," and so on. Still, the most common understanding of cheating may be as a crime, a violation of the social contract but without any religious sense that God is a third party in the covenant. Goodger and Jackson (1985, p. 35), for example, define cheating as "an exploitation of those who compete in good faith. . . . The stealing of advantage in sport is like stealing of any other kind." Indeed, many argue that it is in games and sports that children learn concepts of equality, justice, and "fair play" (Greenberg, Mark, and Lehman 1985).

Bateson makes an interesting point about crime, one that figures later in my ruminations on cheating and creativity. Crime must not be an "act" or "action," he reasons, because crime is not subject to the normal rules of reinforcement. Exploratory behavior in rats is a good parallel; the laboratory psychologist can extinguish a rat's particular exploratory act, but only under the most severe of circumstances can the experimenter extinguish the exploratory behavior itself. Similarly, punishing criminals tends only to make better criminals. So crime must be a class of actions, a class that is a higher logical type than actions themselves. Crime, for Bateson, is one of several "transcontextual syndromes" (like alcohol addiction) that must be understood as cybernetic systems.

Cheating Is a Sickness

On this view, cheating is a technique adopted by a weak or damaged ego (Redl and Wineman 1957). Meeks (1970) played checkers with young clients in therapeutic settings as a way of seeing how the child dealt with the requirements of a highly structured game and with his or her own behavior within that frame. The latency child needs successful adjustment to the reality of the game, both to its rules and to the laws of chance. The latency child who cheats, observed Meeks, "retains the marginal and destructive competitive attitudes which characterize the oedipal child," demonstrating a "marked narcissistic vulnerability" (p. 160).

Although there is no use of the term "addiction" in this literature on cheating as a sickness, Bateson's cybernetic approach to alcoholism might help us see the sense in which a child or adolescent may become "addicted" to cheating as a successful strategy for dealing with certain "testing" frames. Recall, for example, that double-bind communication is a sort of test. I should add that some observers would see this perspective as a symptom of our culture's recent transformation of moral questions into therapeutic ones (Lasch 1979).

Note how these first three views—cheating as sin, as crime, and as sickness—all assume a sort of moral order. Americans are to achieve (or learn or acquire) through hard work, skill, and strategy. Chance is supposed to have little to do with success. Thus, to cheat is to "cut corners" and, thereby, to miss the important steps. A paradigm for this cultural view is the academic examination, a testing context that assumes that skill and strategy are the keys to success. Educators would deny that chance (luck) plays or should play a part in the outcome of the test. A good deal of statistical expertise works on ways to eliminate chance guesses on multiple choice exams, and instructors permit students to bring to tests lucky charms and other aids to chance. Wearing a lucky piece of clothing to an exam or using a lucky pencil is not cheating.

Cheating Is Illegitimate but Functional in Games and in Gamelike Frames

On the functionalist view, cheating is an important element in maintaining the equilibrium of the game frame and, perhaps, of the social system the game may model. This is what Huizinga meant when he claimed that the spoilsport is a much greater threat to the game than is the cheater. The cheater acknowledges the legitimacy of the rules and tries to gain advantage while sustaining an illusion of abiding by the rules.

349

Sociologist Kai Erikson (1966) musters many of the functionalist's arguments in his study of the sociology of deviance in seventeenth-century American Puritan society. Erikson makes the point that any social group must mark its boundaries; this is part of the organizing and meaning making that is social organization. The deviant provides an important service in this boundary marking by moving outside the boundaries and forcing the group to make explicit its understanding of the boundaries. Erikson echoes Huizinga in remarking that "the deviant and his more conventional counterpart live in much the same world of symbol and meaning, sharing a similar set of interests in the world around them" (p. 20).

Erikson states the functionalist case for understanding deviance intolerable enough that the community feels compelled to mark the boundary. But this same view helps us see the continuum of cheating as boundary testing and marking. The individual cheater in a game is like the laboratory rat exploring the boundaries of its environment. The cheater explores the boundaries of permissible behavior in a game. But, for this exploration to be functional for the game frame, the behavior must first be detected and then labeled "cheating."

Some cheating is clearly contrary to the publicly agreed-on rules, and detection in these cases merely reinforces the preexisting rule. But, in many cases, a player may engage in innovative behavior not unambiguously forbidden by the game contract. For the cheating to be functional in these cases, the group must detect the behavior and engage in a period of confrontation and negotiation aimed at defining the innovative behavior as either cheating or as a permissible strategy. Bateson calls these negotiations "metacommunication" about the game frame; it is discourse about the frame and, as such, can be functional in reasserting the collective agreement about the game's rules and boundaries.

Cheating may also be the shared action that bonds the deviating group of adolescents. Baird (1980) discovered in his survey that students preferred cooperative cheating practices to private ones. A university student described for me the organized, cooperative cheating that went on in her competitive, upper-middle-class high school and the strong in-group feelings created by that cooperation. Cooperative cheating may be a central instance of cooperation and bonding for groups like fraternities.

I suppose that the sociobiological view of cheating counts as a version of the sociological functionalist approach. Fagen (1981) briefly describes the sociobiologists' "cheating hypothesis," meant to help explain why animals play at great expense to themselves and to their genes. As an alternative to the competing hypotheses that play is selfish cooperation or that play is damaging competition, the " 'cheating' hypothesis . . . suggests that animals may exploit opportunities to change play into agonistic fighting" (p. 337). The social collectivity benefited by my cheating, in other words, is not my team but my genes.

Cheating Is a Legitimate Strategy in Contest

Whereas the previous, functionalist view sees cheating as illegitimate, this view opines that a player should use any strategy necessary in order to prevail in a contest. Silva (1983, p. 438) suggests that the meaning of "strategy" in sports has become "operationally defined as 'using the rules' or knowing how to circumvent the rules and still gain a tactical advantage." He showed slides of rule-violating behavior to a sample of 203 male and female athletes and nonathletes and discovered support for the idea that there is an in-sport socialization process that breaks down the players' internal prohibitions against cheating and teaches the players to perceive rule violation as legitimate. There are important gender differences in Silva's data; it was the males who demonstrated the strong linear relation between years of participation and level of organized competition, on the one hand, and the perceived legitimacy of rule-violating behavior, on the other.

Another source of insight into the "socialized legitimacy" of cheating in games and sport is the work by Haan (1983) and others on what she calls "the interactional morality of everyday life." Some of the empirical research on cheating addresses the question of interactional moralities and discovers that these moralities are very situational. Forsyth and Berger (1982) found that American college students' ethical ideology was not predictive of their cheating in a laboratory setting. Similarly, Guttmann (1984) used cheating to compare sixth-grade pupils from secular public and religious public schools in Israel and found a low correlation between moral cognition and moral behavior.

A relevant element in the interactional moralities of everyday life is what we might call a sense of "folk justice." Greenberg et al. (1985)

show how players of sports and games learn three forms of justice—distributive, retributive, and procedural—but we might as well look on cheating in the classroom as reflecting students' emergent sense of justice. Students often report on surveys and in university judicial hearings that they cheated on an examination or other assignment because the teacher was not being "fair." If we take this defense at face value, we see at work a view that, once the more powerful party has broken unjustly the "contract" between teacher and students, then justice permits cheating.

Other research on interactional moralities uses sport settings. Goodger and Jackson (1985, p. 39) studied the attitudes of four groups of soccer coaches toward rules and cheating and found that "the attitudes of several coaches were that it was the responsibility of the referee to determine what constituted intentional law infractions and therefore, 'right' conduct." The authors see this as evidence that the coaches operate at a lower level of moral reasoning (i.e., Kohlberg's [1963] type 1, "punishment and obedience orientation") than principled morality (Kohlberg's type 6). Bredemeier and Shields (1984), who are Haan's colleagues at Berkeley, found that their sample of 120 high school and college basketball players, swimmers, and nonathletes used lower levels of moral reasoning to resolve hypothetical dilemmas in sports contexts than in everyday life contexts. "Game reasoning," concluded the authors, "may reflect a special form of bracketed morality in which the competitive strategic setting of sport encourages the temporary adoption of egocentric morality" (p. 356). It seems that even traditional moralities may privilege game frames when it comes to their view of cheating.

Sometimes the advocates of cheating as a legitimate strategy in games will argue for the continuity between the game frame and the more general institutional frames of the society. If this is the case, goes the argument, then learning to cheat well is appropriate "anticipatory socialization" for later life or other frames. Thus, one might take the tack that "all's fair" in the "game" of corporate capitalism, that one may cheat and spy to the extent that one can get away undetected. Everybody does it, after all. Indeed, some studies (Baird 1980; Stevens 1984) show that business majors are more likely to cheat in college than are other majors.

This view makes some sense of the gender differences that seem consistent across studies of cheating in school and in sports. Males cheat more than females. Females are socialized toward a different everyday morality (Gilligan 1982), to be sure, but it is also true that females may see the trajectory of their lives carrying them into adult roles that will not require legitimized cheating. Certainly, some of the management-advice literature aimed at women assumes that a difficulty faced by those managers is the female's greater intolerance for rule violations.

The fact is that we really have very little ethnographic evidence for understanding girls' play (Sutton-Smith 1979), let alone their patterns of cheating in games and contests. In my research on "powder-puff" football, I aim to understand how high school and college women cheat in that game setting normally seen as a theater for the socialization of males for American corporate capitalism.

Of course, the therapist (e.g., Redl and Wineman 1957) might see this perspective as the rationalization by a weak ego striving to account for its own transgressions by arguing that "everybody else does it." But the social psychiatrist might suggest to us that, when these rationalizations and justifications become normal in a society, something else is happening. Otherwise, how are we to account for the fact that a large number of intelligent, nondelinquent young people (e.g., medical school students, West Point cadets, Harvard Law School students) cheat? The answer to this query leads us to the sixth way of looking at cheating.

Cheating Is a Neurotic Response Created by the Nature of Our Civilization

Horney's (1937) *The Neurotic Personality of Our Time* lays out the social psychiatric argument for understanding cheating as a chronic response to the contradictions of American culture. Horney does not mention cheating, but we may construct a reasonable explanation from her general comments. Our cultural principle of competition between individuals, argues Horney, results in " a diffuse hostile tension" between individuals. This hostile tension in turn generates "fear of the potential hostility of others, reinforced by a fear of retaliation for hostilities of one's own." The prospect of failure in this competition further increases anxiety on account of the effect of failure on loss of prestige and, most important, on self-esteem. "According to existing ideologies," writes Horney, "success is due to our own intrinsic merits, or in religious terms, is a visible sign of the grace of God; in reality it is dependent on a number of factors independent of our control—fortuitous circumstances, unscrupulousness, and the like. Nevertheless, under the pressure of the existing ideology, even the most normal person is constrained to feel that he amounts to something when successful, and is worthless if he is defeated. Needless to say, this presents a shaky basis for self-esteem'' (p. 286). The neurotic, then, is caught in a vicious circle. Certain cultural contradictions—such as those between ''competition and success on the one hand, and brotherly love on the other,'' or between ''the stimulation of our needs and our factual frustrations in satisfying them,'' or between ''the alleged freedom of the individual and all his factual limitations''—are, argues Horney, ''precisely the conflicts which the neurotic struggles to reconcile'' (pp. 288–289). Anger, hostility, and impaired self-esteem are the likely responses to these contradictions. The neurotic's self-defense against these feelings is the striving for power, prestige, and possession. But this striving creates its own anxieties as the striving conflicts with the neurotic's need for affection. Thus, the neurotic may recoil from competition while at the same time feeling a need to dominate the other. The neurotic's pursuit of power, therefore, creates ''enhanced superiority feelings (with begrudging envy); enhanced grandiose ideas (with fear of envy); [and] enhanced sensitivity (with renewed tendency to recoil)'' (p. 227). These reactions enhance the neurotic's hostility and anxiety, plunging the person back into the circle. The difference between the neurotic and the normal person's responses to these conflicts is merely quantitative, making every member of the culture a potential candidate for neurosis.

Given Horney's understanding, we might now view cheating as a piece of the neurotic's repertoire for responding to the competitive individualism of American culture. Take the two settings for the empirical investigation of cheating—school examinations and sports contests. When grades become the measure of individual success and a primary source of self-esteem in academic settings, the neurotic experiences the dilemma between the need for affection and the need for prestige. The competitive examination heightens anxiety and fears of the hostility of others. The student may experience a crisis of confidence in the match between potential and actual performance on the examination. The student cheats as a means of succeeding on the examination, but success itself enhances fears of the hostility of others.

The student is caught in Horney's vicious circle of the competing demands for affection and for dominance.

The cheater in the sports contest is enmeshed in a similar web of competition, anxiety, hostility, and fear of the hostility of others. Even when the player is in a team sport, it is often the individual who decides to cheat.

There are two bodies of empirical research relevant to this view of cheating as a neurotic response created by the contradictions of our civilization. One is research aimed at understanding how Rotter's (1966) person variable, "locus of control," interacts with the situation variable of a task or challenge where success is perceived as dependent on skill or chance. As a person variable, "locus of control" is "internal" if the individual believes that the outcomes of events depend on the individual's own skill or effort and "external" if the individual believes that outcomes are beyond control, subject to fate or chance. As a situational variable, "locus of control" refers to the relatively objective conditions for success, internal versus external. Researchers in this area tend to use cheating as the dependent variable, assuming that cheating signals strong motivation to succeed. Srull and Karabenick (1975) predicted that their college student subjects would be more likely to cheat in congruent personality-situation combinations (i.e., internal-skill, external-chance) than in incongruent ones, reasoning that there is a higher reward value in the congruent conditions. The authors found significant relations in the direction they predicted. Moreover, Srull and Karabenick believe that "internals" cheat as a way of approaching success, whereas "externals" cheat as a way of avoiding failure. Later studies by Karabenick and Srull (1978) confirmed their earlier findings.

Kahle (1980) added to the Srull and Karabenick model the notion that people self-select stimulus conditions that match their personalities. Thus, Kahle predicted that "internals and middles will be more likely to select stimulus conditions involving skill, whereas externals will be more likely to select stimulus conditions involving chance," and that, after the "stimulus condition self-selection of a skill or a chance test, subjects who selected a test of skill will be more likely to cheat on a test of skill, whereas subjects who selected a test of chance will be more likely to cheat on a test of chance" (pp. 51–52). Both hypotheses were confirmed in Kahle's sample of 218 male college students.

There are some problems with this "locus of control" research that ought to make us cautious in building an interpretation of cheating on this work. First, this research creates artificial, laboratory conditions for cheating that are almost never paralleled in natural settings, and we have no natural setting studies of cheating and its relation to "locus of control." As Kahle herself warns, the random assignment of subjects to laboratory circumstances may not duplicate the natural settings in which people tend to self-select stimulus situations that suit their motive orientations or in which people tend to modify the situations. Second, and more troubling, this research begins with the "locus of control" person variable without accounting for the social and historical origins of the current distribution of orientations among persons. At least Riesman (1961) provided a theory for the relation between sociohistorical forces and social character types (tradition directed, inner directed, other directed). Without a clear sense of the present distribution of internal/external orientations across gender, race, class, occupation, religion, and so on, and without a model of the sorts of life experiences that create a "locus of control" orientation, the present research is of limited value in elaborating Horney's original insight into cultural patterns and social character.

The second research tradition on social character and cheating is sparser and more ambiguous than the first. This is a research tradition that inquires into the relation between the "need for achievement" motive (McClelland, Atkinson, Clark, and Lowell 1953) and cheating. Fakouri (1972) found no significant difference between the achievement motivation scores of cheaters and noncheaters in a laboratory setting, though he did find proportionally more cheating among the males than among the females. But Johnson (1981, p. 374) found in his laboratory sample of fifty-one males that high-need achievers "were more likely to cheat and cheated more than their low-need counterparts."

Cheating Is a Form of Deliberate Human Resistance against Late Capitalism—in Particular, against Competitive Individualism

The previous perspective sees cheating as a neurotic response to the contradictions of bourgeois capitalism. Let us assume, instead, that the folks who are cheating are not victims of neurosis or "false consciousness" but are choosing cheating as a rational, purposive strategy for resisting the dilemmas and anxieties posed by competitive individualism and by the contradictions enumerated by Horney. From this perspective, cheating is a form of cultural criticism; it is a folk critique of capitalism.

For example, just as Willis (1981) looks at the culture of working-class kids and finds evidence of their critique of capitalism, so we might look at cheating on academic examinations as a form of protest against the system's pitting the students against one another in a competitive situation aimed at making distinctions and attributing value to performances. Sometimes the protest is individual, but often it is collective, the assertion of student *communitas* (Turner 1969) against the structural (hierarchical, differentiating) demands of those in power.

The gender differences in rates and patterns of cheating make sense from this viewpoint since it is males whose social structures (male folk groups, sports) most pressure them toward competitive individualism. The irony here is that males may be cheating for precisely opposite reasons—some because they see it as a legitimate strategy to be learned for succeeding in competitive late capitalism, others because cheating is the only statement they can make that they disdain the culture's values. There very well may be contextual differences between those who cheat alone and those who turn to collective cheating.

Cheating may be a defense mechanism against the alienation that many see as one of the cultural contradictions of capitalism. For example, some analysts (e.g., Gehring, Nuss, and Pavela 1986) argue that students are more likely to cheat when they perceive a lack of appropriateness between an assigned activity and the goals of the course. In the language of cultural criticism, we might say that the students are protesting the separation of means and ends that seems to characterize technology and bureaucracy, the twin forces of the modernization of consciousness (Berger, Berger, and Kellner 1973).

So cheating may be an especially valued tool of resistance for specific underclasses in American society. Rich's (1979) essay "Women: Honor and Lying," for instance, helps us see the relation between lying, cheating, and power in patriarchal society. Children and adolescents are other relatively powerless classes in American society, and their folklore is filled with signs of resistance (Mechling 1986). In my fieldwork at the summer encampment of a California Boy Scout troop, I discovered cheating within their Treasure Hunt, the game that most models capitalism (Mechling 1984).

357

Cheating Is a Member of the Class of Actions Called "Transcontextual Syndromes," Which Also Includes Play and Creativity

I want to argue that we most profitably look at cheating as a variety of "transcontextual syndrome" that shares many of the qualities of play and creativity. The phrase "transcontextual syndrome" is Bateson's (1969), so it is with him and his illustrative example that I begin.

Bateson recounts his experience watching the training of a female porpoise to respond to the sound of a whistle as a "secondary reinforcement" in operant conditioning, which she learns rather quickly. The next training task, however, is to teach her about the class of such training episodes. In the second session, the trainer reinforces not her head raising, as in the first session, but a tail flap. In the third session, the trainer reinforces neither the head raising nor the tail flap but another piece of conspicuous behavior, and so on. At last, the porpoise learns about the class of these training contexts—namely, that she was to offer a new piece of behavior in each session. This sort of learning Bateson calls "deutero learning," the "learning to learn" that involves a higher logical type of learning about the context of learning contexts.

Bateson draws our attention to two important features of this paradigm. First, the trainer sensed several times that the experiment was disturbing the porpoise, so he sometimes gave her unearned reinforcements so as to preserve their relationship. Bateson concludes from this observation that "severe pain and maladjustment can be induced by putting a mammal in the wrong regarding its rules for making sense of an important relationship with another mammal." As for the second feature, I shall let Bateson speak for himself: "Each of the fourteen sessions was characterized by many futile repetitions of whatever behavior had been reinforced in the immediately previous session. Seemingly only by 'accident' did the animal provide a piece of different behavior. In the timeout between the fourteenth and fifteenth sessions, the porpoise appeared to be much excited, and when she came on stage for the fifteenth session she put on an elaborate performance including eight conspicuous pieces of behavior of which four were entirely new— never before observed in this species of animal" (p. 277). Bateson's conclusion, then, is that, if the subject can resist the pathology, the madness lurking behind such exercises in deutero learning, then "the total experience may promote *creativity*." Bateson is calling "creativity" that breakthrough into deutero learning by which an organism deals with paradoxes of logical types in communication, and he coins the term "transcontextual syndromes" to describe the class of strategies human beings employ to deal with such paradoxes. Bateson's list of "transcontextual syndromes" includes play, "nonplay" (whatever he meant by that), fantasy, sacrament, metaphor, humor, falsification, and deutero learning (p. 204).

It is very interesting to consider cheating as a member of the class of "transcontextual syndromes." The claim here is that some adolescents may cheat some of the time as a creative response to the paradoxes of communication in a particular framed activity, in this case academic examinations or games. What might these paradoxes be, and how might we read cheating as a "creative" response to them?

Consider an academic examination. There are many ways in which this framed context is like a game. There are explicit rules, a time limit, a spatial limit or restriction, and a restriction on the sorts of resources and materials to be used within the frame. There is a contest between the players, there are clear criteria for winning and losing, there are scarce and valuable resources for the winners, and success in the contest depends on some mixture of chance, skill, and strategy.

At the same time that an examination is like a game, it is not like other frames in everyday life, including work life. Therein lie the principal paradoxes of the examination frame. The explicit communication by those in power in an exam claims that the exam (or term paper or lab assignment) is aimed at helping the subject learn the material (Learning I). Sometimes there is a claim that the task aims to teach the subject how to be creative, how to "think critically" about certain materials, how to learn creative strategies for problem solving rather than simply learning by rote the solutions to some problems. But the students know, some more consciously than others, that this is not so. Examinations model no other context in life aside from other examinations. Exams generally do not duplicate the conditions under which humans deutero learn, so they do not foster creativity. In no problem-solving context in "real life" are there the restrictions that hold in an examination. In short, most exams are more plausible as a game than as a sacrament.

From this perspective, it is not at all clear that it is more appropriate (or more "healthy," for that matter) to "take" an exam seriously or playfully. There are the serious players, to be sure, but the distinction between those who take an examination "seriously" and those who do not is more like a continuum than a dualism. There is plenty of room in taking an exam for expressive behavior or "style." Sutton-Smith and Kelly-Byrne (1984) write of "the masks of play," by which they mean the ways in which play sometimes masks unacceptable behavior or in which acceptable behavior sometimes masks play. Their examples include ways play masks cruelty, violence, sex, intimacy, power, danger, and even work.

For some students, cheating may be a rewarding form of "deep play." Cheating has danger and risk under circumstances of severe consequences, much like the risk-taking "play" (drunk driving, sex without contraception, hitchhiking with strangers) Sutton-Smith and Kelly-Byrne found among their University of Pennsylvania students. Cheating may offer risks and thrills these adolescents and young adults find in few other places in their lives.

Note that this approach to academic cheating explains several puzzles in the phenomenon. First, teachers observe that some students put a great deal of effort into cheating, so much effort that the teachers wonder aloud whether it would not take less effort simply to study or do the work assigned. Second, some of the research on cheating suggests that cheating is not always correlated with low grades (Roskens and Dizney 1966). Some students choose to cheat not as instrumental behavior aimed at getting better grades but as expressive behavior that is its own reward.

Everything I have said so far about paradoxes of communication and cheating in examinations applies also to games and organized sports. There are many mixed messages about the meaning of athletic contests.

The perspective that I am urging here—that we view cheating as a member of the class of transcontextual syndromes that includes play, humor, falsification, metaphor, and so on—raises an old question about the relation between rules and creativity, between convention and invention. Mozart helped invent an extremely rigid musical form, the sonata-allegro form for the symphony, and then proceeded to display brilliant creativity within the artificial rules of that form. But sometimes he broke his own rules briefly, in part to create a tension in the form, in part to confirm the rules by returning to them, and in part as a way of discovering a musical solution to a compositional problem (Bernstein 1976). Now, there very well might be a developmental question here.

That is, it may be that children of a certain age must learn to keep the rules before learning how to cheat as a form of creativity.

Bateson's story about the porpoise and his several essays taking a cybernetic, communications approach to play, art, schizophrenia, and learning set me to thinking about two cultural settings and the relation between cheating ("cutting corners") and creativity in those settings. The first setting is science. A few years ago, when historian of science Thomas Kuhn visited my campus for a series of lectures and seminars, a group of natural scientists and others of us interested in science and culture gathered over a long lunch to fire questions at the distinguished visitor. The scientists kept coming back to one question. How could they make their graduate students be creative? The problem they faced was one predicted by Kuhn (1969) more than a decade earlier in his justly famous *The Structure of Scientific Revolutions*. Science students "learn" how to do science by replicating the classic experiments in their discipline. The most successful students are those who are best at replicating someone else's work. Suddenly, after six or seven years of university schooling, these bright graduate students are asked to be "creative," to take some risks in their thinking and in their puzzle solving. The professors found most of these students too cautious, too literal, not creative enough. What to do?

Sadly for the gathered scientists, Kuhn had no answer. If anything, he reiterated his gloomy view that the entire structure of science education works against creativity, that the creative scientists are creative in spite of their scientific training rather than because of it. Yet, neither Kuhn nor most of us assembled, I believe, thought that creative scientists were born that way. It was just that those scientists must have had learning experiences in some context outside orthodox science education that taught them how to be creative. The problem faced by my science colleagues, therefore, was much like that facing the trainer of Bateson's porpoise—how could one put the mammal into circumstances such that she would make the breakthrough to Learning II, to learning about the context of contexts? And how could one do this without driving the mammal mad?

Linking the Kuhn visit to Bateson's porpoise led me to wonder whether cheating, as one class of transcontextual syndrome, had anything to do with creativity in science. Koestler (1964) had already argued for the connection between humor, art, and science, and the "flexibility" hypothesis in play studies (e.g., Bruner, Jolly, and Sylva 1976; Fagen 1981) sees play as a crucial experience for innovation and creativity. If cheating is a member of the class of transcontextual syndromes, then it seemed plausible to me that cheating also might be related to creativity.

There is some support for this view in scientific autobiographies. Feynman's (1985) *"Surely You're Joking, Mr. Feynman!"* and Watson's *The Double Helix* (1968) provide plenty of anecdotes about the ways in which these Nobel prize–winning scientists often "cut corners"— cheated, in effect—toward making a breakthrough in their scientific thinking. In fact, *The Double Helix* did more than any other book to show the public how much like a game or contest scientists see their work.

Of course, it may be objected that what I am calling "cheating" in these scientific autobiographies is not cheating but simply "creative problem solving." But that, in a way, is my point. Cheating is wholly contextual, and it is by no means clear that cheating in the contexts of one's science education—by engaging in such practices as sharing lab work, using "crib sheets" during exams, or plagiarizing the work of others—is unrelated to the demands to be creative as a scientist (but see Broad and Wade 1982). The clearest case of this contextual point is that of computer "hackers," who engage in illegal behavior as a game or as a test of their inventive ability to solve puzzles. The exact same behavior praised by a computer science professor may be prosecutable in a different context.

The second setting in which I have been thinking about the connection between cheating (or "cutting corners") and creativity is my fieldwork with a troop of Boy Scouts. The Boy Scouts is a very rule-conscious organization for the eleven- to seventeen-year-old boy, with explicit discourse about honor and trustworthiness. Yet, these boys cheat. In my fieldwork with the troop at their summer encampments in the Sierra Nevada, I witnessed several cases of mild cheating in their games, such as the Treasure Hunt, Capture the Flag, and Nurfball (softball played with a spongey ball and hollow plastic bat). They sometimes cheat on their advancement work toward badges and ranks, though my evidence for this is far less direct and more anecdotal.

The cheating that goes on at a Boy Scout camp is thoroughly comprehensible from the multiple perspectives on cheating discussed above. The cheating in the games serves the rule-testing and rule-affirming functions, and the cheating in their Treasure Hunt seems to be an expected "strategy" in the contest. There are also clear instances of cheating as purely expressive behavior. Since many boys complain that the advancement "classes" and "assignments" are "too much like school," I suspect that the boys' rationalizations for "cutting corners" on some badge requirements would parallel their rationalizations for cheating in school (the Scoutmaster of this troop is, in fact, a high school teacher).

The puzzle for me in the Boy Scout materials is the relation between the ways these boys "cut corners" and the ways they demonstrate creativity in the camp setting. Put differently, one might ask a version of the question my science colleagues put to Kuhn. How does a Scout leader protect and enhance the creativity of adolescent boys within an organization otherwise so structured and conformist? Are there instances of a Scout leader or of the fellow boys themselves putting boys into learning situations similar to the one facing Bateson's porpoise? Are some boys creative because of the Boy Scout experience or in spite of it? These are the sorts of questions I have as I return to my Boy Scout materials.

Conclusions

After reading the existing literature on cheating and working through this thought experiment on the relation of cheating to creativity, I sense that we really know very little about cheating as a class of action. None of the empirical research on cheating and the dialectic between personality and situation is in natural settings. The survey research on cheating captures the outline of self-report on attitudes toward cheating, but none of the subtleties of process and interpretation. Folklorists, sociologists, and anthropologists are just now beginning to include accounts and interpretations of cheating in their study of people at play (e.g., Hughes 1983). There is still only the occasional clinical or therapeutic account of the cheater. Clearly, there is much work to be done on cheating and its multiple meanings.

Finally, I do not want my radical critique of the meanings of cheating to be taken as advocacy for an amoral or relativist attitude toward all behavior labeled as "cheating." As a teacher and writer, I have little sympathy for conscious plagiarism, and, as a patient, I am not sure I would want a personal physician who cheated his or her way through medical school. But I do think that we are missing some wonderful opportunities for understanding the workings of culture if we accept uncritically the current attitudes toward the "problem" of cheating. Only when we appreciate the ways in which public culture is a system of contested interpretations will we unpack fully the ideologies encoded in the current discourse about cheating.

1. As I began work on another project, this time on girls' play in high school "powder-puff" and college coed intramural football, I again became aware of the complex ecology of cheating. Finally, in the course of having our students collect the "folklore" circulating among students, my colleague David S. Wilson and I have amassed a body of student lore on cheating toward a separate essay on cheating in college.

REFERENCES

Baird, J. S. 1980. Current trends in college cheating. *Psychology in the Schools* 17:515–522.

Bateson, G. 1955. A theory of play and fantasy. In *Steps to an Ecology of Mind*. New York: Ballantine, 1972.

Bateson, G. 1969. Double bind. In *Steps to an Ecology of Mind*. New York: Ballantine, 1972.

Berger, P.; Berger, B.; and Kellner, H. 1973. *The Homeless Mind: Modernization and Consciousness*. New York: Vintage/Random.

Bernstein, L. 1976. *The Unanswered Question*. Cambridge, Mass.: Harvard University Press.

Bredemeier, B. J., and Shields, D. L. 1984. Divergence in moral reasoning about sport and everyday life. *Sociology of Sport Journal* 1:348–357.

Broad, W., and Wade, N. 1982. *Betrayers of the Truth*. New York: Simon & Schuster.

Bruner, J. S.; Jolly, A.; and Sylva, K. 1976. *Play: Its Role in Development and Evolution*. New York: Basic.

Erikson, K. 1966. *Wayward Puritans*. New York: Wiley.

Fagen, R. 1981. *Animal Play Behavior*. New York: Oxford.

Fakouri, M. E. 1972. Achievement motivation and cheating. *Psychological Reports* 31:629–630.

Feynman, R. P. 1985. *"Surely You're Joking, Mr. Feynman!"* New York: Bantam.

Forsyth, D. R., and Berger, R. E. 1982. The effects of ethical ideology on moral behavior. *Journal of Social Psychology* 117:53–56.

Gehring, D.; Nuss, E. M.; and Pavela, G. 1986. *Issues and Perspectives on Academic Integrity.* Columbus, Ohio: National Association of Student Personnel Administrators.

Gilligan, C. 1982. *In a Different Voice: Psychological Theory and Women's Development.* Cambridge, Mass.: Harvard University Press.

Goodger, M. J., and Jackson, J. J. 1985. Fair play: coaches' attitudes towards the laws of soccer. *Journal of Sport Behavior* 8:34–41.

Greenberg, J.; Mark, M. M.; and Lehman, D. R. 1985. Justice in sports and games. *Journal of Sport Behavior* 8:18–33.

Guttmann, J. 1984. Cognitive morality and cheating behavior in religious and secular school children. *Journal of Educational Research* 77:248–254.

Haan, N. 1983. An interactional morality of everyday life. In N. Haan, R. Bellah, P. Rabinow, and W. Sullivan, eds. *Social Science as Moral Inquiry.* New York: Columbia University Press.

Horney, K. 1937. *The Neurotic Personality of Our Time.* New York: Norton.

Hughes, L. 1983. Beyond the rules of the game: why are rooie rules nice? In F. Manning, ed. *The World of Play.* West Point, N.Y.: Leisure.

Huizinga, J. 1950. *Homo Ludens: A Study of the Play-Element in Culture.* Boston: Beacon.

Johnson, P. B. 1981. Achievement motivation and success: does the end justify the means? *Journal of Personality and Social Psychology* 40:374–375.

Kahle, L. R. 1980. Stimulus condition self-selection by males in the interaction of locus of control and skill-chance situations. *Journal of Personality and Social Psychology* 38:50–56.

Karabenick, S. A., and Srull, T. K. 1978. Effects of personality and situation variation in locus of control on cheating: determinants of the "congruence effect." *Journal of Personality* 46:72–95.

Koestler, A. 1964. *The Act of Creation.* New York: Dell.

Kohlberg, L. 1963. The development of children's orientations toward a moral order. *Vita Humana* 6:11–33.

Kuhn, T. 1969. *The Structure of Scientific Revolutions.* Chicago: University of Chicago Press.

Lasch, C. 1979. *The Culture of Narcissism*. New York: Norton.

McClelland, D. D.; Atkinson, J. W.; Clark, R. A.; and Lowell, E. L. 1953. *The Achievement Motive*. New York: Appleton-Century-Crofts.

Mechling, J. 1984. Patois and paradox in a Boy Scout treasure hunt. *Journal of American Folklore* 97:24–42.

Mechling, J. 1986. Children's folklore. In E. Oring, ed. *Folk Groups and Folklore Genres: An Introduction*. Logan: Utah State University Press.

Meeks, J. E. 1970. Children who cheat at games. *Journal of the American Academy of Child Psychiatry* 9:157–170.

Redl, F., and Wineman, D. 1975. *The Aggressive Child*. New York: Free Press.

Rich, A. 1979. Women: honor and lying. In *On Lies, Secrets, and Silence: Selected Prose, 1966–1978*. New York: Norton.

Riesman, D., with Glazer, N., and Denney, R. 1961. *The Lonely Crowd*. New Haven, Conn.: Yale University Press.

Roberts, J. M.; Arth, M. J.; and Bush, R. 1959. Games in culture. *American Anthropologist* 61:597–605.

Roskens, R. W., and Dizney, H. F. 1966. A study of unethical academic behavior in high school and college. *Journal of Educational Research* 59:231–234.

Rotter, J. B. 1966. Generalized expectancies for internal versus external control of reinforcement. *Psychological Monographs* 80(whole no. 609).

Silva, J. M. 1983. The perceived legitimacy of rule violating behavior in sport. *Journal of Sport Psychology* 5:438–448.

Srull, T. K., and Karabenick, S. A. 1975. Effects of personality-situation locus of control congruence. *Journal of Personality and Social Psychology* 32:617–628.

Stevens, G. E. 1984. Ethical inclinations of tomorrow's citizens: actions speak louder? *Journal of Business Education* 59:147–152.

Sutton-Smith, B. 1979. The play of girls. In C. B. Kopp, ed. *Becoming Female: Perspectives on Development*. New York: Plenum.

Sutton-Smith, B., and Kelly-Byrne, D., eds. 1984. *The Masks of Play*. West Point, N.Y.: Leisure.

Turner, V. 1969. *The Ritual Process: Structure and Anti-structure*. Ithaca, N.Y.: Cornell University Press.

Watson, J. 1968. *The Double Helix*. New York: New American Library.

Willis, P. 1981. *Learning to Labour: How Working Class Kids Get Working Class Jobs*. New York: Columbia University Press.

22 THE SEMIOTICS OF PLAY FIGHTING AT A RESIDENTIAL TREATMENT CENTER

ROBERT HORAN

Every schoolboy knows that play is a common feature of adolescent social life. Although adolescents are faced with expectations that they prepare for and rehearse adult roles, youngsters who do not play appropriately or who do not play at all are thought to be lacking something. These adolescents are satirized as nerds and geeks or labeled bullies, loners, or deviants. Their marginality suggests a normative center—presumably one in which adolescents play right, go along to get along, and otherwise model the precepts of the parent culture.

Our conception of this normative center is related to our notions of play as "natural" in childhood (Garvey 1977) and to our witness of the "character-building" quality of organized sport (Cavallo 1981; Sutton-Smith 1986). In both cases, play is idealized: the voluntary, joyful, mastery-inducing, and creativity-enhancing aspects of play are promoted while their negatives are denied (Sutton-Smith 1981). The actual result in the home, classroom, or residential center seems to be that, when adolescents are engaging in idealized play forms in an appropriate fashion, they are thought to be playing. On the other hand, when they are play fighting, hanging out, or ritually insulting one another, they are engaged in what might be called nuisance behaviors. The point to be made is that, while these latter activities may well be nuisances to adults, they are not usually considered to be functional. Indeed, it is the unusual teacher or therapist who sees in such activity "the capacity of the ego to find recreation and self-cure in the activity of play" (Erickson 1950, p. 209).

In this chapter, I will argue that these activities are functional, and I will examine several instances of adolescent play masquerading as nuisance behavior. To do this, I will draw on findings of my participant observer study of Boys' Home, a residential treatment center for adolescent males. I will discuss two issues. The first is the invisibility of certain play forms in institutional life; the second is the semiotics of play fighting. I hope to show that play fighting is a structured activity that permits players to explore—physically and nonverbally—issues of sexuality, aggression, and intimacy.

Invisibility

I came to Boys' Home in 1981, armed with a plan to report on the folklore of the institution, and I stayed until 1985.[1] My original purpose was to find a site for dissertation research on adolescent folklore, but, because my wife and I were expecting our first child, I also needed a job. So I entered the Boys' Home community as an employee. My job was to coordinate the activities therapy program; my research goal was to observe the social life I participated in and to discover the community's significant expressive forms. At the time of my study, there were between thirty and forty boys, aged thirteen to eighteen, in residence at Boys' Home, and they, as well as the approximately fifty staff members, knew of my study. While my plans were regarded as an affectation or an improbable fancy, several youngsters were certain that, by letting the world know what they had to say, I would surely make a fortune. These residents were correct about the undiscovered emotional and interpersonal value of their expressive culture, even if they slightly miscalculated its economic value.

I had worked at the Adolescent Treatment Unit at the Institute of Pennsylvania Hospital for several years before returning to graduate school, but two years of graduate work had done much to remove me from the social world of adolescent boys. I was immediately struck by how physical my interactions were with the residents. After a brief sizing up period, I was pushed and pulled, hugged, and grabbed with alarming regularity. I was new and needed to establish my boundaries of personal space, but, even once this was accomplished, it was clear that the adolescents lived in a much more physically intimate world than I did.

This background of physical contact—touching, grabbing, pulling, pushing, and punching—moved to the foreground of our attention through a series of disputes about play. The residents seemed to be constantly bickering among themselves or complaining to staff members about another boy's "playing too much." In turn, staff members were complaining that the residents were "playing too much." Some staff were concerned that the boys were playing too roughly, while others felt that their play was too provocative, that the play was leading to fights. Up to this point, there had been no discussion of the boys' play that did not concern sports. Now, we found ourselves embroiled in distinctions between good and bad play, productive play, trivial play, and so forth. The kind of play we were concerned with was what the residents—along with the ethologists—called "play fighting," and it consisted of boys pushing, pulling, and punching one another or wrestling on the ground. As well as anyone could remember, this type of play had always gone on at Boys' Home, so why had it now become a problem?

In a word, George. A veritable king of play, George was an effervescent fifteen-year-old black boy who, on his arrival at Boys' Home, stood about six foot two and weighed about 220 pounds. At the time George arrived for a preplacement visit, most of the large and all the high-status residents were white; the younger and smaller black residents eagerly anticipated George's admission, hoping that he would redress many of their grievances. They began to defy the white boys who had bullied them, claiming that George "had their back." However, George was coming to Boys' Home because his "fighting" had made him appear unmanageable in his previous placement, and the state social workers had made it clear to George that more fights could well lead to his incarceration. According to George, his "fights" had resulted from his attempting to defend himself against racial slurs at the all-white high school he had been attending. Therefore, while it was in George's interest not to fight, it was also in his interest to oppose racist affronts.

George resisted the efforts of the smaller boys to enlist him in their battles. However, it was also among this group that he sought friends. The smaller residents had wanted George to accede to the role of pack leader; George refused this role. Seemingly because George refused to play the part designed for him by the smaller residents, his efforts to

369

make friends with them were marked by disputes. The smaller boys resented George for not settling old scores for them, while, in turn, George was overly familiar with them. George treated them, he later reported, the way he treated his younger brother.

Meanwhile, the disputes arising from George's play involved the staff as mediators of the residents' play, a role no one seemed to cherish. While most staff held that residents' abilities to negotiate personal relationships were a sign of their relative health, virtually all staff were loathe to become involved in these negotiations and appeared, as a result, determined to avoid taking an active role in them. Moreover, many staff regarded the maintenance of social order to be the most important of their duties. Against this definition of the situation, George's reputation as a fighter, the boys' complaints about George's play, and the occasional fights that arose from these disputes all seemed to be a challenge and contributed to what seemed an emergent crisis. Here is an example from a group counseling session of the grievances lodged against George (Horan 1986, p. 139):

Joe: He [George] came in here and started pluckin snow all over me and I cussed him out.

Teacher: But you been picking on him all morning.

Joe: Who has? Ain't nobody been pickin on him!

Paco: He was pickin on him when he woke up.

Joe: Ever since I woke up, he been pickin on me.

Paco: Yes, true.

Teacher: I don't know. I think you guys have a game going.

Joe: What it is, he like to play when I don't want to play and I tell him to stop playin, right. And he won't stop. Like you know how he be playin, kissin at you and stuff. And I be sayin, "Stop George, man, I think you gay, man." And then, right, I have to tell him for about fifteen minutes, then he decide to stop.

Paco: And then five minutes later he'll start again.

Joe: So when I start playin with *him*, right, he know he bigger than me, so he'll get mad and say, "If you don't stop playin, I'll fuck you up." Then I say, "How about when I be askin you?" And then, when he start grabbin me, I'll bite him.

370

As Joe's remarks suggest, George had disrupted the boys' play frame, and, in the process, he brought the framing, the artifice, the signification of both physicality and play to the center of community attention. As mentioned, the "play" that Joe alludes to is known as "play fighting" by ethologists, and my use of the term is intended to connect this study to related research on children and nonhuman animals (Aldis 1975; Blurton-Jones 1967; Fagen 1981). Unfortunately for human play fighting, the term is imprecise on even a descriptive level: "play fighting" is a play with sexuality as much as it is a play with aggression. Further, the layers of signification and the many possibilities for mixing messages, masking intentions, and alternately understanding and misunderstanding one another should alert us to the rich communicative potential of play fighting.

The nipping and mouthing of animal play fights may indeed "stand for" serious biting and chewing. But human nipping and mouthing connote an erotic aggression, an erotic hunger, at least as much as they connote nonhuman animal dominance rituals or the rehearsal of predatory skills (Neal 1985). Because humans—even juveniles—do not characteristically maintain dominance or acquire food by biting, the extension of the ethological explanation to humans adds "to the layers" of signification even as it claims to penetrate them. Because the functions of biting, mounting, and mouthing are different for humans and nonhuman mammals, the claim that these behaviors in humans are a rehearsal of adult skills is a simile. It consists of saying that human play is like animal play and that animal play seems to be a rehearsal of adult skills. This is the additional level of signification. I am not suggesting that ethological function could not be determined for human play fighting. But we do not have as much "natural history" data of human behavior as we have for the herring gull, to give but one example (Tinbergen 1953). The question of function is further, if not finally, complicated by human history, language, and culture, to say nothing of psychodynamics.

Yet, if we cannot satisfactorily answer the question of function, we have still before us the issue of communication. At the simplest level, play fighting clearly involves messages, senders, and receivers. But at the level above this, where signals are crossed, messages are mixed, and senders and receivers trade places, play fighting is more complex. If play fighting is a form of communication, what kinds of things does it communicate? Past puberty, human play fighting is employed principally by males. My argument is that, for these young men, play fighting both constitutes and reflects their relations with other boys. Conducted "at intimate distance," play fighting evokes reactions to emotional as well as physical closeness. Because the play signals play with agonistic behaviors, players are brought to an awareness of their partner's and their own aggressiveness. Because the play movements, particularly the wrestling, mimic sex play, the players cannot be unaware of the sexual connotations of their activity: when they are perceived to be unaware, their play partner or an observer is sure to bring it to their attention. Finally, because the play depends on each player letting his partner know what is acceptable to do and what is not, players must be cognizant of what they like and what their partner likes, and they will certainly learn where the boundary is that divides what they like and what they do not. In these ways, play fighting serves as a way for boys to play with being close to one another—a way to get close and keep your distance at once.

The Semiotics of Play Fighting

Joe's report about his dispute with George lists several of George's violations, and it also lists Joe's responses to them. Just as their dispute about play violations shows us the boys' expectations of play boundaries, so does Joe's report embody his purpose and his intentions without revealing them:

VIOLATION	RESPONSE
1. "Pluckin snow . . ."	"I cussed him out."
2. "Playin, kissin at you . . ."	"Stop . . . I think you gay, man."
3. "If you don't stop playin . . ."	"How about when I be askin you?"
4. "When he start grabbin me . . ."	"I'll bite him."

This list of violations and responses is "explained" by Joe's categorical description of them: "What it is, he like to play when I don't want to play and I tell him to stop playin, right. And he won't stop."

George's four violations and Joe's responses serve as support for Joe's claim about the nature of the problem. What is not explicit is the rhetorical nature of Joe's complaints. That is, what Joe wants and who he is trying to persuade are not entirely clear.

Joe correctly presumed that his complaints would be treated literally. The staff sided with Joe and subjected George to advice, lectures, and, finally, restriction in order to curb his playing too much. When the boys' play—and the complaints about George—persisted after these usual means of redressing grievances had been employed, the boys' cottage staff responded by outlawing play. In this extreme gesture, the staff declared that anything that looked like fighting would be treated as fighting. This new rule effectively stopped complaints, although it did not stop the play fighting. Faced with the choice of playing without complaints or not playing at all, the residents chose to play. The conflict surrounding the disputes about play subsided as the boys found solidarity in their joint opposition to the staff's decision and in their now-forbidden play.

Interestingly, George adapted to the secretive context of play fighting. Although his play was now considered a violation of the home's rules, George continued to be a popular play partner—even though the other players could no longer complain to the staff about him when he "played too much." Because the staff no longer needed to mediate the disputes about play fighting—the rule permitted them just to issue a restriction whenever a resident looked like he might be fighting—they eventually came to tolerate play fighting. One year after the rule was instituted, it was rarely enforced, and the message of the rule appeared to have been, Don't complain, rather than, Don't play.

For a number of staff members, disputes about play fighting were a bother. The play itself—boys rolling around on top of one another, grabbing, and pushing—appeared to be trivial and valueless. As such, play fighting was at odds with the goals of Boys' Home and the staff's desire to help the boys become productive and self-sufficient. The disputes engendered by the play were impossible to resolve because either complainant could be right or, in an extension of their play with one another, both could be lying. In this way, we justified our prohibition against play fighting. But what we missed was the importance of play as a means of the residents' managing their own affairs. For example, George became "socialized" to the routines at Boys' Home by breaking the rules and play fighting. George's desire to play with his friends and their mutual need to manage their own disputes were more important to his finally displaying appropriate behavior than our discussions, lectures, and warnings to him. Play fighting was significant because it was an arena in which the boys conducted their interpersonal affairs.

If we turn back now to Joe's complaint, we can identify a rhetorical purpose that Joe has not himself identified. Joe wants help in his dealings with George. By making his play fighting appear not to be play, Joe entitles himself to call on adult intervention. Why would Joe seek adult intervention? For present purposes, I will argue that Joe wanted to be protected from the emotional closeness of his relationship with George.

In his complaint, Joe describes himself as capable of responding to George's violations. While he is physically mismatched (Joe was perhaps five foot one and weighed about 110 pounds), Joe is able to employ both verbal (curse, threat, and reference to the rules) and physical (biting) means of defending himself. Although he is describing a series of play rule violations, a literal interpretation of his complaints effectively misses the interpersonal nature of his complaint. The teacher intuits this when she says, "I think you guys have a game going," but, because she is eager to dismiss the whole business as trivial, she does not recognize how right she is. The "game" they have going is their relationship, and they are specifically playing with the boundaries of self and other, reciprocity, and sexual identity. Joe's solicitation of adult intervention can be seen both as a request for help and as an extension of the game to include adults and blur the issue with George. Notwithstanding the play frame and the game analogy, these matters are hardly trivial.

While Joe lists four violations in his complaint, the central issue is, as he states, the lack of reciprocity in his play with George. This refers us to one of the key features of play fighting: the play is a result of the players' desire. At Boys' Home, play fighting occurs among networks of friends; it is primarily, though not exclusively, dyadic. The play fight encounter can be broken into a sequence of framed actions that are marked (and, thus, are likewise masked) by play signs: role reversals, self-handicapping, smiling, laughing, holding punches, kicks, bites, and an alternation between muscular tension and relaxation (Aldis 1975; Horan 1986). In Eco's semiotics (1979), play fighting would appear to be a "fictive sample" in which "part of a gesture [serves] as a sample of the entire gesture." In Bateson's (1972) description, these signs serve to communicate to the players that "this is not combat."

In general, play fights begin when one player pushes or shoves another and then awaits a response. The initiating player may run off a short distance, inviting a chase. The originally passive player chooses whether he wishes to play by returning the push, shove, or punch or by giving chase. Smiles or laughter are outward signs that this is play, but even these signs are dependent on the players' relationship. A smile would not be sufficient to begin a play fight with someone you did not know.

While the use of these signs outwardly resembles that of animal play, an important difference is that the Boys' Home residents masked these signs and otherwise used them as means of managing their relationships with one another. For example, the important smiling or laughing signs may be muted or nonexistent. This seems to force the passive player to interpret the active player's gesture in terms of their relationship. Further, because players are frequently within eyesight of adults whose job it is to understand their behavior, the play fight signs themselves— as well as postplay comments like Joe's complaints—should be seen as signs to nonplaying observers as well as to players. The following example shows George and Joe several months following Joe's complaint; it also introduces Glenn, fifteen and a well-developed 140 pounds (Horan 1986, pp. 168–170):

We had just finished a barbeque dinner outside. Some boys were lingering by the picnic tables talking; a few had drifted over to the basketball court. George was putting his trash in the dumpster. I stopped by to talk; we shook hands, then chatted about the 76ers parade and the celebration at Vet stadium where he'd gone with his class. Glenn came by and I greeted him. The three of us stood by the dumpster, telling stories and passing the time.

Joe came by to throw out his trash. He had two plates, a gob of salad dressing above his mouth, and he was still forking down food as he approached the dumpster. His red doubleknit pants, saggy and with runs in them, were unzipped and unbuttoned at the waist—his boxers showing in front and back, as his pants were sliding down. I asked him what was wrong with his pants. "Nothing," he said. Then I asked him why he didn't pull them up. He ignored me and turned to George and Glenn.

Glenn and George moved out a few steps from the dumpster, toward the yard. George went over to Glenn, grabbed him from behind, and leaned over him, bending Glenn forward. Joe, the salad dressing still on his mouth, circled around them.

George said, "He [Glenn] said he could get you."

Glenn looked over toward me.

Joe started to move in on Glenn, without having said a word. Glenn said, "Naw Joe, we're together." Then Joe punched George in the ribs.

"Cut it out," George complained. His tone was flat and remote.

"Let me go, George," Glenn said. George said nothing. Joe punched George again. Again George complained. Glenn said, "Come on, George, let me go." George was still bending him over forward, holding Glenn's arms behind his back, when Glenn started to walk with George on his back.

George said now in a loud voice, "Come *on,* Glenn. Let me go!" Though I knew this wasn't serious, I actually looked closer to see if George was still in control. Glenn then complained again to which George responded with another complaint that *he* was the one being held.

Joe punched George again. George assumed a hurt look now. He let go of Glenn and ran after Joe. Joe "half-ran" away, looking over his shoulder and smiling as George pursued him. George caught him, grabbed him from behind, and pulled him down. George then climbed on Joe's back and, kneeling over him, seemed to be biting his neck and whispering in his ear. Suddenly Joe shrieked.

Mrs. Moon shouted over for George to stop. I walked over to the two boys. I said to George, "Why are you on top of him? Look how much bigger you are. . . ."

George raised himself up off Joe, put one knee in the small of Joe's back and his hand on Joe's head (covering it entirely). Then George said, "All right Joe," and jumped back away from him.

Joe leaped up in a seeming fury. "You bitch!" he screamed at George. George started to run toward the cottage, smiling, his head turned back at Joe. Joe picked up a tiny stick and threw it at George, hitting him in the back. "So take that," Joe shouted. Then Joe started to walk back toward Glenn and I who were still standing by the dumpster. George followed at a distance. As George approached, Glenn extended his arm toward him, his hand clenched in a fist. Glenn said, "OK George, you want to grab me again?"

"No," George said and started to walk toward the school.

As we see in the example—one that featured players accustomed to each other and treated in this instance to an audience of staff members—all players masked their play signs, blurring the boundary between play and nonplay. It is precisely because play fighting proceeds by virtue of the exchange of signs that those signs can be manipulated: they can be masked, misinterpreted, parodied, exaggerated, and so forth. It is just this openness to a multiplicity of meanings that makes this play a form of communication and not merely an example of behavior in which gestures serve denotative functions. Joe's shrieking when George was atop him effectively drew staff attention to him as a victim; however, it did not result from his actually being hurt or from his desire to stop playing. Furthermore, unlike several months earlier, Joe's protests are not an example of his feeling that George was playing too roughly. Joe's willingness to continue playing with George indicated the degree to which George had learned to compromise in his play. Because it is so physical, play fighting requires the stronger player to handicap himself, to give up some of his strength in order to keep the smaller player involved. George's popularity as a play partner is the clearest evidence that he had learned what his partners wanted and what they did not want and that he had decided to respect their desires. It is perhaps for these reasons—the intensely physical nature of the play, the closeness, the contest, and the importance of knowing and respecting each other's boundaries—that at Boys' Home it was generally the healthier boys who participated. Psychotic residents, those who lacked a network of friends, as well as explosively aggressive boys simply did not engage in the kind of play I have been describing.

The role reversals illustrated in the above example offer yet another example of the structure of play fighting, as they also suggest a feature that permits players of widely discrepant size to play together. Once the two (or more) players contract for the play frame, the active and passive roles assume a status that seems independent of the players. Neither player is confined to one role; instead, they move in and out of the active and passive roles as if they were empty rooms in a house. If play fighting were simply a matter of establishing or confirming physical dominance (Neal 1985), there would be no need for George to play with either Glenn or Joe. The role reversals also work to distinguish play fighting from the serious activities they resemble: real fighting and real sex. At Boys' Home, both actual aggression and sexual activities have their own form and their own rules. In each, serious intentions seem to preclude changing roles and taking turns; in neither are role reversals foregrounded as they are in play fighting (Horan 1986). Just as play fighting takes place in between scheduled activities, in in-between places, so play fighting takes its place in between the serious activities of fighting and sex.

Situating play "in between" a temporal, spatial, or affective reality is a popular—and, in the case of play fighting at Boys' Home, an accurate—place for play theorists to put it (Turner 1967; Winnicott 1971). However, play fighting is also an activity that occurs at what Edward Hall has called "intimate distance": "At intimate distance, the presence of the other person is unmistakable and may at times be overwhelming because of the greatly stepped-up sensory inputs. Sight (often distorted), olfaction, heat from the other person's body, sound, smell, and feel of the breath all combine to signal unmistakable involvement with another body. . . . This is the distance of love-making and wrestling, comforting and protecting. Physical contact or the high possibility of physical contact is uppermost in the awareness of both persons" (Hall 1966, pp. 116–117). Play-fighting boys contend, quite directly, not only with each other's strength (Fagen 1976), but with their physicality and that of their partner. While the physicality described by Hall certainly includes strength, humans absorb information about far more than each other's strength. As I have mentioned, in many cases, there is no question at all of who is the stronger player. In our society, individuals do not get this close with serious intentions unless they are wrestling or making love. Consequently, play fighting among adolescent boys should more properly be viewed as a way to play with aggression, on the one hand, and with sexuality, on the other. It is doubtless because of the power of these feelings and the threat to their control that play fighting evokes that this play belongs to the healthier residents of Boys' Home. While the play was marked by the staff as deviant and bothersome, those residents who were deviant within the residents' social world did not participate.

Conclusions

This process of learning about play fighting, which I have described, constituted in the end a parallel process of learning about the social world of the residents of Boys' Home. The boys' play did not merely reflect their social world any more than it merely reflected their psychodynamic processes. The play was one instance of their social world. When my colleagues and I attempted to interpret their actions strictly in terms of our definition of the situation, we missed our opportunity to engage the residents in their own activity of self-realization. This is inevitably the case not only when we base our interventions on a model of deviance (Matza 1969) but whenever we presume play "stands for" something that is allegedly more serious. Clearly, it is not "deviance" that should be appreciated; rather, it is the reality that play claims as its own: "It is in playing and only in playing that the individual child or adult is able to be creative and to use the whole personality, and it is only in being creative that the individual discovers the self" (Winnicott 1971, p. 54).

NOTES

I would like to thank Harvey Horowitz and two anonymous readers for their helpful comments on an earlier draft of this chapter. Despite their kind help, whatever faults this paper may have are my responsibility. I would again like to thank the residents of Boys' Home for their stories, their play, and their hope.

1. A condition of my study was that the name of the institution and those of its residents remain anonymous. Boys' Home, George, Joe, and the others are fictional names for a real place and real people.

Founded in 1864, Boys' Home is now situated in an idyllic, campus-like setting in an exurban county of a northeastern state. Since the 1930s, the home has struggled to revise its original goal of providing a home away from home in order to care for increasingly poor, increasingly nonwhite, and increasingly disturbed children. Lacking the funding enjoyed by elite child-care institutions and lacking the motivational appeal of church-related institutions, the home has labored to create a therapeutic community with the human and financial resources at hand.

Residents of the home now come from throughout the state; virtually all are funded by the state social service agency. At the time of this study (1981–1985), the racial composition was 50 percent white, 40 percent black, and 10 percent Hispanic. The great majority of the boys come from urban neighborhoods and from the lowest socioeconomic classes. Practically all residents emerge from families that are, by even liberal standards, seriously disturbed. During their stay at the home, they go to on-grounds school and participate in cottage life and a variety of activities. Individual, group, and chemotherapies are provided by psychiatrists, psychologists, and clinical social workers. Family therapy is available, but it has been difficult to get the families to the home. While the residents are all labeled "emotionally disturbed" by child-study teams in the home school districts, few boys, according to the psychiatric consultants employed by the home, would be better served in a mental hospital. Likewise, while most residents have had contact with the police, most of their crimes are status offenses, and few would be better served by juvenile corrections.

REFERENCES

Aldis, O. 1975. *Play Fighting*. New York: Academic Press.

Bateson, G. 1972. *A Theory of Play and Fantasy: Steps to an Ecology of Mind*. New York: Ballantine.

Blurton-Jones, N. G. 1967. An ethological study of some aspects of social behavior of children in nursery school. In D. Muller-Schwarze, ed. *The Evolution of Play Behavior*. Stroudsburg, Pa.: Dowden, Hutchinson, & Ross.

Cavallo, D. 1981. *Muscles and Morals: Organized Playgrounds and Urban Reform, 1880–1920*. Philadelphia: University of Pennsylvania Press.

Eco, U. 1979. *A Theory of Semiotics*. Bloomington: Indiana University Press.

Erikson, E. 1950. *Childhood and Society*. New York: Norton.

Fagen, R. 1976. Exercise, play and physical training in animals. In P. P. G. Bateson and P. Klopfer, eds. *Perspectives in Ecology*. New York: Plenum.

Fagen, R. 1981. *Animal Play Behavior*. New York: Oxford.

Garvey, C. 1977. *Play*. Cambridge, Mass.: Harvard University Press.

Hall, E. 1966. *The Hidden Dimension*. Garden City, N.Y.: Anchor.

Horan, R. 1986. At intimate distance: playfighting, manliness, and social order at Boys' Home. Ph.D. diss., University of Pennsylvania.

Matza, D. 1969. *Becoming Deviant.* Englewood Cliffs, N.J.: Prentice-
Hall.

Neal, S. R. St. J. 1985. Rough-and-tumble and aggression in school-
children: serious play? *Animal Behaviour* 33(4): 1380–1381.

Sutton-Smith, B. 1981. The idealization of play: the relationship between play and sport. Paper delivered at the second annual conference of the North American Society of the Sociology of Sport, Fort
Worth, Texas.

Sutton-Smith, B. 1986. *Toys as Culture.* New York: Gardner.

Tinbergen, N. 1953. *The Herring Gull's World.* London: Methuen.

Turner, V. 1967. *The Forest of Symbols: Aspects of Ndembu Ritual.*
Ithaca, N.Y.: Cornell University Press.

Winnicott, D. W. 1971. *Playing and Reality.* New York: Basic.

PART III

DEVELOPMENTAL AND PSYCHOPATHOLOGICAL ISSUES IN ADOLESCENT PSYCHIATRY

EDITORS' INTRODUCTION

The current interest in the structural criteria in borderline states is of particular importance in the consideration of and the therapeutic efforts for severely disturbed adolescents. From a historical view it clarifies the importance of considering the developmental point of view with longitudinal, observational studies. From a diagnostic point of view, there is gradual general agreement that the borderline syndrome is a personality organization characterized by deficient self and object constancy derived from a developmental defect in ego functions. These formulations, both descriptive and dynamic, pose a serious problem for the clinician attempting to quantify the adolescent patient. The lack of integration makes the adolescent in regressive crisis from internal and external stresses look and act very "borderline." The chapters in this part illustrate developmental and psychopathological issues in adolescent psychiatry and range from the theoretical to clinical and research findings.

Donald B. Rinsley reviews his studies of the pathogenesis of borderline and narcissistic personality disorders and reaffirms his conclusion that the developmental defect related to maternal disjunctive double binding makes its appearance as early as ten to sixteen months. This, Rinsley explains, clarifies why significant oedipal material is not found among borderline and narcissistic cases. Powerful growth-inhibiting injunctions interfere with resolution of "oedipal-triadic and whole-object related dilemmas leading to identity diffusion expressed as a lack of integration of self and object representations and continued use of primitive defenses." Rinsley concludes that the treatment process requires the generation of the object permanency lacking in early development. This is dependent on the generation of mutual trust in the therapeutic relationship and represents establishment of the missing basic trust and eventually a cohesive sense of self.

Cynthia R. Pfeffer examines clinical dilemmas in the prevention of adolescent suicidal behavior. She reviews early recognition of and intervention with those youngsters who may be at risk and discusses prediction of suicidal behavior, assessment of risk factors, repeated suicidal tendencies, and resistance to treatment. Pfeffer concludes that clinical dilemmas are encompassing and involve facets of psychobiological characteristics, social milieu, and the care-giving setting. She advocates early intervention after the important first step of early recognition of the at-risk status of the adolescent.

Max Sugar discusses the battered child from the perspective of subtle forms of emotional abuse and neglect found in the schools, particularly in special education programs. He describes a form of abuse that results in anxiety, insomnia, neurotic symptoms, and psychosomatic disorders and stems from the intense transactions stimulated by transference-countertransference reactions in an adolescent inpatient setting. The author probes the value of psychiatric consultation to teachers and concludes that teachers of emotionally disturbed children and adolescents require practice experience in psychiatric settings.

Ann D. Sigafoos, Carl Feinstein, Marietta Damond, and David Reiss examine progression toward autonomy during adolescence. They studied the development of capabilities that allow for self-direction and a sense of responsibility for the self, behavioral autonomy, critical for self-direction into adulthood. Using a new instrument, the Autonomous Functioning Checklist, the authors summarize research findings that highlight the importance of developmental competence as a significant predictor of favorable psychosocial outcome in adulthood and as a protective factor against psychopathology in childhood.

Rosina G. Schnurr examines the psychological profiles of adolescent girls with trichotillomania using both objective and projective psychometric assessment. Schnurr reports no evidence of severe psychopathology but, rather, concludes that hair pulling may be a manifestation of neurotic reaction.

23 A REVIEW OF THE PATHOGENESIS OF BORDERLINE AND NARCISSISTIC PERSONALITY DISORDERS

DONALD B. RINSLEY

Nearly nine years ago, *Adolescent Psychiatry* asked me to contribute a resource paper on any aspect of my work I might choose. What I settled on was an attempt to provide a coherent historical account of the individual and, later, shared clinical research that had led to the development of Masterson's and my original formulation of the object-relations basis of borderline personality disorder that culminated in our paper on the role of the mother (Masterson and Rinsley 1975). The title of the invited paper that was eventually agreed on was "Borderline Psychopathology: The Concepts of Masterson and Rinsley and Beyond," and the paper found the light of day in 1981.

What follows here has to do with the "beyond," which I shall attempt to elucidate by tracing my own steps backward in time to the many years of experience I was fortunate enough to accumulate in the intensive residential treatment of preadolescent and adolescent children, including the treatment of their families. I began this work in 1959 and departed from it in 1975. During those fruitful years, my coworkers and I had the opportunity to examine in depth and detail the course and natural history of an inpatient therapeutic process directed toward no less than the thoroughgoing rebuilding of our youthful patients' disordered personalities and the restructuring of their dysfunctional family nexuses. In the course of that work, we had the opportunity to study the important contributions of Bettelheim (1950), Bettelheim and Sylvester (1949, 1952), Hendrickson and Holmes (1959), Hendrickson,

Holmes, and Waggoner (1959), Noshpitz (1962), and Redl (1959a, 1959b). Fundamental to our work was an understanding of child development as uniquely provided by psychoanalysis, in particular, the application of the concepts of transference and resistance to the events that were noted to transpire within the complex multidisciplinary milieu. Not surprisingly, we learned that our patients were the victims of traumas, of developmental arrests during the preoedipal years.

To understand these more adequately, we turned to the contributions of Federn (1952) and the British object-relations clinicians. In particular, we immersed ourselves in the writings of Fairbairn (1954), Klein (1975a, 1975b), and Mahler and her colleagues (Mahler, Pine, and Bergman 1975). Fairbairn and Klein provided an understanding of the vicissitudes of the internalized object relations our patients endlessly presented to us. The contributions of Mahler and her associates illuminated the process of separation-individuation. Winnicott's (1951, 1960a) concept of the "good enough" mother and environment and Bion's (1967) concept of the maternal container complemented and deepened our understanding of the earliest features of healthy and pathological child development. Also important for our work were the contributions of Bateson and his colleagues (Bateson 1972; Bateson, Jackson, Haley, and Weakland 1968) to the concept of the disjunctive double bind; of Lidz, Fleck, and Cornelison (1965, 1968), Singer and Wynne (1965a, 1965b), and Wynne and Singer (1963a, 1963b) to an understanding of how dysfunctional families proceed to ruin the developing identities of their offspring; and of Kernberg (1970a, 1970b, 1972, 1975, 1977) to an in-depth understanding of the narcissistically fixated borderline characterology that typified the majority of our young patients and their families. Finally, Bowlby's writings on early childhood grief and mourning (Bowlby 1960a, 1960b, 1961, 1962), Spitz's on anaclitic depression and psychic organizers (Spitz 1945, 1946, 1957, 1965; Spitz and Wolf 1946), and Bergman and Escalona's (1949) on unusual sensitivities in very young children filled out our picture of the effects of early psychological abandonment. We could, in turn, apply this accumulated knowledge to an effort to comprehend the variety of ways in which depersonified children attempt to compensate for the early traumas to which they had been exposed, as exemplified in Winnicott's (1960a) concept of false-self development.

My 1981 paper sought to bring together these various streams of thought as they were noted to contribute to an in-depth understanding of narcissistic psychopathology in adolescence. Included in its discussion was an account of how Masterson and I had independently reached very similar conclusions regarding the internalized object relations of our young patients, and both of us proceeded to extend our findings to include a consideration of these disordered internal states in adult cases as well. This more inclusive, latter-day work proceeded independently and in rather divergent directions. Masterson's evolving contributions pursued a further elaboration of the concept of the "split object-relations unit" (SORU) that we had set out in our 1975 paper, including extensive writings devoted to the psychodynamic psychotherapy of borderline and narcissistic conditions (Masterson 1981, 1983).

My own direction, as it were, carried my thinking beyond our original formulation of the split internalized endopsychic structures embodied in the formulation of the SORU, which I personally found to be simplistic and therapeutically limiting despite its original importance for our earlier theorizing. It had become apparent to me that Fairbairn (1954) had indeed described in a comprehensive fashion what our SORU had encompassed. His so-called basic endopsychic situation, with its emphasis on pristine splitting mechanisms derived in large measure from Klein's formulations regarding the schizoid and depressive positions (Klein 1935, 1940, 1946), very adequately described our patients' internalized object relations. It follows that the borderline patient, whether preadolescent, adolescent, or adult, is developmentally arrested at the level of preoedipal experience, somewhere at or between Fairbairn's late oral stage of infantile dependence and his stage of (transitional) quasi independence (Fairbairn 1954, pp. 28–58). The former of these stages, corresponding with Abraham's oral-aggressive stage of psychosexual development, finds the individual perceiving and responding to whole objects as if they are part objects, and developmental deviation here underlies the pathogenesis of affective disorder; the latter of these stages, in which whole objects are treated as contents, roughly corresponds to Abraham's anal-sadistic and anal-retentive stages, and developmental deviation here underlies the pathogenesis of paranoid and obsessional disorders (Abraham 1912, 1916, 1921, 1924). Further, insofar as hysterical psychopathology is, as it were, the "flip side" of obsessional psychopathology, in accordance with Fairbairn's concept of "transitional mechanisms," then hysterical disorders must be included among these syndromes as well. What we have, then, is the entire range, spectrum, or continuum of psychopathologic syndromes, the pathogenesis of which results, not from regression from unresolved oedipal conflict, but rather from preoedipal trauma, central to which, as Fairbairn cogently pointed out, is the untrammeled operation of the splitting defense.

Enter now the important contributions of Mahler and her colleagues (Mahler, Pine, and Bergman 1975). Her observational-analytic work, beginning with studies of infantile psychosis in the 1960s (Mahler 1968), led eventually to the conclusion (Mahler 1971) that developmental deviation occurring no later than twenty-six to thirty months of age yielded major problems with separation-individuation typical for what we now call borderline personality disorder (and, I perforce add, its more mature manifestation, narcissistic personality disorder). Thus, developmental problems originating during the preoedipal years, arising within the late oral and both anal stages, could be seen to underlie the genesis of major personality disorder as well as the more classical paranoid, obsessional, and hysteriform syndromes.

What was coming together as a result of this work was a synthesis of the major contributions of such divers clinicians as Klein (1975a) on the very early organization of the mind; Fairbairn (1954) on the primacy of splitting; Balint (1968) on "basic fault"; Federn (1952) on the deficiency of unifying energy; Winnicott (1960a, 1960b) on "good enough–ness"; and Kohut (1977) on the failure of early maternal empathy. Additions to our understanding of early trauma were Goldfarb's (1961) writings on parental perplexity and childhood schizophrenia; Jacobson's (1964) and Kernberg's (1966, 1972) on internal representational structures found in healthy and pathological development; Spitz's (1957) on "psychic organizers"; Bowlby's (1969, 1973) on the vicissitudes of attachment and loss; and the epochal work of Piaget (1954, 1963) on the evolution of operational thinking and the sense of reality. The gamut of psychopathological syndromes could indeed be viewed as arrayed along a developmental-diagnostic continuum based on very early developmental arrest, fixation, or deviation resulting from the breakdown or failure of the parent-child nurturant relationship. Such breakdown or failure could in turn be understood in terms of inadequacy or failure of mutual cuing or communicative matching between mother and child, leading to depersonification or appersonation of the child such that the child comes to be perceived and responded to as something or somebody other than what he or she actually is (Rinsley 1980b, pp. 185– 212; Rinsley 1982, pp. 199–215).

Masterson's and my earlier independent and later collaborative work with seriously disturbed in- and outpatient children and adolescents and their families had led to the discovery of a particular form of double-binding mother-child relationship that found peak expression during the rapprochement subphase of separation-individuation. It amounted to a maternal "message" to the child that to grow up, to assert one's ineluctable drive toward separation and individuation, would provoke a critical loss of maternal supplies and, conversely, that remaining dependent, hence essentially symbiotic, would ensure the maintenance of such supplies. We viewed this "message" in terms of an essentially unseparated and unindividuated mother's overdetermined need to perceive her child in terms of, and thereby to project into him or her, the mother's own unresolved separation-individuation dilemma. Put another way, the mother's inability to foster her child's separation-individuation conveyed a recapitulation of her own inability to have separated and individuated in relation to her own mother. The effect, for the child, was a threat of abandonment as a punishment for efforts to grow. It evoked in the child a pervasive form of dysphoric separation anxiety manifested as what Masterson and I termed "abandonment depression." Among the pejorative consequences of the depersonified child's separation-individuation failure are failure of differentiation of self- and object representations, persistent reliance on part-object relations of an essentially transitional nature (Modell 1968), failure to negotiate the tasks of the oedipal period, inadequate development of repression with ongoing reliance on splitting defenses, and inability to mourn. Together, these disabilities represent impairment of individuation, that is, of the development of an endopsychic structure capable of increasingly effectual, age-appropriate adaptation to the demands of one's internal and external environments; they define developmental arrest at, hence failure healthily to negotiate, the depressive position (Klein 1935, 1940).

The pathogenetic effect of such failure is an endopsychic condition characterized by what Kernberg (1966) terms a predominance of negative introjections; conversely, it implies a relative deficiency of positive introjections. Adler (1985) collectively refers to these positive introjections as the "soothing introject." As the function of this introject is to ease or allay the powerful affectomotor storms, the autonomic visceral instability to which all infants are otherwise subject (Mahler 1965; Rinsley 1987), its deficiency or inadequacy leaves the young child, and later the adult, deficient in the capacity to summon up or evoca-tively to recall those internal images that are necessary for the miti-gation or modulation of the internal disruptions of which all of us are episodic victims (Adler 1985). The borderline individual's defective evocative recall thus leads to a condition characterized by both object impermanency and object inconstancy (Rinsley 1984, 1985), which forms the basis for much of his or her symptomatology.

During the 1960s and 1970s, it became evident to a number of psy-choanalytic investigators that there exists a range of personality dis-orders that, irrespective of their descriptive symptomatology or their state-determined nosology, share a psychodynamics and internalized object relations that may be considered to be borderline in nature, that is, midway, as it were, between psychosis and what had generally been thought of as psychoneurosis. The factor-analytic studies of Grinker and his colleagues (Grinker and Werble 1977; Grinker, Werble, and Drye 1968) pointed toward the existence of a spectrum or continuum of borderline disorders that found support in the later writings of such investigators as Adler (1985), Kernberg (1980, 1984), Kohut (1977), Meissner (1984), Rinsley (1982), and Stone (1980). The idea thus evolved that the range of diagnosable personality disorders, including the three syndrome "clusters" set forth in the DSM-III and DSM-III-R (*Diag-nostic and Statistical Manual of Mental Disorders* 1980 and 1987, re-spectively), could be subsumed under either of two major diagnostic categories of personality disorder, namely, the (lower-level) borderline and the (higher-level) narcissistic. Indeed, Adler (1981) published a key paper aptly entitled "The Borderline-Narcissistic Personality Disorder Continuum."

The question naturally arose concerning how to account for the gen-erally more coherent, more stable, and often higher-achieving func-tioning of the narcissistic personality as compared with the less adequately functioning borderline personality. Analysis of the former cases soon provided at least a partial answer. What we found was that there indeed had been a double-binding maternal message to the de-veloping child who would later emerge as suffering from narcissistic personality disorder, differing in one major respect, however, from that communicated to the future borderline. That message was to the effect that one could indeed go through the motions of emancipatory growing up, but if and only if everything to be accomplished was inevitably in relation to the maternal figure. Thus did a powerful, controlling maternal introject foster a developmental state of affairs in accordance with which a significant degree of individuation could occur without a concomitant degree of separation (Rinsley 1980b, pp. 287–293; Speers and Morter 1980). This dissociation of the individuation subprocess from the separation subprocess seemed to characterize the developmental history of the narcissistic personality. As a result of the presence in such cases of the powerful maternal introject, there resulted no defect in evocative recall, no failure of object permanency, as occurred in the case of the borderline personality; but the fearful price that the narcissistic personality had to pay could be counted in failed and blighted interpersonal relationships, riven by ambivalence and typified by exploitiveness and emotional detachment. Inasmuch as the evocative recall of the maternal image or its perceptual equivalents called up powerful charges of ambivalence in view of its preclusion of other, healthy relationships, it failed ultimately to serve as a "soothing introject"; hence, it failed to provide what Anna Freud (1960, 1968) termed object constancy. In both borderline and narcissistic cases, the ever-present threat of abandonment underlies all else. In the case of the borderline personality, the threat concerns overall growth apart from the symbiotic mother; in the case of the narcissistic personality, the threat concerns achievement and relationships apart from her. It is this maternal introject in all its varied endopsychic manifestations that provides for the narcissistic personality what Kohut (1977) terms stable, archaic self and self-objects in contrast to what he terms fragmented archaic self and self-objects that typify the borderline personality.

In 1984 and 1985, I had the opportunity to publish two papers in which these matters were considered in some detail. The latter paper presented an account of the developmental pathogenesis of the narcissistic personality based on extensive experience with prior and current juvenile and adult cases. What emerged from this experience was the fact that the form that the depersonification of the future narcissistic child had originally assumed amounted to a profound adultomorphization, which had spurred the child on toward the development of an essentially obsessional personality organization with its defensive isolation of cognition from affect. The basis for this proved not difficult to determine: it resulted from the mother's powerful need to get rid of what appeared to her as a needy but persecutory infantile object, the projected image of the mother's own neediness and the aggression stemming from it; paradoxically, in addition, it resulted from the mother's equally powerful need to create, as it were, an adult "container," a nurturing, succoring figure who would, at last, slake her long-unrequited thirst for supplies. All this the unfortunate child proceeded to internalize, setting up this maternal introject within the self as a harshly devaluing and expectantly demanding superego forerunner that could provide the services of a quasi-soothing introject only if its ultimately symbiotic demands were met. This, it became apparent, was the origin of the narcissistic personality's object inconstancy that could be seen to exist alongside an otherwise well-preserved object permanency (Rinsley 1982, pp. 153–169; Rinsley 1984; Rinsley 1985).

The etiology of the narcissistic personality's chronic depressive dysphoria also became clear: it stems from the maternal superego's unremittent demands and devaluations. The ego's response to these is to mount the range of manic defenses against them: *grandiosity,* conveyed by persistent infantile omnipotence, a by-product of adultomorphization that endows the child's nascent ego with enormous power that drives it to fuse with and temporarily vanquish the maternal-superego introject (identification with the superego), resulting in episodic, triumphant, manic states; *devaluation* of others, viewed as persecutors, resulting from the projection of hostile impulses into them; *pathological idealization* as a way of denying others' persecutory nature; *persistent splitting,* conveyed by an all good–all bad worldview and the essentially unintegrated self- and object representations common to borderline and narcissistic personalities; *manic restitution,* with its variety of self-sacrificial actions derived from the need to restore the powerful introject perceived as damaged by one's aggression directed toward, and identification with, it; and, of course, the *denial* common to all these. Added to them are the isolation of affect, overintellectualization, and guilt-laden undoing that characterize the obsessional component of the narcissistic personality. Together, all these account for the often-puzzling mixture of autoplastic and alloplastic symptomatology that typifies this "higher-level" borderline personality.

Developmental Chronology and Its Critics

No discussion of these matters could be deemed thorough unless some reference was made to the dimension of time in relation to pathogenesis. It was Margaret Mahler herself who, in 1971, drew attention to the rapprochement subphase of separation-individuation, that is, the

394

period roughly spanning sixteen to thirty months postnatally, as significantly related to the etiology of borderline disorder. This is the period of what she termed the "rapprochement crisis," that is, the toddler's first significant awareness of separateness from the person of the mother with its mixture of pleasure and separation anxiety that accompany that awareness in both mother and child. Masterson and I (1975) could readily confirm Mahler's hypothesis. We found that the depersonifying, disjunctive maternal message of reward for dependency and abandonment for growth, so critical for the genesis of borderline personality disorder, reached the apex of its effect during the rapprochement subphase and, further, that it actually fueled the rapprochement crisis that, it turns out, finds disruptive symptomatic expression in those children who are the victims of depersonifying parenting.

It was again Mahler herself, together with Louise Kaplan and others, who took Masterson and me to task for what seemed to suggest, in our earlier writings, that borderline disorder could be traced to events specific or limited to the rapprochement subphase per se (Kaplan 1980; Mahler and Kaplan 1977). I must admit that our writings did indeed leave the reader open to such an inference. Two criticisms, each of which centered on this issue, were directed toward us.

The first of these concerned what Mahler and Kaplan termed "subphase adequacy." Kaplan (1980) wrote, "To focus . . . on the dominance of one subphase manifestation in the content of treatment material, whether as transference or actual life behavior, serves to obscure that there are always corrective or pathogenic influences from other phases of separation-individuation which will also have left their imprint on oedipal organization" (p. 41). Again, "Mahler's findings on *normal* subphase adequacy will eventually illuminate facets of the Oedipus complex which have remained obscure—for example, the effects of separation-individuation on narcissism, the fate of the libidinal and aggressive drives, and the differential outcomes of gender identity in men and women" (p. 40). Inherent in this criticism one may discern a resurgence of the knotty problem of developmental arrest or fixation versus regression, the latter representing the classical view of pathogenesis as epitomized in Arlow and Brenner's (1964) monograph and in Abend, Porder, and Willick's (1983) concept of borderline pathogenesis and treatment. This conflict, in turn, represents a manifestation of the even knottier problem that besets contemporary psychoanalytic theorizing, involving devotees of the so-called drive-defense and deficit approaches (Greenberg and Mitchell 1983). Of course, oedipal material is abundant in the lives and therapeutic experience of borderline and narcissistic personalities since everyone, including psychotics who present such material in more fragmented form, "passes through" an oedipal stage, and it is almost a platitude to assert that major difficulties with separation-individuation inevitably exert a most baleful effect on the child's ensuing efforts to negotiate the oedipal task and, hence, to achieve healthy repression, whole-object relations, and the capacity to mourn. It is my view, however—and clinical experience with primitively organized personalities and their families affirms this—that such oedipal material constitutes an epiphenomenon engrafted on prior traumas resulting from the depersonifying experiences to which I have referred, leading to primary developmental arrest. I, for one, find it impossible to understand the borderline patient's notable problems with self-identity, with the vicissitudes of "raw" aggression and sexuality, with failure of sublimation, and with alloplastic symptomatology in terms of regression from traumas associated with oedipal tasks, not to mention the signal failure of "classical" analytic technique with these patients, Abend, Porder, and Willick (1983) to the contrary notwithstanding. Essentially the same holds true for the borderline's less immature sibling, the narcissist.

The second criticism of our work has to do with the role of the mother in the pathogenesis of borderline personality disorder (and, of course, narcissistic personality disorder by latter-day extension). Put succinctly, Esman (1980) accuses us of "mother baiting," of blaming it all on Mom when, for example, there is significant evidence that many borderline people come into the world with cognitive-perceptual deficits that pave the way for major problems with separation-individuation. A related criticism has to do with objections to Masterson's and my original inference that the mothers of borderline juveniles and adults themselves suffer from borderline personality disorder.

So far as the "mother-baiting" criticism is concerned, suffice it to say that our awareness of pathogenic mothering patterns, and specifically of the disjunctive communications to which I have referred, grew both from direct observation of family interactions during treatment and from patients' descriptions and accounts of the events of their early childhood and ensuing years. In all fairness, it must be conceded that, in many cases of individual analytic treatment, an adequate differentiation could not be made between what had actually taken place and the patients' inferential accounts and fantasies of actual occurrences and patterns. Still, the reported occurrences and patterns of interaction showed a notable consistency across cases. Of course, the role of the father, if indeed there was one in the home during the patient's prelatency years, was noted to exert a very important influence on the mother's parenting patterns; although a comprehensive discussion of such a role and influence is beyond the scope of this chapter, reference needs to be made to dysfunctional mate selection, and parental interactional patterns as these affect the mother's capacity to mother her children (Rinsley and Rinsley 1987).

The criticism to the effect that not all mothers of borderline children and adults can be validly diagnosed as borderline themselves (Chatham 1985, p. 206; Shapiro 1978; Shapiro, Zinner, Shapiro, and Berkowitz 1975; Singer 1977) becomes an arguable issue when one focuses not on nosology but on parenting patterns. Diagnostically, the matter comes down to which of the many extant state- or trait-related criteria one chooses to use, including those set forth in the DSM-III and DSM-III-R. Thus, while all swans are not white and all mothers of borderline patients may well not be diagnosable as themselves suffering from borderline personality disorder depending on the criteria employed, it can be said that Masterson and I had not discovered one who had not recapitulated with her unfortunate offspring the very abandonment-depressive issues so evident in the latter.

Conclusions

I might summarize these considerations by reaffirming the evident fact that preoedipal as well as oedipal determinants and experiences play significant roles in the psychic economy of borderline and narcissistic personalities. Thus, while the parental depersonifications destined to bring about major personality disorder certainly do not appear de novo during the rapprochement subphase, they nonetheless become egregiously apparent during that time when, as Mahler has pointed out, the child mounts a sustained if ambivalent effort toward separation. It is also clear that the maternal disjunctive double binding of the child makes its appearance no later than the antecedent practicing subphase (ten to sixteen months), when the now bipedal, binocular toddler "falls in love with the world" and proceeds aggressively to explore it. I have no doubt that the problem has even earlier roots, although our clinical data do not provide adequate support for this inference.

Again, as I have already noted, significant oedipal material is hardly to be unexpected among borderline and narcissistic cases, and the reason for this is not difficult to determine. Already saddled with powerful growth-inhibiting injunctions, these patients come to further grief as the inexorable push of development thrusts them into oedipal-triadic and whole-object-related dilemmas that they are incapable of resolving. Freud's redoubtable "queen of the neuroses" is hardly the issue with them.

Finally, there is no end of objections to the concept of so-called critical stages or periods with its implication of functions or achievements forever undeveloped or lost unless experienced at those particular times (Esman 1980). Most of these objections correctly point out that postulated developmental chronologies are usually too rigid and that the timing of children's expanding masteries is both highly flexible and idiosyncratic. The most quoted of these recent critics is Stern (1985), who disputes Mahler's concept of phases and, in particular, throws out her concept of the autistic phase. But even Stern cannot escape some notion of phasic development—witness his so-called emergent self (zero to two months), core self (two to seven months), subjective self (up to eighteen months), and verbal self (eighteen months and beyond). And Mahler never disputed the fact, central to object-relations theory, that infants seek objects ab initio—witness the immediate rooting and sucking reflexes. It needs to be remembered that Mahler regarded her phases, and, in particular, the symbiotic phase, essentially as metaphors (Mahler 1968; Mahler, Pine, and Bergman 1975).

If the notion of some sort of continuum finds fruitful expression in the domain of developmental diagnosis, should we expect to find it applicable as well to treatment? We should, and it is. It was none other than Freud himself (1913) who suggested an analogy between the course of psychoanalytic treatment and the phasic games of chess. Lewis (1970) and Masterson and I (Masterson 1972; Rinsley 1980a, 1980b) applied it to the course of intensive residential treatment, and Adler (1985) applied it to the psychoanalytic treatment of adult borderline cases. In particular, Adler correctly concluded that the successful treatment of borderline personality resulted in the emergence of the (higher-level) narcissistic personality. The key to this transmutation is to be found in the generation of object permanency where, before, it was lacking. In Adler's terms, the transmutation hinges on the formation of the "soothing introject," initially organized around the person of the therapist or analyst. Once this has occurred, the basis for a genuine therapeutic alliance has been formed.

The establishment of the soothing introject is predicated on the generation of mutual trust in the therapeutic relationship. It is not difficult to see that such trust represents the "basic trust" (Erikson 1963) that was lacking very early in the patient's mother-child relationship. Stated in terms of "empathy," this is the major point of treatment as practiced by the followers of self psychology (Kohut 1977, 1982). It is inherent in Langs's (1976) notion of the "bipersonal field," in Bion's (1967) notion of the "container-contained," and in Winnicott's (1950–1955, 1960a, 1960b) concept of the "good enough" mother and environment.

Once object permanency has been established, the pathway is open to the generation of true object constancy with its capacity for the evocative recall of genuinely soothing (affecto-motor tension-reducing) self-object representations, now apart from the immediacy of the therapeutic relationship. With that, a cohesive self proceeds to come together, the hallmark of psychological health.

NOTE

This chapter was presented at the meeting of the American Society for Adolescent Psychiatry Institute V, "Adolescent Psychotherapy: Clinical Approaches and Research Perspectives," Seattle, Washington, February 27, 1988.

REFERENCES

Abend, S. M.; Porder, M. S.; Willick, M. S. 1983. *Borderline Patients: Psychoanalytic Perspectives*. Kris Study Group of the New York Psychoanalytic Institute, Monograph no. 7. New York: International Universities Press.

Abraham, K. 1912. Notes on the psycho-analytical investigation and treatment of manic-depressive insanity and allied conditions. In *Selected Papers on Psycho-Analysis* (*Selected Papers of Karl Abraham, M.D.*). London: Hogarth, 1927; 1953.

Abraham, K. 1916. The first pregenital stage of the libido. In *Selected Papers on Psycho-Analysis* (*Selected Papers of Karl Abraham, M.D.*). London: Hogarth, 1927; 1942.

Abraham, K. 1921. Contributions to the theory of the anal character. In *Selected Papers on Psycho-Analysis* (*Selected Papers of Karl Abraham, M.D.*). London: Hogarth, 1927; 1942.

Abraham, K. 1924. A short study of the development of the libido, viewed in the light of mental disorders. In *Selected Papers on Psycho-Analysis* (*Selected Papers of Karl Abraham, M.D.*). London: Hogarth, 1927; 1942; 1953.

Adler, G. 1981. The borderline-narcissistic personality disorder continuum. *American Journal of Psychiatry* 138:46–50.

Adler, G. 1985. *Borderline Psychopathology and Its Treatment*. New York: Jason Aronson.

Arlow, J., and Brenner, C. 1964. *Psychoanalytic Concepts and the Structural Theory*. New York: International Universities Press.

Balint, M. 1968. *The Basic Fault: Therapeutic Aspects of Regression*. London: Tavistock.

Bateson, G. 1972. *Steps to an Ecology of Mind*. New York: Ballantine.

Bateson, G.; Jackson, D.; Haley, J.; and Weakland, J. 1968. Toward a theory of schizophrenia. In D. Jackson, ed. *Communication, Family and Marriage*. Palo Alto, Calif.: Science & Behavior Books.

Bergman, P., and Escalona, S. 1949. Unusual sensitivities in very young children. *Psychoanalytic Study of the Child* 3/4:333–352.

Bettelheim, B. 1950. *Love Is Not Enough*. Glencoe, Ill.: Free Press.

Bettelheim, B., and Sylvester, E. 1949. Milieu therapy: indications and illustrations. *Psychoanalytic Review* 36:54–68.

Bettelheim, B., and Sylvester, E. 1952. A therapeutic milieu. *American Journal of Orthopsychiatry* 22:314–334.

Bion, W. R. 1967. *Second Thoughts: Selected Papers on Psychoanalysis*. New York: Basic.

Bowlby, J. 1960a. Grief and mourning in infancy and early childhood. *Psychoanalytic Study of the Child* 15:9–52.

Bowlby, J. 1960b. Separation anxiety. *International Journal of Psycho-Analysis* 41:89–113.

Bowlby, J. 1961. Processes of mourning. *International Journal of Psycho-Analysis* 42:317–340.

Bowlby, J. 1962. Childhood bereavement and psychiatric illness. In D. Richter, J. M. Tanner, L. Taylor, and O. L. Zangwill, eds. *Aspects of Psychiatric Research*. London: Oxford University Press.

Bowlby, J. 1969. *Attachment*. Vol. 1 of *Attachment and Loss*. New York: Basic.

Bowlby, J. 1973. *Separation: Anxiety and Anger*. Vol. 2 of *Attachment and Loss*. New York: Basic.

Chatham, P. M. 1985. *Treatment of the Borderline Personality*. New York: Jason Aronson.

Diagnostic and Statistical Manual of Mental Disorders (DSM-III). 1980. 3d ed. Washington, D.C.: American Psychiatric Association.

Diagnostic and Statistical Manual of Mental Disorders (DSM-III-R). 1987. 3d ed., rev. Washington, D.C.: American Psychiatric Association.

Erikson, E. H. 1963. *Childhood and Society*. Rev. ed. New York: Norton.

Esman, A. H. 1980. Adolescent psychopathology and the rapprochement process. In R. F. Lax, S. Bach, and J. A. Burland, eds. *Rapprochement: The Critical Subphase of Separation-Individuation*. New York: Jason Aronson.

Fairbairn, W. R. D. 1954. *An Object-Relations Theory of the Personality*. New York: Basic.

Federn, P. 1952. *Ego Psychology and the Psychoses*. New York: Basic.

Freud, A. 1960. Discussion of Dr. John Bowlby's paper. *Psychoanalytic Study of the Child* 15:53–62.

Freud, A. 1968. Panel discussion held at the 25th Congress of the International Psycho-Analytical Association, Copenhagen, July, 1967. *International Journal of Psycho-Analysis* 49:506–512.

Freud, S. 1913. On beginning the treatment (further recommendations on the technique of psycho-analysis, I). *Standard Edition* 12:123. London: Hogarth, 1958.

Goldfarb, W. 1961. *Childhood Schizophrenia*. Cambridge, Mass.: Harvard University Press.

Greenberg, J. R., and Mitchell, S. A. 1983. *Object Relations in Psychoanalytic Theory*. Cambridge, Mass.: Harvard University Press.

Grinker, R. R., and Werble, B. 1977. *The Borderline Patient*. New York: Jason Aronson.

Grinker, R. R.; Werble, B.; and Drye, R. 1968. *The Borderline Syndrome: A Behavioral Study of Ego Functions*. New York: Basic.

Hendrickson, W. J., and Holmes, D. J. 1959. Control of behavior as a crucial factor in intensive psychiatric treatment on an all-adolescent ward. *American Journal of Psychiatry* 115:969–973.

Hendrickson, W. J.; Holmes, D. J.; and Waggoner, R. W. 1959. Psychotherapy of the hospitalized adolescent. *American Journal of Psychiatry* 116:527–532.

Jacobson, E. 1964. *The Self and the Object World.* New York: International Universities Press.

Kaplan, L. J. 1980. Rapprochement and oedipal organization: effects on borderline phenomena. In R. F. Lax, S. Bach, and J. A. Burland, eds. *Rapprochement: The Critical Subphase of Separation-Individuation.* New York: Jason Aronson.

Kernberg, O. F. 1966. Structural derivatives of object relationships. *International Journal of Psycho-Analysis* 47:236–253.

Kernberg, O. F. 1970a. Factors in the psychoanalytic treatment of narcissistic personalities. *Journal of the American Psychoanalytic Association* 18:51–85.

Kernberg, O. F. 1970b. A psychoanalytic classification of character pathology. *Journal of the American Psychoanalytic Association* 18:800–822.

Kernberg, O. F. 1972. Early ego integration and object relations. *Annals of the New York Academy of Sciences* 193:233–247.

Kernberg, O. F. 1975. *Borderline Conditions and Pathological Narcissism.* New York: Jason Aronson.

Kernberg, O. F. 1977. The structural diagnosis of borderline personality organization. In P. Hartocollis, ed. *Borderline Personality Disorders: The Concept, the Syndrome, the Patient.* New York: International Universities Press.

Kernberg, O. F. 1980. *Internal World and External Reality: Object Relations Theory Applied.* New York: Jason Aronson.

Kernberg, O. F. 1984. *Severe Personality Disorders: Therapeutic Strategies.* New Haven, Conn.: Yale University Press.

Klein, M. 1935. A contribution to the psychogenesis of manic-depressive states. In *Melanie Klein: Love, Guilt and Reparation and Other Works, 1921–1945.* New York: Delacorte/Seymour Lawrence, 1975.

Klein, M. 1940. Mourning and its relation to manic-depressive states. In *Melanie Klein: Love, Guilt and Reparation and Other Works, 1921–1945.* New York: Delacorte/Seymour Lawrence, 1975.

Klein, M. 1946. Notes on some schizoid mechanisms. In *Melanie Klein: Envy and Gratitude and Other Works, 1946–1963.* New York: Delacorte/Seymour Lawrence, 1975.

Klein, M. 1975a. *Melanie Klein: Envy and Gratitude and Other Works, 1946–1963.* New York: Delacorte/Seymour Lawrence.

Klein, M. 1975b. *Melanie Klein: Love, Guilt and Reparation and Other Works, 1921–1945.* New York: Delacorte/Seymour Lawrence.

Kohut, H. 1977. *The Restoration of the Self.* New York: International Universities Press.

Kohut, H. 1982. Introspection, empathy and the semi-circle of mental health. *International Journal of Psycho-Analysis* 63:395–407.

Langs, R. J. 1976. *The Bipersonal Field.* New York: Jason Aronson.

Lewis, J. M. 1970. The development of an adolescent inpatient service. *Adolescence* 5:303–312.

Lidz, T.; Fleck, S.; and Cornelison, A. R. 1965. *Schizophrenia and the Family.* New York: International Universities Press.

Lidz, T.; Fleck, S.; and Cornelison, A. R. 1968. Schism and skew in the families of schizophrenics. In N. W. Bell and E. F. Vogel, eds. *A Modern Introduction to the Family.* New York: Free Press.

Mahler, M. S. 1965. On early infantile psychosis: the symbiotic and autistic syndromes. *Journal of the American Academy of Child Psychiatry* 4:554–568. Reprinted in *The Selected Papers of Margaret S. Mahler.* New York: Jason Aronson, 1979.

Mahler, M. S. (in collaboration with M. Furer). 1968. *Infantile Psychosis.* Vol. 1 of *On Human Symbiosis and the Vicissitudes of Individuation.* New York: International Universities Press.

Mahler, M. S. 1971. A study of the separation-individuation process and its possible application to borderline phenomena in the psychoanalytic situation. *Psychoanalytic Study of the Child* 26:403–424. Reprinted in *The Selected Papers of Margaret S. Mahler.* New York: Jason Aronson, 1979.

Mahler, M. S., and Kaplan, L. J. 1977. Developmental aspects in the assessment of narcissistic and so-called borderline personalities. In P. Hartocollis, ed. *Borderline Personality Disorders: The Concept, the Syndrome, the Patient.* New York: International Universities Press.

Mahler, M. S.; Pine, F.; and Bergman, A. 1975. *The Psychological Birth of the Human Infant: Symbiosis and Individuation.* New York: Basic.

Masterson, J. F. 1972. *Treatment of the Borderline Adolescent: A Developmental Approach.* New York: Wiley-Interscience.

Masterson, J. F. 1981. *The Narcissistic and Borderline Disorders: An Integrated Developmental Approach.* New York: Brunner/Mazel.

Masterson, J. F. 1983. *Countertransference and Psychotherapeutic Technique: Teaching Seminars on Psychotherapy of the Borderline Adult.* New York: Brunner/Mazel.

Masterson, J. F., and Rinsley, D. B. 1975. The borderline syndrome: the role of the mother in the genesis and psychic structure of the borderline personality. *International Journal of Psycho-Analysis* 56:163–177.

Meissner, W. W. 1984. *The Borderline Spectrum: Differential Diagnosis and Developmental Issues*. New York: Jason Aronson.

Modell, A. H. 1968. *Object Love and Reality: An Introduction to a Psychoanalytic Theory of Object Relations*. New York: International Universities Press.

Noshpitz, J. D. 1962. Notes on the theory of residential treatment. *Journal of the American Academy of Child Psychiatry* 1:284–296.

Piaget, J. 1954. *The Construction of Reality in the Child*. New York: Basic.

Piaget, J. 1963. *The Origins of Intelligence in Children*. New York: Norton.

Redl, F. 1959a. The concept of a "therapeutic milieu." *American Journal of Orthopsychiatry* 29:721–736.

Redl, F. 1959b. Strategy and technique of the life space interview. *American Journal of Orthopsychiatry* 29:1–18.

Rinsley, D. B. 1980a. Principles of therapeutic milieu with children. In G. P. Sholevar, R. M. Benson, and B. J. Blinder, eds. *Emotional Disorders in Children and Adolescents: Medical and Psychological Approaches to Treatment*. New York: SP Medical & Scientific Books.

Rinsley, D. B. 1980b. *Treatment of the Severely Disturbed Adolescent*. New York: Jason Aronson.

Rinsley, D. B. 1981. Borderline psychopathology: the concepts of Masterson and Rinsley and beyond. *Adolescent Psychiatry* 9:259–274.

Rinsley, D. B. 1982. *Borderline and Other Self Disorders: A Developmental and Object-Relations Perspective*. New York: Jason Aronson.

Rinsley, D. B. 1984. A comparison of borderline and narcissistic personality disorders. *Bulletin of the Menninger Clinic* 48:1–9.

Rinsley, D. B. 1985. Notes on the pathogenesis and nosology of borderline and narcissistic personality disorders. *Journal of the American Academy of Psychoanalysis* 13:317–328.

Rinsley, D. B. 1987. A reconsideration of Fairbairn's "original object" and "original ego" in relation to borderline and other self disorders. In J. F. Grotstein, M. F. Solomon, and J. A. Lang, eds. *The Bor-

derline Patient: Emerging Concepts in Diagnosis, Psychodynamics and Treatment. Hillsdale, N.J.: Analytic.

Rinsley, D. B., and Rinsley, C. 1987. Incest: its developmental and familial context. *Seminars in Adolescent Medicine* 3:9–16.

Shapiro, E. R. 1978. The psychodynamics and developmental psychology of the borderline patient: a review of the literature. *American Journal of Psychiatry* 135:1305–1315.

Shapiro, E. R.; Zinner, J.; Shapiro, R. L.; and Berkowitz, D. A. 1975. The influence of family experience on borderline personality development. *International Review of Psycho-Analysis* 2:399–411.

Singer, M. T. 1977. The borderline diagnosis and psychological tests: review and research. In P. Hartocollis, ed. *Borderline Personality Disorders: The Concept, the Syndrome, the Patient*. New York: International Universities Press.

Singer, M. T., and Wynne, L. C. 1965a. Thought disorder and family relations of schizophrenics. III. methodology using projective techniques. *Archives of General Psychiatry* 12:186–200.

Singer, M. T., and Wynne, L. C. 1965b. Thought disorder and family relations of schizophrenics. IV. results and implications. *Archives of General Psychiatry* 12:201–212.

Speers, R. W., and Morter, D. C. 1980. Overindividuation and underseparation in the pseudomature child. In R. F. Lax, S. Bach, and J. A. Burland, eds. *Rapprochement: The Critical Subphase of Separation-Individuation*. New York: Jason Aronson.

Spitz, R. A. 1945. Hospitalism: an inquiry into the genesis of psychiatric conditions of early childhood. *Psychoanalytic Study of the Child* 1:53–74.

Spitz, R. A. 1946. Hospitalism: a follow-up report. *Psychoanalytic Study of the Child* 2:113–117.

Spitz, R. A. 1957. *No and Yes: On the Genesis of Human Communication*. New York: International Universities Press.

Spitz, R. A. 1965. *The First Year of Life: A Psychoanalytic Study of Normal and Deviant Development of Object Relations*. New York: International Universities Press.

Spitz, R. A., and Wolf, K. M. 1946. Anaclitic depression: an inquiry into the genesis of psychiatric conditions of early childhood. II. *Psychoanalytic Study of the Child* 2:313–342.

Stern, D. N. 1985. *The Interpersonal World of the Infant: A View from Psychoanalysis and Developmental Psychology*. New York: Basic.

Stone, M. H. 1980. *The Borderline Syndromes: Constitution, Personality, and Adaptation*. New York: McGraw-Hill.

Winnicott, D. W. 1950–1955. Aggression in relation to emotional development. In *Collected Papers: Through Paediatrics to Psycho-Analysis*. London: Tavistock, 1958.

Winnicott, D. W. 1951. Transitional objects and transitional phenomena. In *Collected Papers: Through Paediatrics to Psycho-Analysis*. London: Tavistock, 1958.

Winnicott, D. W. 1960a. Ego distortion in terms of true and false self. In *The Maturational Processes and the Facilitating Environment: Studies in the Theory of Emotional Development*. New York: International Universities Press, 1965.

Winnicott, D. W. 1960b. The theory of the parent-infant relationship. In *The Maturational Processes and the Facilitating Environment: Studies in the Theory of Emotional Development*. New York: International Universities Press, 1965.

Wynne, L. C., and Singer, M. T. 1963a. Thought disorder and family relations of schizophrenics. I. a research strategy. *Archives of General Psychiatry* 9:191–198.

Wynne, L. C., and Singer, M. T. 1963b. Thought disorder and family relations of schizophrenics. II. a classification of forms of thinking. *Archives of General Psychiatry* 9:199–206.

CYNTHIA R. PFEFFER

The following example of a suicidal adolescent points out a variety of factors associated with suicidal risk and the clinical dilemmas in planning treatment. Two psychiatrists were responsible for planning this patient's care, and they had different opinions about how to manage the initial treatment. Such a varied clinical perspective is not unusual; yet the patient's outcome may be different depending on the type of initial care provided.

William, an eighteen-year-old college student, left school in the middle of the first semester because he felt deeply despondent and anxious and thought about killing himself. He described having a difficult adjustment at college and, especially, trouble getting along with his two roommates. He felt ostracized by them and worried that they ridiculed him. His academic work was poor, and he complained about not being able to concentrate. He felt sad, homesick, and lonely, and he was initially preoccupied with ending his life. He began to drink and use marijuana heavily within the two months after the college semester began. The drug seemed to have a tranquilizing effect on him, although he experienced agitated feelings at other times.

William felt particularly angry with his family. His parents divorced when he was ten years old, and his father remarried when William was fifteen. His mother was depressed and embittered about being abandoned by her former husband. William felt a strong loyalty to his mother and was enraged at his father. While at school, William worried about his mother's emotional health and felt guilty about being away from home. He repeatedly worried that his mother might take an overdose of pills as she had done one year after her divorce.

William had been home for three weeks after he left school. During this time, he felt increasingly more irritable and on several occasions had overwhelming feelings of wanting to destroy the home. In fact, he broke the bathroom mirror by throwing his boot at it. He thought of shooting himself but realized that he wanted to live. Yet his despair and anger were uncontrollable and seemed to overpower him.

Realizing how distraught her son was, William's mother called on his father for help. It was the first time in years that William's mother overcame her bitterness and called for help from her former husband. William's parents discussed their son's situation with a family friend who was a physician. The friend suggested that, since William was so depressed and out of control, he would be better treated in a psychiatric hospital. Frightened by this suggestion, but willing to help their son in any way possible, his parents brought William to the nearby psychiatric hospital for admission.

William was reluctant and angry about being admitted to the hospital. Although he wanted help, he was angry at his parents for uniting in their opinion about wanting to hospitalize him. He refused to be hospitalized. As a result, two psychiatrists were asked to evaluate William for admission. Their opinions differed. One psychiatrist thought that a trial of outpatient treatment was indicated. He based his opinion on the fact that William had not shown any suicidal acts, that he wanted help, and that the family was concerned and cooperative. The second psychiatrist felt strongly that William should be hospitalized for a comprehensive diagnostic assessment. This psychiatrist believed that William was at high risk for a suicidal act and that his safety was in jeopardy.

This case study highlights a number of clinical dilemmas that beset the clinician who must make decisions about formulating a treatment plan for the suicidal adolescent. This example illustrates that many options are possible and that the clinical dilemmas encountered often involve the primacy of appreciating the degree of life threat to the patient.

A Statement of the Issues

Although the rapid increase in youth suicide began in the late 1960s, clinicians and researchers directed their attention only minimally to

408

understanding this problem. However, in the 1970s, systematic re-search on suicidal behavior in children and adolescents began to emerge. Presently, there is not only an urgent need to study the phenomenology of youth suicidal behavior but also a necessity to educate clinicians to be effective in early recognition of and intervention with youngsters who may be at risk.

One of the most important tasks for the practicing clinician is to plan a course of intervention that can prevent morbidity and mortality as-sociated with suicidal ideation. The assessment of suicide risk is a complex issue beset by the influences of the clinician's reactions to and knowledge of suicidal impulses in youths and the multifaceted underpinnings of suicidal behavior. Yet a comprehensive assessment of risk is the most important factor in developing an intervention and prevention plan. Such a plan is often not easy to actualize. With these thoughts considered, this chapter will discuss factors that require clin-ical attention and especially those issues that contribute to clinical dilemmas that may hamper effective prevention of youth suicidal behavior.

For the sake of this discussion, a clinical dilemma will imply a clinical situation for which conclusive information based on empirical research about a phenomenon does not exist. As a result, the clinician is faced with a situation in which a best-judgment approach based on existing information must be utilized. The dilemmas are many with regard to treatment of suicidal youths, especially because relatively little empir-ical research on this issue has been conducted. Nevertheless, the data for this chapter are based on those research findings that may provide insights in developing a treatment plan. The issues to be discussed involve prediction of suicidal behavior, risk factors, repeated suicidal tendencies, and resistance to treatment. Furthermore, it must be ap-preciated that, given the paucity of research data on youth suicidal behavior, many clinical dilemmas exist. As a result, at present the treatment planning for suicidal youths must be conceptualized within the realm of a balance between the art and the science of general psychiatric practice.

Prediction of Suicidal Acts

One important issue on which to base a recommendation for treat-ment is the feasibility of predicting future suicidal behavior. In fact, this is one of the greatest clinical dilemmas for the practicing clinician.

From an epidemiological perspective, it is not possible to predict which individuals will commit suicide. The main reason for this is the low sensitivity and specificity of available identification procedures and the low base rate of suicidal behavior (Pokorny 1983). Although over 5,000 adolescents and young adults commit suicide every year, this is a relatively low incidence. Nevertheless, from a clinical perspective, the dilemma can be refocused so that a clinician attempts to make the best estimate possible over a short period of time about the likelihood that a given patient may carry out a suicidal act. Pokorny (1983) noted that, in the usual clinical situation, "diagnosis in clinical practice (in contrast to a prospective research project) typically consists of a sequence of small decisions. . . . in each case, the decision is not what to do for all time, but rather what to do next, for the near future" (p. 257). For the sake of this discussion, one may call the time between one assessment and the next the predictive interval. Pokorny suggests that the clinical predictive interval be brief.

In the clinical illustration of William, one psychiatrist believed that William should be hospitalized so that he could be observed and treated intensively. This psychiatrist opted to manage William by means of an extremely brief predictive interval. In the hospital situation, a nurse/ therapist would be with William constantly and thereby be available to offer assistance at the moment that William felt distressed or suicidal. The other psychiatrist considered that the likelihood that William would carry out a suicidal act was sufficiently low and that William could therefore be safe in treatment on an outpatient basis. This psychiatrist opted to utilize a longer predictive interval.

Another issue related to prediction is whether adolescents who exhibit nonfatal suicidal acts are similar to those adolescents who commit suicide. The importance of this is in the ability of the clinician to determine the relative risk of suicide occurring if specific characteristics known to be associated with suicide are evident in a given adolescent. The clinical dilemma is whether there is a continuous spectrum of suicidal behavior that ranges from nonsuicidal behavior, suicidal ideas, nonfatal suicidal acts, and suicide.

Currently, there are those who believe that individuals who commit suicide can be distinguished from those who attempt suicide (Stengel and Cook 1958). This belief has not been evaluated empirically for adolescents, but studies of nonfatal suicidal behavior of children and adolescents suggest that there is a continuous spectrum of nonfatal suicidal behavior. This range of nonfatal suicidal tendencies includes nonsuicidal behavior, suicidal ideas, and nonfatal suicidal acts. Some studies suggest that the severity of suicidal tendencies is directly related to degrees of intensity of specific factors (Brent, Kalas, Edelbrock, Cosello, Dulcan, and Conover 1986; Pfeffer, Solomon, Plutchik, Mizruchi, and Weiner 1982). For example, increasing severity of depression is associated with greater severity of suicidal tendencies. The importance of this concept of continuity of suicidal tendencies is that a clinician can expect that an adolescent who exhibits suicidal ideas may move into a state of increased risk for expressing suicidal acts. The likelihood of this happening will depend on the severity of associated risk factors such as the intensity of depression.

Another issue regarding the evaluation of the likelihood to carry out a serious suicidal act involves the relation between intent to kill oneself and the seriousness of the act. Robbins and Alessi (1985), in a recent study of sixty-four adolescent psychiatric inpatients who were interviewed with semistructured interviews following the format of the Schedule for Affective Disorders and Schizophrenia (SADS), elucidated this issue. The SADS contains four items describing suicidal feelings and behavior: preoccupation with suicide, intent to die, number of previous suicide attempts, and the lethality of the most recent suicide attempt. The results of the study indicated that all four items correlated highly with each other. The importance of these data is that the clinician can gather data about one of these factors and thereby have a firmer basis for making inferences about the other three factors.

In summary, prediction of a future suicidal act in a given individual is not possible with statistical certainty. From a clinical perspective, one way of dealing with this clinical dilemma is to take precautions to minimize the time between assessment and application of intervention when an adolescent is in a phase of an acute suicidal episode (Pfeffer 1986). This issue involves planning a brief predictive interval. Furthermore, since there appears to be a continuous spectrum of suicidal tendencies ranging from nonsuicidal behavior, to suicidal ideas, to nonfatal suicidal acts, a clinician should view any communication by an adolescent of suicidal ideation seriously and realize that an adolescent may be likely to express an intention to commit a suicidal act. As an associated feature of this, communication of suicidal intent by an adolescent should be viewed very seriously by the clinician, especially since suicidal intent is highly correlated with seriousness of suicidal acts.

Assessment of Risk Factors

Adolescent suicidal behavior is associated with a variety of factors. A significant clinical dilemma is that the relative weight of these factors for risk of suicidal behavior is yet to be determined. The associated factors that are important are those that raise the probability that suicidal behavior will occur. Conversely, protective factors also need to be evaluated. These factors are ones that decrease risk for expression of suicidal impulses. Although the suicidal episode usually does not exist for a long period of time, risk factors can be present for an extensive time, and as they either intensify or become more numerous, the probability of a suicidal act occurring becomes more elevated (Pfeffer 1986).

Risk factors can be clustered into intrinsic and external factors. The intrinsic factors involve psychobiological variables; the external factors include family and environmental variables. A clinician must be skilled in recognizing the protective and risk factors, particularly among adolescents. A clinician must be especially alert to knowing how these factors, found in adolescents, may differ from those factors found in adults. Thus a developmental perspective on adolescent suicidal behavior and its associated risk and protective factors is important. In William's case, the psychiatrist who wanted to hospitalize William believed that the severity of risk factors, and the fact that there were a large number of them, made it very likely that William would carry out a suicidal act. The other psychiatrist did not believe that the risk factors were severe enough to create an imminent risk of life-threatening acts. In fact, this psychiatrist focused mostly on the weight of protective factors such as concerned parents and the willingness of the adolescent to agree to treatment. As a result, the second psychiatrist opted to work in a less intensive way with this suicidal adolescent.

PSYCHOBIOLOGICAL RISK FACTORS

Studies of suicide fatalities and nonfatal suicidal behavior among adolescents have shown that depression is associated with suicidal behavior. Among those adolescents who attempt suicide, the presence of both major depressive disorder and borderline personality disorder significantly increases the severity of suicidal behavior (Friedman, Arnoff, Clarkin, Corn, and Hurt 1983). Features of affective disorder and/or antisocial symptomatology were identified among young adolescent

412

suicide victims (Shaffer 1974). Shafii, Carrigan, Whittinghill, and Derrick (1985), utilizing the psychological autopsy method, evaluated twenty adolescents who committed suicide and compared them to nonsuicidal adolescents who were matched for sex, age, race, and social status. There was a significantly higher prevalence of suicidal ideas and acts, use of drugs or alcohol, antisocial behavior, and loneliness among the suicide victims. The role of drugs and alcohol in risk for suicidal behavior was also found to be a major factor of youth suicide in the San Diego Suicide Study (Fowler, Rich, and Young 1986). In this study, 53 percent of the 133 consecutive young suicides who were less than thirty years old had a principal DSM-III diagnosis of substance abuse.

Although more research is needed to delineate psychological risk factors for fatal and nonfatal youth suicidal behavior, it is apparent that certain factors have been consistently identified: depression, antisocial symptoms, and substance abuse. Currently, there is little information about biological correlates of youth suicidal behavior. However, research evidence from studies of adults indicates that factors associated with serotonin functioning (Lidberg, Tuck, Asberg, Scalia-Tomba, and Bertilsson 1985; Mann, Stanley, McBride, and McEwen 1986) appear to be promising areas for research among adolescents.

The clinical dilemma regarding psychological risk factors for youth suicide involves the clinician's ability to recognize the signs and symptoms that are associated with these factors and to appreciate their importance in raising the risk for suicidal behavior. William's example indicated that he was experiencing serious signs of depression involving sadness, loneliness, hopelessness, social withdrawal, poor concentration, and sleep problems. As suggested by Robbins and Alessi (1985) in their study of sixty-four adolescent inpatients, symptoms of depression such as depressed mood, negative self-evaluation, anhedonia, insomnia, poor concentration, indecisiveness, lack of reactivity of mood, and psychomotor disturbance were associated with suicidal behavior. It must also be appreciated that antisocial symptomatology such as lying, stealing, violence, and truancy has been associated with serious suicidal behavior among youths. Studies of suicidal adolescents and adults indicate that an increase in aggression is an important factor (Lidberg et al. 1985; Pfeffer, Newcorn, Kaplan, Mizruchi, and Plutchik 1985; Shaffer 1974). In fact, a clinician should realize that the presence of aggressive and depressive symptoms is a significant combination associated with seriousness of suicidal behavior. Alcohol and drug abuse

413

have shown a marked increase among adolescents. Although substance abuse has become so widespread, its association to suicidal risk must be considered seriously. In fact, any attempt to decrease drug or alcohol abuse is an important method for suicide prevention.

FAMILY RISK FACTORS

Environmental influences have a profound effect on the potential for adolescent suicidal behavior. Shaffer (1974) noted that, among thirty young adolescent suicide victims, the suicide was provoked by an immediate family or peer crisis. Pfeffer et al. (1985) identified a number of environmental factors that were associated with suicidal acts in 200 adolescents, age thirteen to nineteen years, who were psychiatrically hospitalized: problems with a boyfriend/girlfriend, sexual and violent abuse, school changes, and family violence. These studies suggest that multiple experiential factors are linked to fatal and nonfatal adolescent suicidal behavior.

More specifically, parental psychopathology is a key component for risk of adolescent suicidal tendencies. The clinical dilemma facing the clinician is to evaluate the family in the initial phase of an assessment of a suicidal adolescent. Gathering extensive history about relatives with depression, suicidal behavior, alcoholism, drug abuse, and violent behaviors that include physical and sexual child abuse is necessary. Adolescent suicide is associated with experiences with suicidal relatives and friends and with emotional problems of family members (Shafii et al. 1985).

Another clinical dilemma is the early recognition of adolescents at risk even if they do not manifest suicidal tendencies. For example, research indicates that children and adolescents who have parents with major depressive disorders are at a threefold risk for psychopathology that specifically involves major depression, attention deficit disorder, and separation anxiety (Weissman, Prusoff, Gammon, Merikangas, Leckman, and Kidd 1984). In fact, in a study of 194 youngsters with parents who have a major affective disorder, 6.5 percent of the youngsters were shown to express suicidal ideation (Weissman et al. 1984). Thus a psychiatrist working with adults with affective disorders, substance abuse disorders, and a history of violence should be aware that the children of such adults may be at risk for psychopathology that includes suicidal tendencies. In fact, it can be suggested that such children be screened for evidence of psychiatric disorder. This is especially pertinent for the children of parents who require psychiatric hospitalization. With respect to this, research findings suggest that suicidal youngsters, compared to nonsuicidal depressed youngsters or youngsters with other forms of psychiatric problems, have more family stresses such as parental separation, death, and divorce (Cohen-Sandler, Berman, and King 1982). Separation of parent and child because of parental hospitalization may be an important stressor in addition to the effect of parental emotional disorder. Thus, whether youth suicidal behavior is determined by genetic or environmental influences, clear evidence exists for suicidal behavior to be manifest in multiple family members. An important aspect of primary prevention is to recognize individuals at risk before suicidal tendencies are evident.

SOCIOCULTURAL RISK FACTORS

Two socioculturally determined factors are particularly relevant for suicidal youths: imitation of suicidal behavior and use of firearms as a suicidal method. These factors are socioculturally determined because they are promoted by cultural sanctions. For example, possession of firearms is culturally accepted in the United States; and, in the last several decades, not only has there been an increase of firearms in the household, but also efforts to control gun sales have been significantly opposed. On a more individual level, studies have shown that adolescents who commit suicide are aware of others who have shown suicidal acts or have committed suicide (Shafii et al. 1985). The effect of such knowledge is to diminish inhibitions toward self-destructive acts and to increase the likelihood that a teenager will commit a suicidal act. For example, this effect is seen most prominently when a teenager commits suicide and an epidemic of subsequent suicide or suicide attempts occurs within the same town or school district. A recent illustration of this was in Omaha, Nebraska. Newspaper reports (Robbins 1986) stated, "Third Suicide Stuns Students In Omaha. Grieving students walked the halls and filled the classrooms of Bryan High School today wearing yellow buttons to show their concern. Many others left the campus to attend the funeral of the third of their classmates to commit suicide in 5 days."

An important issue illustrated by such newspaper reporting is the complexity of the effects of media reporting of suicidal behavior on both the local and the national levels. Thus cultural sanctions for extensive reporting of adolescent suicide have a catalytic effect on increasing adolescent suicidal behavior (Phillips and Carstensen 1986). An important question is, Did the newspaper report of the Omaha suicides stimulate additional suicidal acts in Omaha as well as in other, even distant, locations? Recent research has provided evidence suggesting that newspaper reports of teenage suicide or general discussion about suicide in the news can precipitate suicidal behavior (Phillips and Carstensen 1986). In addition, fictional accounts of suicide in the media have a similar suicide-promoting effect (Gould and Shaffer 1986).

A clinician must evaluate whether an adolescent who is at risk has knowledge of another suicidal person or has been preoccupied by an immediate presentation about suicide. The clinical dilemma is to develop an approach that will counteract the effects of knowledge about a specific adolescent suicide as well as the effect of media presentations about the death. Counteracting culturally sanctioned behavior is a difficult venture. Intervention geared to discussing preoccupations about the suicides of others may help an adolescent to gain insight into his or her own motivations involving personal suicidal ideas as well as to gain some distance from the imagery and fantasies about the deceased youths. The dilemma is increased when a clinician, as is usually bound to happen, is asked to consult to a community in which there has been a suicide of a teenager. The most effective aspect of such a consultation is if the clinician can help the community form a network of people who will be available to speak with teenagers about the death of a peer. As with individual treatment, this community effort provides an opportunity for many adolescents to talk about their fears, fantasies, temptations, and inhibitions about suicidal behavior. Specifically, romanticizing the suicide of a peer should be avoided. Small group or individual discussions with teenagers are advisable. It must be realized that the effect of the event is greatest within several weeks after the death but that a longer-range effort must be utilized to prevent the potential later suicide or suicidal act of a teenager. Therefore a plan of intervention-prevention should be formulated with a long-range perspective.

REPETITION OF SUICIDAL ACTS

One of the important dilemmas encountered during the therapeutic work with a suicidal adolescent is having to estimate who may be likely

416

to repeat a suicidal act. Certainly, it has been documented that those who attempt and those who complete suicide have frequently exhibited previous suicidal behavior. Shaffer (1974) reported that approximately 46 percent of thirty young suicide victims had previous evidence of suicidal behavior. These findings were supported by the study by Shafii et al. (1985) in which 40 percent of suicide victims had previous suicidal attempts compared with 6 percent of teenagers who did not commit suicide. Pfeffer et al. (1985) determined that, among 200 consecutively admitted adolescent psychiatric inpatients, 34 percent made suicide attempts. Among these suicidal youngsters, 19.5 percent committed multiple suicidal acts within the six months before the index suicidal episode under investigation.

Further studies are needed to determine differences between adolescents who repeat suicidal acts and those who do not. Most information about this is derived from clinical populations who were in psychiatric or emergency room settings. Stanley and Barter (1970) studied thirty-eight adolescent psychiatric inpatients who had attempted suicide and compared them to thirty-eight nonsuicidal adolescents who were hospitalized. In a follow-up study, these clinicians noted that 50 percent of the index attempted suicides were followed by a repeat suicide attempt. The factors that distinguish the adolescents who showed repeat suicidal acts from those who never were suicidal and also from those who were suicidal only at the time of the initial assessment were that the repeat suicidal adolescents had greater problems in their social network: they had poorer peer relationships, were less likely to be living with parents, and had poor school records.

In a study of adolescent inpatients who had attempted suicide, Motto (1984) found several factors that were associated with adolescents who committed suicide within ten years after an initial suicide attempt. In this study of 122 male adolescents who had attempted suicide and who were ten to nineteen years old at the time of hospitalization, the adolescents who committed suicide had the following characteristics at the time of their index suicide attempt: they communicated intent to make the suicide attempt, they had a fear of losing their minds, they sought help before the suicide attempt but had a mixed or negative attitude toward the care giver, they had an increased need for sleep, they had feelings of hopelessness and psychomotor retardation, they were able to communicate with others, and they had financial resources. This study did not evaluate at the time of follow-up the clinical features of those adolescents who did not commit suicide. Therefore

417

there was no information reported on the prevalence of repeat, nonfatal suicidal behavior.

Goldacre and Hawton (1985) studied adolescents who took overdoses and were evaluated in medical settings. These researchers indicated that repetition of an overdose occurred most frequently within a few months after admission. Within 2.8 years after the initial admission, 9.5 percent of the 2,492 individuals age twelve to twenty years who were studied repeated a suicidal act. Six of the ten subjects who died probably committed suicide. This study also indicates that overdose is a serious suicidal behavior and does result in death.

These studies suggest that there are factors that distinguish between repeat suicidal adolescents and those with no subsequent suicidal behavior. However, the amount of information is not comprehensive because of the relative paucity of systematic research about this issue. What appears evident is that a clinician must be alert to appraising the interpersonal system of a suicidal adolescent. Therapeutic efforts should focus on enhancing a consistently supportive network of individuals who are able to help the adolescent effectively at a moment of distress. Thus an important task for the clinician is to be a consultant to and a coordinator of people specified as key individuals in the adolescent's social sphere. Furthermore, a clinician working alone with a suicidal adolescent will be less effective than one who works within a team framework. Such a team effort should include moment-to-moment communication between the suicidal adolescent, the therapist, and key individuals within the therapeutic network.

RESISTANCE TO TREATMENT

There are few empirical studies assessing the effects of treatment on suicidal adolescents. Thus the types of treatment and the time needed to maximize effectiveness require investigation. However, clinicians often report that many suicidal adolescents are difficult to engage in a treatment process. Often there is resistance to following through with a treatment recommendation. There are some empirical data about this also. For example, Mattsson, Seese, and Hawkins (1969) reported that, among seventy-five adolescents evaluated in an emergency service for suicidal behavior, 50 percent did not follow up on the recommendation for additional intervention. Some of the factors influencing resistance to participation in treatment have been specified. Taylor and Stansfeld

(1984) reported that, among fifty adolescents who took overdoses, twenty-eight kept an appointment for psychiatric treatment. The most important factors associated with whether the youngster went for treatment were parental attitudes and the parents' cultural background. Other factors that may affect the willingness of an adolescent to remain within a treatment process may involve the diagnostic profile of the adolescent and the treatment system in which the adolescent is initially seen. For example, do adolescents with major depressive disorder and borderline personality disorder engage less in treatment than those adolescents with a major depressive disorder alone? Do therapist factors, such as sex, personality, and treatment philosophy, determine how well an adolescent will follow through with treatment? Is there a difference in the type of emergency services offered that affect the likelihood that an adolescent will develop a willingness to continue in treatment? These and other questions remain unanswered and account for many clinical dilemmas experienced by clinicians who provide care for suicidal adolescents.

Conclusions

This chapter highlighted some of the clinical dilemmas that exist in therapeutic work with suicidal adolescents. There is a great need to study these issues by means of empirical research. Perhaps with added information, some of the clinical dilemmas may be lessened. Nevertheless, clinical dilemmas are encompassing and involve facets of the psychobiological characteristics of the suicidal adolescents, the social milieu of the adolescent, and the care-giving setting.

It is apparent that our understanding of suicidal youths is increasing, and, in keeping with the amount of new information generated from ongoing clinical research, it is mandatory for psychiatrists and other clinicians to be current in their knowledge about youth suicidal behavior. Sharing clinical experiences among colleagues provides an essential professional support so needed by clinicians who work with acutely suicidal adolescents.

This chapter selected certain clinical issues that affect the clinician's decision about planning treatment for the suicidal adolescent: the prediction of suicidal risk, knowledge of risk factors, repetition of suicidal acts, and resistance to treatment. It advocated that an important foundation of prevention of adolescent suicidal behavior is early intervention for an adolescent considered to be at risk. Thus the early recognition of suicidal risk is the most important first step in prevention efforts for the practicing clinician.

REFERENCES

Brent, D. A.; Kalas, R.; Edelbrock, C.; Costello, A. J.; Dulcan, M. K.; and Conover, N. 1986. Psychopathology and its relationship to suicidal ideation in childhood and adolescence. *Journal of the American Academy of Child Psychiatry* 25:666–673.

Cohen-Sandler, R.; Berman, A. L.; and King, R. A. 1982. Life stress and symptomatology: determinants of suicidal behavior in children. *Journal of the American Academy of Child Psychiatry* 21:178–186.

Fowler, R. C.; Rich, C. L.; and Young, D. 1986. San Diego Suicide Study. II. substance abuse in young cases. *Archives of General Psychiatry* 43:962–965.

Friedman, R. C.; Arnoff, M. S.; Clarkin, J. F.; Corn, R.; and Hurt, S. W. 1983. History of suicidal behavior in depressed borderline inpatients. *American Journal of Psychiatry* 140:1023–1026.

Goldacre, M., and Hawton, K. 1985. Repetition of self-poisoning and subsequent death in adolescents who take overdoses. *British Journal of Psychiatry* 146:395–398.

Gould, M. S., and Shaffer, D. 1986. The impact of suicide in television movies: evidence of imitation. *New England Journal of Medicine* 315:690–694.

Lidberg, L.; Tuck, J. R.; Asberg, M.; Scalia-Tomba, G. P.; and Bertilsson, L. 1985. Homicide, suicide and CSF5-HIAA. *Acta Psychiatrica Scandinavia* 71:230–236.

Mann, J. J.; Stanley, M.; McBride, A.; and McEwen, B. S. 1986. Increased serotonin and B-adrenergic recepter binding in the frontal cortices of suicide victims. *Archives of General Psychiatry* 43:954–959.

Mattsson, A.; Seese, L. R.; and Hawkins, J. W. 1969. Suicidal behavior as a child psychiatric emergency. *Archives of General Psychiatry* 20:100–109.

Motto, J. A. 1984. Suicide in male adolescents. In H. S. Sudak, A. B. Ford, and N. B. Rushford, eds. *Suicide in the Young*. Boston: Wright.

Pfeffer, C. R. 1986. *The Suicidal Child*. New York: Guilford.

Pfeffer, C. R.; Newcorn, J.; Kaplan, G.; Mizruchi, M. S.; and Plutchik, R. 1985. Suicidal behavior in adolescent psychiatric inpatients. Paper presented to the annual meeting of the American Psychiatric Association, Dallas.

Pfeffer, C. R.; Solomon, G.; Plutchik, R.; Mizruchi, M. S.; and Weiner, A. 1982. Suicidal behavior in latency-age psychiatric inpatients: a replication and cross validation. *Journal of the American Academy of Child Psychiatry* 21:564–569.

Phillips, D. P., and Carstensen, L. L. 1986. Clustering of teenage suicides after television news stories about suicide. *New England Journal of Medicine* 315:685–689.

Pokorny, A. D. 1983. Prediction of suicide in psychiatric patients: report of a prospective study. *Archives of General Psychiatry* 40:249–257.

Robbins, D. R., and Alessi, N. E. 1985. Depressive symptoms and suicidal behavior in adolescents. *American Journal of Psychiatry* 142:588–592.

Robbins, W. 1986. Third suicide stuns students in Omaha. *New York Times* (February 11).

Shaffer, D. 1974. Suicide in childhood and early adolescence. *Journal of Child Psychology and Psychiatry* 15:275–291.

Shafii, M.; Carrigan, S.; Whittinghill, J. R.; and Derrick, A. 1985. Psychological autopsy of completed suicide in children and adolescents. *American Journal of Psychiatry* 142:1061–1064.

Stanley, E. J., and Barter, J. T. 1970. Adolescent suicide behavior. *American Journal of Orthopsychiatry* 40:87–96.

Stengel, E., and Cook, N. G. 1958. *Attempted Suicide.* Maudsley Monograph no. 4. London: Chapman & Hall.

Taylor, E. A., and Stansfeld, S. A. 1984. Children who poison themselves. II. prediction of attendance for treatment. *British Journal of Psychiatry* 145:132–135.

Weissman, M. M.; Prusoff, B. A.; Gammon, G. D.; Merikangas, K. R.; Leckman, J. F.; and Kidd, K. K. 1984. Psychopathology in the children (ages 6–18) of depressed and normal parents. *Journal of the American Academy of Child Psychiatry* 23:78–84.

25 SUBTLE CLASSROOM ABUSE IN AN ADOLESCENT INPATIENT PROGRAM

MAX SUGAR

In the past twenty-five years, child abuse and neglect have become almost household words. First described as the battered child syndrome (Kempe, Silverman, Steele, Droegemueller, and Silver 1962), physically and sexually abused children are now recognized more readily. Emotional abuse, however, is difficult to catalog. This chapter focuses on subtle forms of emotional abuse and neglect found in a special education classroom in an adolescent inpatient program.

Emotional abuse has been defined as the willful destruction or significant impairment of a child's competence (Gabarino 1978). This, however, seems limiting since emotional abuse often occurs without the conscious awareness of the perpetrator, who may deny or rationalize. Further, competence is not always affected overtly since there may be no changes in school behavior, but the youngster suffers from marked anxieties, insomnia, neurotic symptoms, various psychosomatic disorders, or worse. This may occur even after just one trauma, more so in the dependent and vulnerable.

Paulson (1983) described such covert maltreatment in preschools as excessive reliance on packaged educational materials, nonuse of materials that have intrinsic interest for children, and dislike of children or particular ones. Overt forms of maltreatment described were regular and frequent occurrences of emotional abuse, physical coercion, and direct verbal attack. For instance, Paulson describes a three-year-old boy who came out of the bathroom pulling up his pants. The teacher shouted: " 'Aren't you ashamed to come out like that?' Child does not know what he has done and begins to cry. Teacher shouts, 'stop crying.' The child is now sobbing. Teacher: 'if you don't stop crying, your mother won't pick you up' '' (p. 51). Another illustration is that of a two-and-a-half-year-old boy who, when tasting sand, was asked by the teacher, "Why didn't you eat your breakfast? Only pigs eat dirt!" (p. 51).

Krugman and Krugman (1984) described emotional and physical abuse by a teacher in third- and fourth-grade classes that led to symptomatic behavior. The teacher upset the classes by his behavior, which was reported by students and observed by some parents. This consisted of harassment, pejorative labeling ("stupid"), inconsistency, screaming, threatening, allowing some children to harass and belittle others, demanding unrealistic academic goals, and physical pain (pinching, slapping, shaking, and pulling ears). The majority of youngsters' symptoms were resolved by the removal of the teacher.

That there are good teachers, such as those portrayed in *Goodbye, Mr. Chips* and *To Sir, with Love,* is well known. That good teachers may have their bad moments is not news. The position involves expectations by the community of an exalted level of continuous professional behavior. By and large, teachers are interested in doing the best job possible, and most of the time they do so.

When devoted professionals act out against children in their charge, it behooves us to try to examine and learn from the situation to forestall or better manage such situations in the future. All too often, the major source of the difficulty is unavailable to provide data to help us further. Nevertheless, it seems worthwhile to attempt a review and dissection of such matters, especially if we can approach it from all possible views, including transference and countertransference features.

Case Illustrations

CASE 1: THE GUILD RESPONSE TO SEXUAL ABUSE

The inappropriate behavior by a teacher on an inpatient adolescent unit was confirmed by all patients. Daily, she greeted every student, male and female, with a hug and a kiss on the cheek. Her favorites also received a kiss on the neck, a pat on the buttocks, and a long embrace. In class, she asked male patients who were going on a pass if they "were going to get a piece." On return from a pass, she again asked them in class if they had any sex. The males felt ''she was coming on'' to them. She derogated absent patients and their doctors. When discipline with understanding was required, she did not attempt to deal with the youngsters' difficulties but simply threatened to send them back to the psychiatric unit.

When the matter was brought by the adolescent program psychiatrists to the head teacher, principal, and school board, they all reacted as if it were an attack on all teachers, and they closed ranks in her defense. This occurred despite a gentle approach by the medical director. The working situation with the teachers, medical staff, and administration of the hospital shifted from one of mutual respect and cooperation to a battleground where teachers stopped talking to physicians and would not give any reports to the physicians for staffings. They behaved as if they were completely autonomous in their function instead of team members in a psychiatric hospital. The school board found no fault with the individual teacher, but, eventually, she was placed in another school, apparently without concern by the board for her inappropriate behavior. Much later, it was learned that one of the teachers, whose written report had confirmed the students' complaints, had been intimidated into silence and that her report had been squelched by her supervisor.

CASE 2: DIVIDED LOYALTIES

The teachers at a psychiatric hospital often took the adolescents for outings as part of the educational-socialization program. Some of the outings seemed to be duplicating preexisting occupational or recreational therapy programs and appeared to be meeting the teachers' personal needs. After some unscheduled outings, an inquiry by the unit medical director led him to conclude that the trips were noneducational. He ordered that the patients were not to be taken off the unit except as part of unit or special educational programs. At this point, the educational and psychiatric staffs entered a period of disagreement and friction. A mediation conference was held, and everyone agreed to schedule outings only for educational-therapeutic reasons.

Then another area of conflict emerged, namely, the issue of autonomy of the educator. The teachers were under direct contract with the school board of the city on loan to the hospital, but for the summer session the teachers were paid by the hospital. School reports were to be given to the patient's psychiatrist, who then shared the material with the patient's family and integrated the findings with the overall therapeutic plan. One of the teachers provocatively chose to send his regular assessment directly to parents on a monthly basis or after each report card, bypassing the psychiatrists.

Yet a third area of difficulty occurred when there were severe classroom disruptions by some of the youngsters. It was considered useful to have a member of the unit staff sit passively in the classroom as a teacher's aide and to help support the teachers to maintain control in the classroom. It was thought this might obviate confrontations and prevent the youngsters from going out of control. One teacher had no objections to this, but the aforementioned educator did. When asked about his objection to this plan, however, he was sullen, withdrawn, and would not explain.

The teacher's attitudes and actions continued to be at variance with the desired therapeutic ward program. For example, during the course of the year, he had various difficulties with one particular youngster who had problems with authority. The teacher responded in a very authoritarian and rigid fashion. He also did not give the youngsters their full teaching time since he dismissed the class to the dayroom if they behaved well. He continued to take patients off the unit for outings on his own, although the objections to this had been discussed repeatedly at staff meetings. Further, despite the teenagers' complaints, he refused to turn on the air conditioning in his class because he liked it hot.

These items were discussed in a multidisciplinary staff meeting in an effort to help the teacher understand the unit policies and heal any rift or difficulty between him, the director of the unit, and the particular patient. The teacher continued to be sullen and withdrawn and refused to discuss the matters at hand.

After the complaints surfaced concerning the teacher's incompetence and emotional abuse and neglect of the youngsters, he was not offered the summer school post. Later, it was learned that he had taken no education courses and had worked as a probation officer before teaching. When he was offered the opportunity to take his teacher certification and extra university education courses, he declined since he had failed twice previously.

Discussion

As part of the medical tradition, mental health professionals are imbued with having supervision as needed, without casting aspersions on the therapist. When teachers have someone "looking over their shoulders" after their student practice-teaching days, they are usually considered to be in serious trouble. Having a psychiatric aide or nurse in the special education teacher's class to help the youngsters with control and as an aid to the teacher is, therefore, seen as a threat to many teachers and is often resisted. Contrary to the supervisory approach, a consultant to the teacher may be viewed as a reflection of the teacher's incompetence instead of as a potential benefit to help obtain a clearer understanding of the youngsters and group phenomena in the class or to examine countertransferences and their effect on students' learning.

From the cultural perspective (Korbin 1980), we have to consider that some teachers may come from backgrounds in which children are not inherently valued as individuals and are viewed only as able to provide something for the adults' personal world, such as the adults' acquisition of things or the adults' triumphs. Other teachers' backgrounds may be such that the need to contribute to the family is based on an approach from the medieval or early industrial age when children were used to provide labor. In such a setting, youngsters are raised with harshly punitive and rigid authoritarian attitudes and behavior. They are punished for misdeeds as if they are adults, and, if they do well, they are given rewards for good behavior. Good behavior might be simply doing the ordinary or usual social things for which no reward would be forthcoming in families holding middle-class values. However, to such a teacher, this is something of importance because it means an absence of vandalizing, burglarizing, and so on, which is the common way of life for street children.

In these situations, there are numerous levels of abuse—sexual, emotional, cognitive, social, and cultural—that are harmful to youngsters. This involves the social system, the school administration, and the teachers. Perhaps many of the teachers had been abused as children and were now doing unto others what had been done to them (Steele 1970). For the injured youngsters the abuse promotes increased distrust of and hostility toward authority, retaliation, confusion, lowered self-esteem, and identification with the aggressor (becoming an abuser).

426

A problem of possible adversarial polarities arises in a hospital setting since the physician has medical responsibility and his focus is on treatment of the youngster, while teachers focus on teaching. The input to special education postgraduate programs about the special situations of hospitalized psychiatric patients is generally limited. The teacher is taught to be in sole charge of his domain, meeting specified curriculum goals and answering only to an administrative hierarchy. The physician is trained under supervision to be the one in charge of the treatment of his patient and to work with ancillary disciplines, including supervising them. Thus, the stage is set for misunderstanding unless these polarities and different tasks are recognized and clarified.

TRANSFERENCE AND COUNTERTRANSFERENCE

That the teacher's position is of inescapable and exaggerated importance to students has long been noted. Freud (1914) observed that there was a "perpetual undercurrent in all of us, and that in many of us the path to the sciences led only through our teachers. Some of us stopped half-way along that path, and for a few—why not admit as much?—it was on that account blocked for good and all" (p. 242). It seems that the youngsters' transference to the teachers led to idealization since being mistreated, misled, and undermined by the teachers was similar to the behavior of many of the patients' parents. Many of the adolescents had been involved in mutual splitting, bribery, and exploitation with their parents, and many were in a symbiosis with a parent or parent substitute. They were thus primed to find other authorities with whom to continue these conflicts. Therefore, it should come as no surprise that the patients did not report these behaviors of the teacher. Had it not been for one particular patient in each case who was negatively involved with each teacher and revealed the situation, it might have continued longer. It seems that the two youngsters who spoke up were acting out of their own hostile negative transference reactions or rivalry with other patients and not out of idealistic notions.

We have to consider the teacher as having identified with the patients against authority figures and having their hostile transferences combined. Additionally, they may have been having pathologically managed countertransference reactions.

Frequently, the medical director (and other psychiatrists) sits in on various functions on the adolescent service. On reviewing the discussed situations, it was apparent that the physicians, administrators, nurses, and staff did not enter the classrooms to observe a typical hour, which they often do in other areas of the adolescents' daily activities in the hospital. This finding of avoidance was strange. But we must consider that all the professionals—administrators, physicians, nurses, and recreational therapists—had had many years of schooling, with mostly positive transferences to their teachers. If this is so, then we may postulate that they had some residuals of this and showed great and unrealistic deference to the teachers, leading to avoidance of the usual inspection and observation procedures.

These two teachers may have been having their own unresolved negative transferences to the physicians as authorities and as rivals. Perhaps the school board members had an institutional rivalry with the hospital brought forth by these teachers, which promoted their protective reaction.

Long and Newman (1965) have written sensitively of the teacher's mental health, countertransference reactions, and use of inservice training or consultation service to help educators deal with their feelings more suitably. They comment, "A teacher who knows he has acted crabby all the morning, because of a squabble at home, can pull himself together and keep the squabble where it belongs. He can proceed to make something more pleasant for the rest of the day. The teacher with awareness knows that when too many people have been sent to detention hall that week, something may well be wrong not with the class but with himself" (p. 307).

Special education teachers may be in somewhat more of a risk position to abuse than other teachers since they deal with a more troubled group of children with very primitive impulses, fewer controls, and impaired boundaries. These emotions may be more likely to evoke a teacher's harmful countertransference reactions and behavior. For special education teachers, especially in a psychiatric hospital, there is an exponential increase in all these factors.

A crucial issue for administrators of psychiatric programs for children and adolescents is whether to have special education teachers under contract to the hospital or to the local education authority. In the latter case, complications may arise between the hospital and the school board with scrutiny of credentials, conflicts of loyalties, and questions as to who is the final authority. On the other hand, if the hospital

428

employs the teacher, there is the possible problem of hiring educators who are unaware of current educational techniques. It is a question as to which arrangement would better serve the patients' therapeutic and educational needs.

Psychiatrists can be very helpful to the individual by clarifying the issues, supporting, and acting as advocates for the individual. Group intervention (Sugar 1986) and consultation efforts with schools (Berkovitz and Sinclair 1984) are additional areas for consideration.

Special education teachers may be better prepared with more practice training in psychiatric hospitals, beginning with their postgraduate courses. Special educators in hospitals should be prepared for the turmoil brought on by emotionally disturbed youngsters and their effect on others. Toward this end, ongoing consultation services, group discussions, and continued inservice training programs should be considered necessary for all teachers, but especially for hospital special education teachers.

Children are now being taught about "good versus bad touch" to alert them to and avoid potential sexual abuse. Perhaps students should be taught to pursue their rights and charge teachers with abuse and neglect when that is the case just as they may do to parents. This might help decrease some teachers' abuse, promote teachers' awareness of internal problems and countertransference issues, and decrease underachievement, school dropouts, and school vandalism. Thus, it is unwise to assume that the student is simply manipulating or fabricating to malign the teacher after some mischief by the youngster. Rather, one should consider the opposite possibility—that the teacher is maligning the child and is the perpetrator of mischief for which the youngster retaliates.

Parents need to listen and investigate their children's complaints without becoming caught up in a polarized position. Parents should inquire, check with other parents, and, when action is indicated, confront the teacher or principal about the unwarranted behavior. If the teacher has been abusive, then a first requirement would be an apology and redress by the teacher to the student.

With an open-minded approach, perhaps subtle, devious abuse and neglect by teachers may be decreased through helping the student to report the facts. These should be sifted and dealt with properly, after which the teacher is helped with consultative, administrative, or therapeutic intervention.

429

Conclusions

This chapter presents situations of subtle emotional abuse that may occur in classrooms in an adolescent inpatient service and the deterrent effect on education as well as the emotional damage it does to the students. Multiple transference and countertransference aspects are explored. The students' dependent position should not be equated with an inability to observe and report accurately what is transpiring. Therapeutic efforts for abused students and abusing teachers with this problem deserve more attention. Suggestions are made to offer more training, consultation, and inservice experiences to all teachers—and particularly special education teachers—to try to minimize emotional abuse.

REFERENCES

Berkovitz, I. H., and Sinclair, R. E. 1984. Teaching child psychiatrists about intervention in school systems. *Journal of Psychiatric Education* 8:240–245.

Freud, S. 1914. Some reflections on schoolboy psychology. *Standard Edition* 13:239–244. London: Hogarth, 1953.

Gabarino, J. 1978. The elusive "crime" of emotional abuse. *Child Abuse and Neglect* 2:89–99.

Kempe, C. H.; Silverman, F. M.; Steele, B. F.; Droegemueller, W.; and Silver, H. K. 1962. The battered child syndrome. *Journal of the American Medical Association* 181:17–24.

Korbin, J. E. 1980. The cross-cultural context of child abuse and neglect. In C. H. Kempe and R. E. Helfer, eds. *The Battered Child*. 3d ed. Chicago: University of Chicago Press.

Krugman, R. D., and Krugman, M. A. 1984. Emotional abuse in the classroom. *Archives of Diseases of Children* 138:284–286.

Long, N. T., and Newman, R. G. 1965. The teacher and his mental health. In H. J. Long, W. C. Morse, and R. G. Newman, eds. *Conflict in the Classroom*. Belmont, Calif.: Wadsworth.

Paulson, J. S. 1983. Covert and overt forms of maltreatment in the preschools. *Child Abuse and Neglect* 7:45–54.

Steele, B. F. 1970. Parental abuse of infants and small children. In E. J. Anthony and T. Benedek, eds. *Parenthood: Its Psychology and Psychopathology*. Boston: Little, Brown.

Sugar, M. 1986. Defusing a high school critical mass. In M. Sugar, ed. *The Adolescent in Group and Family Therapy*. Chicago: University of Chicago Press.

26   THE MEASUREMENT OF BEHAVIORAL
      AUTONOMY IN ADOLESCENCE: THE
      AUTONOMOUS FUNCTIONING CHECKLIST

ANN D. SIGAFOOS, CARL B. FEINSTEIN, MARIETTA DAMOND,
AND DAVID REISS

The concept that human development involves a progression from dependence on others for care and guidance to self-care and self-direction has been addressed from many empirical and theoretical perspectives. While progression toward autonomy is a component of development over several stages of the lifespan, it is of central importance in the adolescent period. During the adolescent stage of life, the development of capabilities that allow for self-direction and a sense of responsibility for the self are critical for successful transition into adulthood. One component of adolescent autonomy is behavioral autonomy—the behaviors and skills that allow for self-care and self-reliance in adulthood. While the development of these skills is of central importance, adolescent behavioral autonomy is rarely assessed in adolescent psychiatry.

In the first portion of this chapter, we will briefly review the concept of autonomy as it applies to adolescent development. We will then introduce the concept of behavioral autonomous functioning as a synthesis of adaptive and psychological dimensions of autonomy that has the potential to serve as an index of developmental competence in adolescence. Following this, we will summarize research findings that highlight the importance of developmental competence as a significant predictor of favorable psychosocial outcome in adulthood and as a protective factor against psychopathology in childhood.

© 1988 by The University of Chicago. All rights reserved.
0-226-24061-4/88/0015-0027$01.00

In the second portion of this chapter, we will review existing measures of adaptational competence in childhood. We will describe a new instrument, the Autonomous Functioning Checklist, that is designed to measure behavioral autonomous functioning in adolescence. This description will include findings from a preliminary psychometric study.

Introduction

"Autonomy" is a frequently cited term to which a multiplicity of meanings have been attached (Steinberg and Silverberg 1986). The fact that both psychological and adaptive elements are intertwined in this construct may contribute to this profusion of usages.

From the psychological perspective, the progression toward inner autonomy during adolescence has been widely discussed and can be only touched on here. The classic psychoanalytic position, as stated by Anna Freud (1958), emphasized emotional autonomy, that is, the loosening and ultimate detachment of the child's libidinal ties to the parent. Blos (1967) emphasized the separation/individuation process with regard to the development of autonomy in adolescence, stating that it "implies that the growing person takes increasing responsibility . . . rather than depositing this responsibility onto the shoulders of those under whose influence and tutelage he has grown up" (p. 168).

Hartmann (1958) added to the psychoanalytic theory of ego development by postulating a conflict-free ego sphere of adaptive functioning, autonomous from the drives and directed toward pragmatic mastery of the outside world. Erikson (1968) incorporated the adaptational perspective into his theory of adolescent development by emphasizing the importance of identity development, a concept that integrates both psychological and adaptive processes.

From a more purely adaptational perspective, adolescence is the psychosocial stage in which the transition from childhood dependence on caretakers to independent, self-sustaining, self-initiating adulthood occurs. A key developmental task of this stage, therefore, involves the application of physical, cognitive, and social skills learned earlier in childhood, as well as those acquired during the teenage years, to the goal of self-sufficiency in the social surround. The many elaborations of this developmental tendency in adolescence are precursors of the adult's capacity to live independently and to achieve social and vocational competence.

Since the furtherance of autonomy and autonomous functioning is so central to the adolescent process, an effective means of measuring it could serve as an index of stage-specific developmental competence. Harter (1982) has developed a child and adolescent self-report measure that reflects "perceived competence." There is, in fact, some indirect evidence that "competence" is associated with the experience of psychological well-being in adolescence. Reviewing his extensive research on normal adolescence, Offer (1986) noted that the most highly endorsed item in the Offer Self-Image Questionnaire was, "A job well done gives me pleasure," indicating the importance of work accomplishments as a source of personal satisfaction.

However, a subjective awareness or valuation of competence by the adolescent is not a sufficiently reliable indication of its actual presence. Nor does it help us determine how well the teenager is doing in each of the several developmental arenas—such as self-help, school, social, or prevocational—in which it must be achieved. We believe a more direct approach, involving the definition and measurement of actual behaviors, is needed.

In particular, it has seemed to us that this might be possible by integrating Blos's formulation of adolescent autonomy with the actual measurement of adaptive behaviors. This approach would consist of identifying a body of activities that implicitly require some measure of autonomy in order to be performed and that are acquired and gradually made routine during the course of adolescence. Such activities would be a manifestation of an adaptational autonomy or, what we feel is a more apt term, "behavioral autonomous functioning."

The various activities of behavioral autonomous functioning would be those that, by their very nature, require a sense of personal responsibility, self-direction, or self-reliance, in addition to specific skills, for their routine accomplishment. Since autonomy in adolescence is the forerunner of adult autonomy, the activities included in this construct should include personal physical care, management of responsibilities and obligations, utilization of community resources, initiative in social involvement and recreational activities, and the early stages of vocational or income-generating pursuits. The Autonomous Functioning Checklist (AFC), described in the Appendix to this chapter, is a product of this approach.

Numerous factors, both internal and external, may influence the degree and quality of the expansion in autonomous functioning for a given adolescent (Zinn 1979). Internal factors, for example, might include such attributes as ability, temperament, and internalized values. External factors might include such elements as the range of experiences available in a particular environment and the manner in which the family system negotiates issues of dependence/independence and individuality/conformity. These sorts of issues are, at times, addressed in detailed diagnostic evaluations of adolescent patients. However, information obtained about these issues has traditionally been utilized to explain symptom patterns rather than level and profile of stage-appropriate developmental competencies.

Despite the prevailing diagnostic emphasis on symptoms, a growing body of research suggests that developmental competence is a potent variable in its own right. Such research, both longitudinal and cross sectional, has demonstrated that certain personality attributes related to functional competence are associated with greater resilience in the face of childhood adversity, lower vulnerability to psychopathology, and more favorable outcome in adult life.

Longitudinal studies, recently reviewed by Garmezy (1985) and Rutter (1985), have pinpointed specific coping styles, temperamental traits, or special competencies in childhood that function as protective factors against psychopathology or other adverse psychosocial outcomes in high-risk children. Indeed, the term "competence" pervades many of the multiproblem family membership and all other childhood variables in predicting adult mental health and capacity for interpersonal relationships.

From a cross-sectional perspective, Pellegrini, Kosisky, Nackman, Cytryn, McKnew, Gershon, Hamovit, and Cammuso (1986) have recently shown that "personal resources," a construct closely related to autonomous functioning, operate as a powerful protective or resilience factor in children at risk for bipolar affective disorder. They found that a composite score, reflecting social problem-solving ability, internality, self-esteem, and self-perceived competence, was inversely correlated with psychopathology in these children.

Achenbach and Edelbrock (1981) have developed a scale of social competence, administered as a companion to their Child Behavior Checklist, a measure of psychopathology in childhood and adolescence. The Social Competence Scale contains relatively few items, but two of the subscales, Activities and Social, contain items such as participation in sports, other activities, social organizations, and number

435

of jobs. These items, particularly in adolescence, imply some element of initiative and social, vocational, and avocational direction. Thus, the Social Competence Scale may be seen as a very abbreviated presentation of a measure of autonomous functioning. Achenbach and Edelbrock (1981) found that clinically referred children scored significantly lower than demographically matched nonreferred children on each item of the Social Competence Scale. Although the direction-of-effect relation between psychopathology and social competence, as operationalized in these measures, cannot be determined from this study, it strongly supports the notion that autonomy, as a subcomponent of psychosocial adaptation, is a highly significant attribute.

MEASUREMENT OF BEHAVIORAL AUTONOMOUS FUNCTIONING

In view of the fact that adaptive behavior is an inextricable component of autonomous functioning, it is necessary to review briefly the history, general assumptions, and methodology that have grown up around the substantial body of work done in this area. Historically, both the construct of adaptive behavior and its measurement grew out of the process of defining mental retardation. From this perspective (Heber 1959), adaptive behavior is considered to have two facets: the ability of the individual to maintain himself independently and the degree to which the individual meets culturally imposed demands of personal and social responsibility. Deficits in adaptive behavior have been defined, along with subnormal intelligence, as critical to the correct assessment and classification of mental retardation (Grossman 1983).

Although this definition of adaptive behavior would seem to be universal in application, the instruments designed to assess this construct have been directed almost exclusively toward mentally retarded or developmentally disabled individuals. Constricted by the dual necessities of measuring functioning beginning with infancy and of capturing the deficits of severely impaired individuals, these tests emphasize basic activities of daily living and the more rudimentary motor, social, and cognitive skills. Most of their items measure skills far below those that would apply to a normal or unselected adolescent population (Bruininks, Woodcock, Weatherman, and Hill 1984; Nihira, Foster, Shellhaas, and Leland 1974). Since few of the more complex skills are assessed, the elements of initiative, self-reliance, and self-direction involved in such skills are not included. Because the focus is on whether specific skills have been attained, parental estimates of the child's capabilities are utilized for measurement instead of the regularity with which the skills are performed.

The Vineland Adaptive Behavior Scale (Sparrow, Balla, and Cicchetti 1984), although also measuring adaptive behavior from infancy and deriving from the assessment of mental retardation, is significantly different from other instruments in this area by virtue of its broader range of applicability ("whenever an assessment of an individual's daily functioning is required"). The Vineland's wider scope results in the inclusion of some more highly complex skills, relevant to normal adolescents. An additional advantage of the Vineland, in contrast to other measures of adaptive behavior, is that it defines adaptive behavior as typical performance, not ability or estimates of ability.

Since some Vineland items appropriate to the adolescent age range involve complex activities, this instrument, in fact, possesses a limited capacity to assess autonomous functioning. However, the Vineland remains fundamentally more concerned with skills. The selection and ordering of the items follow multiple, sequential lines of development, with each item assigned to the age by which it is normatively established. The scoring is basically a process of determining how far along these chronologically based continuums the individual has progressed.

Rehabilitation indicators are a group of instruments designed to provide information about disabled individuals' level of functioning (Brown, Diller, Gordon, Fordyce, and Jacobs 1984; Brown, Gordon, and Diller 1983; Diller, Fordyce, Jacobs, Brown, Gordon, Simmens, Orazem, and Barrett 1983). They include a wide range of functions, reflecting overall quality of life, using as a standard all activities available to nondisabled individuals. Thus, recreational pursuits are as legitimate an area of concern in defining the quality of functioning as behaviors more concerned with survival. These instruments, furthermore, distinguish between an individual's capability to perform an activity (Skill Indicators) and the extent over time that an individual actually performs these behaviors (Activity Pattern Indicators). This distinction between the ability to perform and the routine performance of any given activity parallels the Vineland's insistence that adaptive behavior be defined by routine performance rather than potential.

Rehabilitation indicators, while offering considerable potential for the rating of competence in adults, are not designed with children or adolescents in mind. Furthermore, they are intended not as a unified scale applicable to all individuals but rather as a resource for developing individualized evaluations, tailored to a given individual's disability. This instrument, however, served as an important basis for our initial efforts toward developing the AFC.

In summary, most instruments for measuring adaptive behavior include items related to competence in childhood, although largely at levels too low for adolescents. The Vineland, by requiring routine performance rather than estimates of ability as the criteria for rating adaptive behavior, contributes significantly to the methodology for assessing developmental competence. However, current measures of adaptive behavior are fundamentally more concerned with defining deficits. They cannot serve well as assessment procedures for positive measures of developmental competence in adolescence because they do not take into account the stage-specific psychosocial tasks of this phase of development and do not assess a wide enough range of activities.

The Autonomous Functioning Checklist

In this section, we present some considerations that directed the development of the AFC. Following this, we will review the AFC and the findings from research to date on its psychometric properties.

GENERAL CONSIDERATIONS FOR MEASURING BEHAVIORAL AUTONOMY

Our purpose is to study the unfolding of autonomy in adolescence rather than to describe the development of specific skills. Therefore, the activities that compose the ratings are those that require the attributes of personal responsibility, initiative, self-regulation, and self-direction. It is important to note that these attributes in no way imply that the activities must be performed independently or in isolation. Autonomous functioning includes help-seeking and cooperative activities that are based on the initiative and self-directedness of the adolescent.

Since the attributes of personal responsibility and self-regulation are stressed, it follows that a positive rating for any activity is based on typical performance. The simple capacity to perform an activity in the absence of actually doing it does not indicate autonomy. In this respect, we adhere to the methodology of both the Vineland Adaptive Behavior Scales and the Rehabilitation Indicators. We believe, in addition, that reliance on observed behavior is fundamentally more sound than estimates of ability.

Autonomous functioning behavior develops in the context of stage-specific environmental and social demands, opportunities, and experiences to which adolescents in our culture are normatively exposed. It is manifested by the routine activities, responses, and initiatives taken by the adolescent in response to this psychosocial context. Therefore, the activities rated in an index of functional autonomy, although derived from a developmental theory, should generally be routine, familiar, and normative. Since, in addition, the ratings are based on observable behavior, such an instrument lends itself well to a wide variety of clinical or research purposes and is, in this sense, atheoretical.

The dimension of autonomy we are studying concerns the transition from reliance on parents for caretaking to self-reliance. This, along with the requirement that a wide variety of activities be rated, many of them in the home, points to parents as the most appropriate raters of adolescents' autonomous functioning. There is, however, nothing inherent in the construct of autonomous functioning that prohibits ratings by parent substitutes or, if the adolescent is living away from home, the adults in loco parentis.

DESCRIPTION OF THE AFC

The AFC is a parent-completed checklist designed to measure behavioral autonomous functioning in adolescents between the ages of twelve and eighteen (see the App.). It contains seventy-eight items and is subdivided into four conceptually distinct subscales: Self- and Family Care, Management, Recreational Activity, and Social and Vocational Activity. Each item in the first three subscales is a short description of a behavior. The parent rates the adolescent in relation to each item on a five-point scale ranging from 0 (does not do) to 4 (does every time there is an opportunity). The items on the fourth subscale, Social and Vocational Activity, are rated by the parent on a dichotomous, yes/no scale. For each scale, high scores indicate that the adolescent routinely performs many of the activities listed.

The Self- and Family Care subscale contains twenty-two items that measure the extent to which basic daily maintenance activities are carried out by the adolescent. These items include routine personal care as well as family-oriented functions. Examples of this include meal preparation, care of possessions, performance of household chores and simple repairs, transportation, and shopping. Possible scores on this subscale range from 0 to 88.

The Management subscale contains twenty items that measure the extent to which the adolescent independently handles his or her interaction with the environment. Self-management is conceptualized as the adolescent's use of social/organizational resources as well as the assumption of personal responsibility for commitments and obligations. Scores may range from 0 to 80.

The Recreational Activity subscale contains sixteen items that measure the ways in which the adolescent chooses to use free time. Subscale scores may range from 0 to 64.

The Social and Vocational Activity subscale contains twenty items that measure social involvement and pursuit of vocational directions. Items are scored dichotomously. Subscale scores may range from 0 to 20.

Written instructions to the parent enable most parents or caretakers to complete the AFC. The presence of a professional or paraprofessional may be required for some parents with low literacy levels, visual impairment, or lack of comprehension of either the instructions or any of the checklist items. If necessary, the instructions and questions may be read to the parent. Wording of any oral instructions must closely follow the wording of the written instructions that accompany the AFC.

Psychometric and Normative Evaluation of the AFC

SAMPLE

The AFC was administered to a sample of 349 families. In each family, one parent or caretaker completed the AFC about his or her adolescent between the ages of twelve and eighteen. In fifty-two of these families, both caretakers completed the AFC on the same adolescent for purposes of estimating interrater reliability. However, only one parent's AFC scores were used for all other data analysis. Of the families, 89 percent were two-parent households, and 11 percent were single-parent households. The number of children in these families ranged from one to eight, with a median of two. Nine percent of the target adolescents were single children in the family; 37 percent were youngest children; and 44 percent were the oldest children in the family. Eighty-four percent of the parents reported that they were currently married and in their first marriages; 7 percent were remarried; and 9 percent were not married (divorced, widowed, or never been married). The noncorrespondence between marital status figures and reports of single- and two-parent households probably resulted from the absence of a category for "separated" in the background questionnaire and from lack of provision for coding second parents or caretaking figures, who may have been living in the household but not married to the responding parent.

The parents ranged in age from twenty-six to sixty-five years, with a median age of forty-three. Less than 1 percent of the sample had completed elementary school only; 9 percent had completed high school only; 44 percent had completed college or technical school only; and 46 percent had completed graduate or professional school. Total household income ranged from less than $25,000 per year to more than $100,000 per year. Since precise incomes were not obtained, we can report only that the median income was between $50,000 and $75,000 per year. Thus, the study population came from the middle-class population with a degree of affluence ranging from modest to wealthy.

ADOLESCENT CHARACTERISTICS

The normative sample composition, by age and sex of adolescent, is presented in table 1. The distribution of the age and sex of the adolescents is relatively uniform. However, the age-eighteen group is relatively balanced on sex but has less than half the total number of adolescents in comparison to most of the other age groups.

PROCEDURE

Families with at least one adolescent child were recruited through local parent-teacher associations and YMCAs. Except for a few families

TABLE 1

SAMPLE COMPOSITION: NUMBER OF ADOLESCENTS IN EACH AGE-BY-SEX GROUP

Sex	Age							
	12	13	14	15	16	17	18	Total
Male	19	30	30	28	36	29	12	184
Female	21	29	27	26	28	25	9	165
Total	40	59	57	54	64	54	21	349

recruited individually, families were recruited through a (geographically) stratified selection of organizations. The selection process was aimed at obtaining as broad a representation as possible of income and style of living (e.g., urban, suburban, and rural). Through these organizations, families were asked to participate in a study of adolescent development, for which they would complete several questionnaires. Compensation consisted of small donations to the sponsoring organization for each set of questionnaires returned. In the few instances in which families were not recruited through an organization, payment was made directly to the family.

Parents were asked to complete a ninety-five-item version of the AFC. In addition, they signed a consent form and filled out a background questionnaire eliciting information about marital status, family composition, income and level of education, and the index adolescents' age, sex, grade-point average, leadership experience, and number of extracurricular activities. Because many families had more than one adolescent between the ages of twelve and eighteen, a method of selecting the index adolescent was developed in order to prevent the parents from choosing the adolescent themselves. Half the questionnaires distributed instructed the parent to select the oldest child in the family between the ages of twelve and eighteen, while the other half instructed the parent to select the youngest child in this age range. For the subsample of families in which two parents completed the AFC, additional instructions were included to ensure that both parents selected the same adolescent.

Data analyses included psychometric and normative evaluations. Preliminary psychometric analyses indicated that seventeen of the ninety-five items on the original form of the AFC had inadequate distributions and/or low correlations with their subscale totals. Therefore, these items were eliminated from further psychometric and normative analyses, resulting in a seventy-eight-item checklist.

Results

For each of the subscale scores and for the total score, the median and the first and third percentile scores by the age of the adolescent are presented in figures 1–5. In general, the median scores increase with age for all the subscale scores and the total score.

T-tests on the subscale and total scores by sex of adolescent indicated significant differences between males and females for three of the subscales and the total score: Self- and Family Care, $t(324) = 2.16$, $p < .05$; Recreation, $t(346) = 3.13$, $p < .01$; Social and Vocational Activity, $t(347) = 3.24$, $p < .01$, and total score, $t(346) = 3.16$, $p < .01$. In each case, the mean of the female adolescents' scores is higher than that of the males' scores. Subscale means and standard deviations are presented by age and sex of adolescent in table 2. The subscale means for females are higher than those for males in almost every age group.

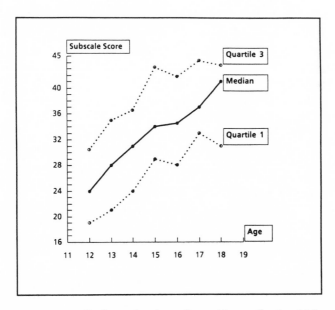

FIG. 1.—Self- and Family Care subscale medians with quartiles 1 and 3 by age of adolescent.

443

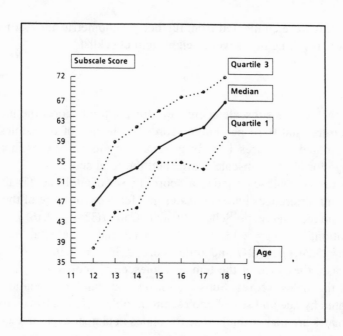

FIG. 2.—Management subscale score medians with quartiles 1 and 3 by age of adolescent

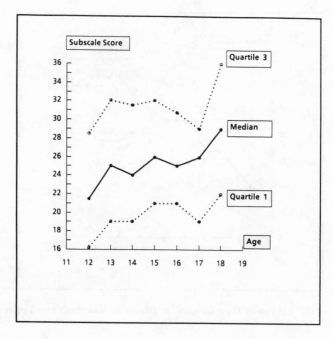

FIG. 3.—Recreation subscale median scores with quartiles 1 and 3 by age of adolescent

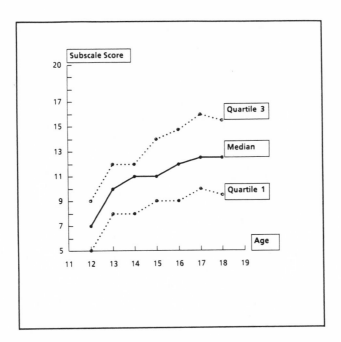

FIG. 4.—Social and Vocational Ability subscale median scores with quartiles 1 and 3 by age of adolescent.

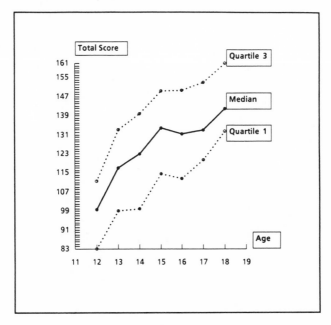

FIG. 5.—Total AFC scale median scores with quartiles 1 and 3 by age of adolescent

445

TABLE 2
Means and Standard Deviations by Age and Sex of Adolescents for Each Subscale

Subscale	12 M	12 SD	13 M	13 SD	14 M	14 SD	15 M	15 SD	16 M	16 SD	17 M	17 SD	18 M	18 SD
Self- and family care:														
Female	25	10.38	29.59	9.58	33.48	11.26	36.04	10.58	36.25	11.74	41.24	11.99	38.89	8.72
Male	24.89	7.80	27.67	8.57	29.10	11.16	34.57	9.67	31.19	10.30	37.31	6.86	37.67	8.37
Management:														
Female	45.38	10.71	52.14	9.05	55.0	10.06	60.73	9.91	60.64	9.85	64.12	8.83	69.78	7.24
Male	43.89	10.22	52.37	11.64	50.57	12.71	58.29	7.52	60.28	9.56	56.79	13.68	61.33	12.78
Recreation:														
Female	22.76	6.98	26.79	7.17	28.41	9.57	27.24	7.77	28.93	7.25	26.76	8.05	33.67	6.94
Male	21.53	8.19	25.53	9.48	23.80	9.53	26.29	9.48	23.55	9.32	24.59	9.47	25.58	9.64
Social and vocational activity:														
Female	7.0	2.61	10.03	2.73	11.44	2.19	11.81	3.41	13.57	4.78	13.08	3.24	14.33	3.46
Male	8.0	3.23	9.43	2.72	9.77	3.36	10.79	3.74	10.44	3.50	11.34	4.08	10.17	3.74

PSYCHOMETRIC EVALUATIONS

ITEM ANALYSES

The results of the item analyses are presented in table 3. The sub-scales have high levels of internal consistency, with coefficient alpha of .76–.86. In addition, within the possible spread of scores for each subscale, the range is quite broad, suggesting that the subscales are sensitive to individual differences.

INTERRATER RELIABILITY

For purposes of estimating interrater reliability, the AFC was distributed to a small sample of two-parent households, in which both parents were asked to complete the AFC on the same adolescent in the family. Fifty-two couples completed and returned the AFC. Inter-rater reliability was assessed by means of Pearson correlations of the parents' subscale scores. The results are presented in table 4. The coefficients are relatively high and statistically significant. Since it is unlikely that both parents would have absolutely identical standards for and assessments of their adolescents' functioning, the fact that interparent reliability was not even higher probably reflects naturally occurring parental variations in perception rather than a limitation of the instrument.

VALIDITY

Preliminary studies concerning the validity of the AFC were undertaken by studying the relations between AFC subscale scores and the additional data collected in the questionnaires. Table 5 summarizes these analyses.

The findings provide preliminary evidence on concurrent validity. All the subscales are highly correlated with the age of the adolescent, except for Recreational Activity, which has a lower but statistically significant correlation. This indicates that the constructs being measured reflect a developmental progression. The Recreational Activity subscale has a weaker correlation with age. Examination of the data suggests that, for the middle years of adolescence, there may not be significant changes in patterns of recreational activity but that, in the

447

TABLE 3

ITEM ANALYSIS RESULTS BY SUBSCALE

Subscale	Possible Minimum and Maximum Scores	Observed Minimum and Maximum Scores	M	SD	Coefficient Alpha	M interitem r
Self- and family care (22 items)........	0–88	6–86	32.64	10.98	.82	.19
Management (20 items).............	0–80	23–80	55.86	12.18	.86	.25
Recreation (16 items).............	0–64	8–54	25.59	8.62	.79	.19
Social and vocational activity (20 items)	0–20	1–19	10.66	3.68	.76	.14

TABLE 4

INTERRATER (Parental) RELIABILITY: PEARSON
CORRELATION COEFFICIENTS

Subscale	
Self- and family care	.46**
Management	.57**
Recreation	.62**
Social and vocational activity	.53**

NOTE.—N = 52 pairs.
** $p < .01$.

TABLE 5

VALIDITY MEASURES: PEARSON CORRELATION OF SUBSCALE SCORES WITH MEASURES
OF ADOLESCENT AND FAMILY CHARACTERISTICS

	Self- and Family Care	Management	Recreational Activity	Social and Vocational Activity
Age of adolescent...........	.38**	.44**	.11*	.36**
Sex of adolescent	.11*	.10	.16**	.17**
Adolescent's grade-point average	−.05	.28**	.26**	.21**
Adolescent's leadership experience	.21**	.26**	.21**	.36**
Honors awarded to adolescent	−.04	.19**	.18**	.22**
Number of adolescent's extracurricular activities ...	.11*	.34**	.28**	.45**
Parental education	−.07	.07	−.18**	.003
Household income	.008	.15**	−.11*	.04
Number of children in the family	.17**	.05	.03	.10
Parental marital status	−.08	.06	.12*	.07

* $p < .05$.
** $p < .01$.

spans from twelve to thirteen and from sixteen to eighteen, more change occurs. Among the possibilities of why this may be so are the timing of onset of puberty and the obtaining of a driver's license, for example.

Academic grade-point average is strongly associated with the subscale scores in the expected directions. Adolescents who maintain high grade-point averages also had high scores on the Management, Recreation, and Social and Vocational subscales. Grade-point average, however, was not correlated with Self- and Family Care. A similar pattern is evident for honors awards, which is a composite of special academic and extracurricular recognition. Devotion to extrafamilial activity would not be expected to be associated with high levels of intrafamilial or self-directed care. Associations between extracurricular activities and the subscale scores also adhere to this pattern, with the exception that a low but still significant correlation with the Self- and Family Care subscale is present. This could possibly indicate that the factors involved in extracurricular participation (although they, by definition, occur outside the home) are not as much out of synchrony with Self- and Family Care as those supporting academic achievement.

In contrast, few relations between family characteristics and the AFC subscale scores are evident. Parents' education is not related to any of the subscale scores, except for a moderate inverse correlation with Recreational Activities, possibly the result of more educated parents' emphasis on academic achievement at the expense of recreation activity. A moderate positive relation exists between household income and Management, possibly explained by greater opportunities to engage in certain types of activities (such as handling money) in these families. However, family income is not correlated with Self- and Family Care or with Social and Vocational Activities and has a modest negative correlation with Recreational Activities. The positive correlation between number of children in the family and Self- and Family Care is expected, given that adolescents in these families would have both more opportunities and more pressure to undertake such activities.

Conclusions

The results of this study indicate that the AFC measures a developmentally progressive process, that it has acceptable reliability, and that it shows some good early indications of both concurrent and discriminant validity.

The finding of significant sex differences in behavioral autonomous functioning suggests an area for further research. Research in related areas of adolescent functioning has yielded inconsistent results regarding sex differences. For example, Dusek and Flaherty (1981) and Flaherty and Dusek (1980) noted that adolescent self-concept development differs for males and females, with females scoring higher than males on factors related to congeniality and sociability. Males were found to score higher on achievement/leadership factors.

450

Groth (1972), however, found that females scored higher than males on leadership measures, while Enright, Lapsley, Drivas, and Fehr (1980) found lower autonomy scores for females. A partial explanation for these apparent discrepancies may lie in the nature of the measures used. Autonomy as assessed by attitudinal measures may differ from autonomy as measured by behavioral measures. What an adolescent reports about his or her feelings of competence may or may not be in correspondence with what the adolescent actually does in daily life. An important question becomes the extent to which the adolescent's reported self-concept is in correspondence with his or her actual behavioral autonomous functioning, as assessed by the AFC. Further, what are the factors that may intervene in this process?

A limitation in the development of this instrument to date is the small amount of data regarding very low income families as well as a lack of information regarding ethnic and subcultural distinctions. In addition, the scoring method used as the basis for data analysis in the normative study relies on a composite of the number of positively rated items and the number rating of these items. It would be of considerable interest to reexamine these data to see if, using this scoring procedure, there were separate and distinct patterns of autonomous development not presently evident. For example, some adolescents might develop functional autonomy by exploring a wide variety of experiences at a low level of intensity, and others might pursue a few areas more deeply. We plan to pursue this question in a subsequent report. In addition, there is a pressing need to perform a normative study on a larger, more diverse population. This would enable us to employ factor analytic approaches to subscale information. It is also of great importance to examine the AFC in relation to existing scales of adaptive behavior, social competence, and locus of control.

The AFC is easily and briefly administered and scored. Since it is based on parental report, it can be readily used as a research or assessment tool for a wide variety of adolescents, without problems in administration secondary to physical, cognitive, or emotional disability on the part of the adolescent. It is thus particularly well suited to explore research questions of great interest to developmentally oriented psychiatrists. Among these are the study of the relation between non-symptom-oriented dimensions of adolescent personality and the occurrence of psychopathology and the search for predictors in adolescence of both successful adaption and emotional health in adult life.

451

AUTONOMOUS FUNCTIONING CHECKLIST

The purpose of the Autonomous Functioning Checklist (AFC) is to learn about what your teenager does every day. There are no "right" or "wrong" things for your teenager to do. Teenagers of different ages do many different things. These questions are simply for the purpose of getting an idea of your teenager's daily activity.

When you answer these questions, *first,* read the question and think about whether or not it describes what you see or have seen your teenager do. You should answer the questions in relation to what you *know* your teenager does or does not do rather than what you *believe or think* he or she *could* do or *could not* do.

Second, tell us how the question describes what your teenager does by choosing one of alternatives "0," "1," "2," "3," or "4" from the scale and *placing that number in the space to the right* of the item. Here is how to use the rating scale with a sample question.

0	1	2	3	4
DOES NOT DO	DOES ONLY RARELY	DOES ABOUT HALF THE TIME THERE IS AN OPPORTUNITY	DOES MOST OF THE TIME THERE IS AN OPPORTUNITY	DOES EVERY TIME THERE IS AN OPPORTUNITY

Sample Item

My teenager picks up trash in the yard.   _____

0.—You should mark "0" if you have *never seen* your teenager do this, even though he or she may not have done it because there has never been a chance. (For the sample item you may mark "0" because, for example, you live in an apartment and do not have a yard.)

1.—You should mark "1" if you have seen your teenager do this when there has been a chance; but there have been many more times that he or she has not done it.

452

2.—You should mark "2" if your teenager does this about half the time there is a chance but if he or she does not do it readily or comfortably.

3.—You should mark "3" if there are more times that your teenager does this than does not do it, given the chance, and if he or she does it readily.

4.—You should mark "4" if your teenager does this whenever there is a chance and if he or she does it readily.

Your teenager will not have had a chance to participate in some of the activities the questions describe. These items should be answered as "*does not do*," even though you may feel that your teenager could or would do this if he or she were given the chance. Please mark "0" for the questions that describe activities that your teenager has *never had the chance* to do. Some of the questions describe things that your teenager may do with help from others. Answer these questions after you think about who has the most responsibility for *completing* the activity. For example, your teenager may cook the family meals and may be helped by other family members who set the table or chop vegetables. If your teenager is the family member with the *most* responsibility for cooking *every* meal that the family eats together, your answer would be "4," which stands for "does every time there is an opportunity." On the other hand, if your teenager helps other family members by doing jobs that they tell him or her to do and *never* has the *most responsibility* for fixing dinner, your answer would be "0" or "does not do."

Please write the age of your teenager here: _____ .

Self- and Family Care Activity

My teenager:

1. Keeps own personal items and belongings in order (for example, makes bed, puts away own clothing and belongings).   _____

2. Prepares food that does not require cooking for himself/herself (for example, cereal, sandwich).   _____

3. Cares for his/her own clothing (for example, laundry, simple repair, shoe cleaning). _____

4. Travels to and from daily activities (for example, rides bikes or walks, takes bus, arranges for transportation, drives car). _____

5. Prepares food that requires cooking for himself/ herself (for example, hamburger, soup). _____

6. Performs simple first aid or medical care for himself/ herself (for example, bandages, takes own temperature). _____

7. Purchases his/her own clothing and personal items that are used on a daily basis (for example, underwear, toiletries). _____

8. Performs minor repair and maintenance in his/her own environment (for example, changes bulbs, hangs pictures). _____

9. Shops for and purchases his/her own groceries. _____

10. Responds to his/her own medical emergency by calling parent. _____

11. Responds to his/her own medical emergency by calling doctor or hospital. _____

12. Does designated household maintenance chores involving family living areas (for example, cleans, takes out trash, does simple yard work). _____

13. Performs routine daily personal care for another family member (for example, dresses, feeds). _____

14. Keeps personal items and belongings of another family member in order (for example, makes bed, puts away clothing and belongings of another family member). _____

15. Prepares meals for other family member(s). _____

16. Transports (or arranges for transport of) another family member to and from daily activities. _____

17. Purchases clothing and personal items (that are used on a daily basis) for other family members. _____

18. Shops for and purchases family groceries. _____

19. Performs minor repair and maintenance in family living areas (for example, changes light bulbs, hangs pictures). _____

20. Repairs and maintains (or makes arrangement for repair and maintenance of) major household needs (for example, plumbing, yard work, electrical wiring). _____

21. Responds to household emergency (for example, stove fire, plumbing problem) by calling parent or neighbor. _____

22. Responds to household emergency (for example, stove fire, plumbing problem) by calling fire department, using fire extinguisher, calling repair service, or shutting off water). _____

Management Activity

My teenager:

23. Uses the telephone and telephone directories. _____

24. Carries out transactions with salespeople (for example, listens to information, asks questions, gives payment, receives change). _____

25. Uses postal services (for example, uses postage, mails letters, packages). _____

26. Uses bank (for example, fills out deposit or withdrawal slips, uses passbook). _____

27. Uses travel-related services for short trips (for example, taxi, bus, subway). _____

28. Uses travel-related services for long trips (for example, airline, train, bus). _____

29. Uses library services (for example, checks out books or uses copying machine). _____

30. Maintains and uses his/her own savings account. _____

31. Maintains and uses his/her own checking or charge account. _____

32. Maintains adequate personal care and grooming (for example, bathes, trims fingernails and toenails when needed). _____

33. Maintains his/her routine general health and fitness (for example, has adequate eating, sleeping, exercise habits). _____

34. Selects clothing that is suited to the weather (for example, raincoat if raining, warm clothes in winter). _____

35. Plans and initiates activity for himself/herself in everyday unscheduled free time (for example, chooses to watch television or work on hobby if bored). _____

36. Plans activity for his/her long-term free time (for example, makes plans for summer vacation, mid-semester vacation). _____

37. Initiates friendships with peers (for example, plans or attends parties, outings, games, club meetings). _____

38. Meets nonacademic social obligations or commitments (for example, keeps appointments for family and peer-related social events arranged by self or others). _____

39. Meets academic obligations and commitments (for example, completes homework assignments on time, brings necessary supplies to class). _____

40. Plans transportation to and from special activities (for example, arranges for rides with friends or family, plans car or bus route and schedule). _____

41. Manages his/her own budget from allowance or income (for example, saves money for large purchases, pays for routine expenses throughout week without running out of money). _____

42. Makes long-term educational and/or career plans (for example, selects courses, investigates colleges or technical schools). _____

Recreational Activity

When my teenager is *free* to *choose* how he/she will spend his/her unscheduled time, he/she chooses to:

43. Listen to music (for example, radio or stereo). _____

44. Read for relaxation (for example, books, newspapers, magazines). _____

45. Play games or puzzles (for example, cards, crossword puzzles, jigsaw puzzles, computer games). _____

46. Write letters to friends, relatives, acquaintances. _____

47. Work on or take lessons in crafts or hobbies (for example, cooking, collections, pet care, sewing, model building, car repair). _____

48. Practice or take lessons that involve a trained artistic or academic skill (for example, piano or other musical instrument, ballet, singing, creative writing, foreign languages). _____

49. Go to movies, rock concerts, dances. _____

50. Go to plays, theater, lectures. _____

457

51. Pursue activities that are related to his/her career interest(s) (for example, run a business, work with computers, practice piano for professional preparation). _____

52. Go for walks. _____

53. Go shopping or spend time at shopping centers or in shopping areas. _____

54. Attend club meetings or other organized social group meetings. _____

55. Work for pay (for example, babysit, play in a band, do yard work, walk dogs, work at a part-time job, deliver papers). _____

56. Clean and/or maintain living environment or belongings (for example, clean house, wash or repair clothes, wash car, make household repairs). _____

57. Work on schoolwork (for example, spend extra time on homework, make special preparations for class projects, spend time in the library). _____

58. Spend time with family (for example, work on family projects, have discussions or casual conversations, attend family gatherings such as picnics or parties). _____

Social and Vocational Activity

On these final items, please circle "YES" or "NO" in response to each description: "YES" if the description fits your teenager; "NO" if it does not.

My teenager:

59. Has casual friendships with teenagers of the opposite sex.   NO   YES

60. Has close friendships with teenagers of the opposite sex.   NO   YES

61. Has casual friendships with adults outside the family (for example, teachers, neighbors, coaches, Scout leaders).

NO   YES

62. Has close friendships with adults outside the family (for example, teachers, neighbors, coaches, Scout leaders).

NO   YES

63. Has casual friendships with younger children.

NO   YES

64. Has close friendships with younger children.

NO   YES

65. Is active in casual/recreational groups of teenage friends.

NO   YES

66. Has many friendships.

NO   YES

67. Is active in one or more organized extracurricular groups (for example, French club, student council, sports team).

NO   YES

68. Has a leadership position in one or more organized extracurricular groups (for example, president of the student council, captain of a sports team).

NO   YES

69. Has a close friendship with an adult member of the extended family (for example, uncle, aunt, or grandparent).

NO   YES

70. Works or has worked either for pay or as a volunteer in an area of particular career interest (for example, in science lab or legal office, as a teacher's aid or candystriper).

NO   YES

71. Works or has worked to earn money by providing a service on a regularly scheduled basis (for example, contracts for yard work, dog walking, babysitting).

NO   YES

459

72. Works or has worked to earn money by using a special skill (for example, musical performance, typing, tutoring).   NO   YES

73. Works or has worked to earn money in a self- or peer-run organization or business.   NO   YES

74. Works or has worked to earn money fundraising for an organization or charity (for example, Scouts, church groups, political organizations).   NO   YES

75. Does or has done volunteer work without pay for a service (for example, a school or political organization; a social agency; a club; a church; or a hospital).   NO   YES

76. Participates or has participated in prevocational (career) or vocational (career) classes or training (for example, a technical training or career development class).   NO   YES

77. Has explored career interests by visiting work sites or interviewing people in that job or career.   NO   YES

78. Has spent time reading, researching, or "finding out" about a career that particularly interests him/her.   NO   YES

REFERENCES

Achenbach, T. M., and Edelbrock, C. S. 1981. Behavioral problems and competencies reported by parents of normal and disturbed children aged 4 through 16. *Monographs of the Society for Research in Child Development* 46(Serial no. 188).

Blos, P. 1967. The second individuation process of adolescence. *Psychoanalytic Study of the Child* 22:162–186.

Brown, M.; Diller, L.; Gordon, W. A.; Fordyce, W.; and Jacobs, D. F. 1984. Rehabilitation indicators and program evaluation. *Rehabilitation Psychology* 29:21–35.

Brown, M.; Gordon, W. A.; and Diller, L. 1983. Functional assessment and outcome measurement: an integrative review. *Annual Review of Rehabilitation* 3:93–120.

Bruininks, R. H.; Woodcock, R. W.; Weatherman, R. F.; and Hill, B. K. 1984. *Scales of Independent Behavior: A Manual*. Allen, Tex.: Teaching Resources.

Diller, L.; Fordyce, W.; Jacobs, D.; Brown, M.; Gordon, W.; Simmens, S.; Orazem, J.; and Barrett, L. 1983. Final report: rehabilitation indicators project. Grant no. G008003039. Washington, D.C.: U.S. Department of Education, National Institute of Handicapped Research.

Dusek, J. B., and Flaherty, J. F. 1981. The development of the self-concept during the adolescent years. *Monographs of the Society for Research in Child Development* 46(Serial no. 191).

Enright, R. D.; Lapsley, D. K.; Drivas, A. E.; and Fehr, L. A. 1980. Parental influence on the development of adolescent autonomy and identity. *Journal of Youth and Adolescence* 9:529–545.

Erikson, E. H. 1968. *Identity: Youth and Crisis*. New York: Norton.

Flaherty, J. F., and Dusek, J. B. 1980. An investigation of the relationship between psychological androgeny and components of the self-concept. *Journal of Personality and Social Psychology* 38:984–992.

Freud, A. 1958. Adolescence. *Psychoanalytic Study of the Child* 13:255–278.

Garmezy, N. 1985. Stressors of childhood. In N. Garmezy and M. Rutter, eds. *Stress, Coping, and Development in Children*. New York: McGraw-Hill.

Grossman, H. J. 1983. *Classification in Mental Retardation: 1983 Revision*. Washington, D.C.: American Association on Mental Deficiency.

Groth, N. J. 1972. Achievement of autonomy and other developmental tasks in bright and average adolescents. *Gifted Child Quarterly* 16:290–292.

Harter, S. 1982. The perceived competence scale for children. *Child Development* 53:87–89.

Hartmann, H. 1958. *Ego Psychology and the Problem of Adaption.* New York: International Universities Press.

Heber, R. F. 1959. *A Manual on Terminology and Classification in Mental Retardation. American Journal of Mental Deficiency* 64(monograph suppl.).

Nihira, K.; Foster, R.; Shellhaas, M.; and Leland, H. 1974. *AAMD Adaptive Behavior Scale.* Rev. ed. Washington, D.C.: American Association on Mental Deficiency.

Offer, D. 1986. Adolescent development: a normative perspective. In A. J. Francer and R. E. Hales, eds. *Psychiatry Update: The American Psychiatric Association Annual Review,* vol. 5. Washington, D.C.: American Psychiatric Press.

Pellegrini, D.; Kosisky, M. A.; Nackman, D.; Cytryn, L.; McKnew, D. H.; Gershon, E.; Hamovit, J.; and Cammuso, K. 1986. Personal and social resources in children of patients with bipolar affective disorder and children of normal control subjects. *American Journal of Psychiatry* 143(7): 856–861.

Rutter, M. 1985. Stress, coping, and development: some issues and some questions. In N. Garmezy and M. Rutter, eds. *Stress, Coping, and Development in Children.* New York: McGraw-Hill.

Sparrow, S.; Balla, D.; and Cicchetti, D. 1984. *Vineland Adaptive Behavior Scales: Survey Form Manual.* Interview ed. Circle Pines, Minn.: American Guidance Service.

Steinberg, L., and Silverberg, S. 1986. The vicissitudes of autonomy in early adolescence. *Child Development* 57:841–851.

Zinn, D. 1979. A developmental preventative approach to problems of psychopathology in adolescence. In J. Noshpitz, ed. *Basic Handbook of Child Psychiatry,* vol. 4. New York: Basic.

27 PSYCHOLOGICAL ASSESSMENT AND DISCUSSION OF FEMALE ADOLESCENTS WITH TRICHOTILLOMANIA

ROSINA G. SCHNURR

The incidence of trichotillomania, an irresistible urge to pull out body hair (Hallopeau 1889), is reported to be considerably higher in females than in males (Greenberg and Sarner 1965; Mannino and Delgado 1969) and greatest during adolescence (Krishnan, Davidson, and Guajardo 1985). Greenberg and Sarner suggest that adolescent girls afflicted with the disorder form a distinct categorical group. Trichotillomania in this group is described as a malignant affliction that may in time progress to grievous physical and psychic damage. Sorosky and Sticher (1980) present the opposite view, that trichotillomania in the adolescent is a multidetermined habit disorder that may not necessarily be viewed as a poor prognostic sign.

Psychological assessment of patients with trichotillomania has not been extensive. Limited subject population combined with historical antecedents (dermatology vs. psychiatry) and philosophy of etiology (e.g., psychoanalytic [Buxbaum 1960; Meyer and Haag 1984; Monroe and Abse 1963] vs. behavioral [Azrin, Nunn, and Franz 1980; De L'Horne 1977; Jillson 1983]) has resulted in few good opportunities for psychological assessment. Reports that are available, which have employed psychometric assessment, have shown that patients diagnosed with trichotillomania showed more severe emotional disturbance and psychopathology than other causes of hair loss, such as alopecia areata (Toback and Rajkumar 1979). Other reports have concentrated more on diagnoses (Greenberg and Sarner 1965; Zawadzki 1971).

The following case reports examine the psychological makeup of three adolescent girls who presented with trichotillomania by using both objective and projective psychometric assessment procedures.

Case Reports

Three adolescent girls were referred for psychological assessment. Sarah T. was referred for nonattendance at school, and Joan H. and Kelly C. were referred specifically because of their hair loss. According to school and parental reports, all three children ranged in intellectual ability from at least average to above average and came from middle- to upper-middle-class families.

All three girls completed the Minnesota Multiphasic Personality Inventory (MMPI—Hathaway and McKinley 1983) and a sentence completion inventory (Adams 1982). The Thematic Apperception Test (Murray 1938) and the Rorschach ink blots (Rorschach 1942) were administered to them. Drawings were also obtained of a house, a tree, and a person. In addition, Sarah and Kelly also completed depression inventories (Birleson 1981; Kovacs 1980–1981) and anxiety inventories (Reynolds and Richmond 1985), and a Child Behavior Checklist (Achenbach and Edelbrock 1979) was completed by the mothers for these two girls.

Sarah, aged thirteen, was referred for nonattendance at school following a social incident. She had experienced an upset with her two only friends, and the loss was perceived as intolerable. The hair-pulling symptoms involved her eyelashes and, later, the hair on her head. Testing showed distress related to the familial situation as well as the current social situation. There was no evidence of depression, increased anxiety, acting out, or psychotic symptoms. Rather, Sarah tended to be passive, indecisive, and conscientious. The symptom of hair pulling did not seem to be important to her. The hair loss was considered to be only an incidental aspect. The parental report confirmed these characteristics.

Joan, aged sixteen and adopted, was referred for hair loss that had not responded to medical treatment and whose resources had been explored in depth. Three years prior, her closest girlfriend had moved away. Approximately six months after the move, the symptoms of trichotillomania were present. When the friend returned for a four-week visit, Joan's hair began to grow again. Biting her nails was a long-standing problem as well. Although Joan stated her concern with her hair loss, she never seemed to be sufficiently concerned to wear a wig or a hat to cover her scalp, the entire top of which was exposed. In fact, she actively participated in school activities and had a boyfriend. Psychological testing showed her to be a very strong and determined person who could use manipulation to obtain her wishes. She had great difficulty in facing anything that might cause psychological pain. There were no indicators of depression, anxiety (other than biting her nails), acting out, or psychotic symptoms.

Kelly, aged twelve, was referred for hair pulling that began at age five. Trichotillomania of the scalp hair began approximately ten months prior to this evaluation. There were a number of losses in her life at the age of five—two grandparents had died, and a long-term foster child to whom Kelly was quite attached had left the family. At this time, only the eyelashes were affected. There was some evidence to suggest that an eye infection may also have been present. Various behavioral programs had been attempted, with limited success, over the following five years. Prior to being seen, Kelly had experienced some knee problems that prevented her from being as active in sports as she would have preferred (perceived as a loss). Behavioral programs had again been tried without achieving success, mainly owing to the fact that Kelly would misrepresent the facts when monitoring was required. Psychological assessment showed her to be a very socially dependent person who was actively interested in sports. She had great difficulty facing any family conflict; for example, she would become very upset if her parents argued, however minimal the conflict. She acknowledged her hair problems but gave no importance or emphasis to the difficulty during the assessment. There were no indications of familial stress, depression, increased anxiety, delinquency, or severe psychopathology.

Discussion

Psychological assessment of these three female adolescents shows some similarities and some major differences. There was no evidence of severe psychopathology. Rather, the difficulties presented at the level of neuroses. This is in agreement with Sorosky and Sticher (1980) but not with Toback and Rajkumar (1979).

The hair loss, in all three cases, could be associated with the experience of a severe personal loss, for example, a friend or family member. This would be in agreement with Irwin's (1953) suggestion that hair pulling may be an aggressive reaction with the associated emotions of grief and rage. Krishnan, Davidson, and Miller (1984) have treated trichotillomania as an atypical variation of depressive illness. The use of monoamine oxidase (MAO) inhibitor therapy was found to be successful. Krishnan et al. (1985) illustrate trichotillomania as related to object loss, often the unavailability of the mother. The mothers of all three girls were very available to their daughters, perhaps too much so. A certain dependency was observed in that, for example, the girls wished to have their mothers present at the initial interview.

Greenberg and Sarner (1965) have described the majority of mothers of children who develop trichotillomania as highly pathological individuals. Fathers were characterized as aloof, withdrawn, and passive aggressive. Delgado and Mannino (1969) also suggest significant parental characteristics that contribute to the hair-pulling symptom. The parents of the girls in this study could not be described as such. The mothers presented as capable and competent and the fathers as interested and involved. Sarah's father traveled extensively, and there was reported conflict between them when he was at home. Nevertheless, they played together in sports activities. He also made a special effort to come for an interview. The fathers of Joan and Kelly readily presented for the evaluation with a concerned attitude and a sincere willingness to help their daughters. The parent who spent the most time with the daughter and who expressed the most concern about the symptoms of trichotillomania was the mother in each case. While the mothers did present as strong individuals, there was no evidence to suggest aggressive or ambivalent tendencies. While the fathers presented as less involved than the mothers, they were not perceived as extremely passive or inadequate.

The onset of hair pulling in these three adolescents tended to be associated with what the child may have perceived as an unsolvable problem, that is, a loss. Being either unable or unwilling to look at the difficult and frustrating situation resulted in hair loss. This may be seen as an internalizing symptom, and it is possible that the expression of their discomfort or distress became an automatic behavior, that is, a habit that fluctuated with anxiety producing external events (Delgado and Mannino 1969). Oranje, Peereboom-Wynia, and De Raeymecker (1986) speak of this aspect as a "trigger point" (precipitating factor) and of how the behavior then becomes conditioned and maintained.

Trichotillomania of the scalp was seen by the parents of both Sarah and Kelly as a more severe symptom than the eyelash pulling. Ilan and Alexander (1965) discuss eyelash and eyebrow pulling in two adolescent girls. They suggest that eyelash and eyebrow pulling is different than general trichotillomania in that it is related to a different stage of psychosexual development.

Kelly differed from Sarah and Joan in that the onset (i.e., involvement of the eyelashes) was preadolescent while the onset of scalp-hair involvement occurred during adolescence. As the difficulty persisted into adolescence, it does not appear to be of the self-limited and benign variety of childhood as described by Greenberg and Sarner (1965). It is possible that there may be two groups of preadolescent children who present with trichotillomania: those who have a "habit" type of behavior, which is treatable by behavioral intervention, and those who may have more severe difficulties that carry over into adolescence. Sticher, Abramovits, and Newcomer (1980) state that hair plucking that begins in childhood and extends into adolescence and adulthood may represent a more complex psychopathological condition.

Differences can be most clearly seen in the MMPI profiles. The response sets (i.e., the approach that each girl took in completing the test) were quite different. Also, there were differences in degree of reported unhappiness, hysterical symptoms, activity levels, and social involvement.

Sorosky and Sticher (1980) describe their two cases of adolescent girls as being nonpsychotic and passive dependent with hysterical features. These symptoms could be applied to the three cases presented here. Although their MMPI profiles show differences, they all presented as very dependent on others, lacking in insight, unable to face and accept what was perceived as an intolerable situation, and quite capable of passively manipulating their family situations. They could be further described as repressive, indifferent, and showing no anxiety related to their symptom of hair loss.

Greenberg and Sarner (1965) conceptualize trichotillomania in adolescence as an ongoing compromise between the patient's drives for self-assertion and mastery and the parents' needs to maintain an unhealthy status quo. The three female adolescents addressed in this chapter can be seen as involved in the process of self-assertion and mastery. However, there was no evidence to suggest a strong desire by their mothers to maintain an unhealthy status quo. Rather, it would appear that other personality characteristics (e.g., hysterical tendencies) contributed to the trichotillomania as well. It is well documented (e.g., Delgado and Mannino 1969) that hair pulling does not occur as an isolated symptom.

Conclusions

While there are similarities in adolescent girls who present with symptoms of trichotillomania, there are also differences. The question of whether they represent a specific category or grouping cannot be answered on the basis of the results reported in the literature or on the results of analysis of small numbers of cases. A well-controlled and comprehensive study of trichotillomania, as it unfolds developmentally, is needed.

REFERENCES

Achenbach, T. M., and Edelbrock, C. S. 1979. The child behavior profile. II. boys aged 12–16 and girls aged 6–11 and 12–16. *Journal of Consulting and Clinical Psychology* 47:223–233.

Adams, P. L. 1982. *A Primer of Child Psychotherapy.* 2d ed. Boston: Little, Brown.

Azrin, N. H.; Nunn, R. G.; and Frantz, S. E. 1980. Treatment of hair pulling (trichotillomania): a comparative study of habit reversal and negative practice training. *Journal of Behavior Therapy and Experimental Psychiatry* 11:13–20.

Birleson, P. 1981. The validity of depressive disorder in childhood and the development of a self-rating scale: a research report. *Journal of Child Psychology and Psychiatry and Allied Disciplines* 22:73–88.

Buxbaum, E. 1960. Hair-pulling and fetishism. *Psychoanalytic Study of the Child* 15:243–260.

Delgado, R. A., and Mannino, F. V. 1969. Some observations on trichotillomania in children. *Journal of the American Academy of Child Psychiatry* 8:229–246.

De L'Horne, J. J. 1977. Behavior therapy for trichotillomania. *Behavioral Research and Therapy* 15:192–196.

Greenberg, H. R., and Sarner, C. A. 1965. Trichotillomania, symptom and syndrome. *Archives of General Psychiatry* 12:482–489.

Hallopeau, M. 1889. Alopecie par grattage (trichomanie ou trichotillomanie). *Annales de dermatologie et syphiligraphie* 10:440–441.

Hathaway, S. R., and McKinley, J. C. 1983. *Minnesota Multiphasic Personality Inventory*. Minneapolis: University of Minnesota Press.

Ilan, E., and Alexander, E. 1965. Eyelash and eyebrow pulling (trichotillomania) treatment of two adolescent girls. *Israel Annals of Psychiatry and Related Disciplines* 3:267–281.

Irwin, D. 1953. Alopecia. In B. G. Russell and E. D. Wittkower, eds. *Emotional Factors in Skin Disease*. New York: Hoeber.

Jillson, O. F. 1983. Alopecia. II. trichotillomania (trichotillohabitus). *Cutis* 31:383–389.

Kovacs, M. 1980–1981. Rating scale to assess depression in school-aged children. *Acta Paedopsychiatrie* 46:305–315.

Krishnan, K. K. R.; Davidson, J. R. T.; and Guajardo, C. 1985. Trichotillomania—a review. *Comprehensive Psychiatry* 26:123–128.

Krishnan, R. R.; Davidson, J.; and Miller, R. 1984. MAO inhibitor therapy in trichotillomania associated with depression: case report. *Journal of Clinical Psychiatry* 45:267–268.

Mannino, F. V., and Delgado, R. A. 1969. Trichotillomania in children: a review. *American Journal of Psychiatry* 126:87–93.

Meyer, A. E., and Haag, A. 1984. Psychosomatics of trichotillomania and related states or disorders. *Psychotherapy and Psychosomatics* 42:119–123.

Monroe, J. R., and Abse, D. W. 1963. The psychopathology of trichotillomania and trichophagy. *Psychiatry* 26:95–103.

Murray, H. A. 1938. *Explorations in Personality*. New York: Oxford University Press.

Oranje, A. P.; Peereboom-Wynia, J. D. R.; and De Raeymaecker, D. M. J. 1986. Trichotillomania in childhood. *Journal of the American Academy of Dermatology* 15:614–619.

Reynolds, C. R., and Richmond, B. O. 1985. *Revised Children's Manifest Anxiety Scale (RCMAS)*. Los Angeles: Western Psychological Services.

Rorschach, H. 1942. *Psychodiagnostics*. Translated by Paul Lemkau and Bernard Kronenberg. 2d ed. Bern: Huber.

Sorosky, A. D., and Sticher, M. B. 1980. Trichotillomania in adolescence. *Adolescent Psychiatry* 8:437–454.

Sticher, M.; Abramovits, W.; and Newcomer, V. R. 1980. Trichotillomania in adults. *Cutis* 26:90–101.

Toback, C., and Rajkumar, S. 1979. The emotional disturbance underlying alopecia areata, alopecia totalis and trichotillomania. *Child Psychiatry and Human Development* 10:114–117.

Zawadzki, Z. 1971. A rare case of persistent trichotillomania in an adult case report. *Bulletin of Polish Science and History* 14:77–78.

PART IV

PSYCHOTHERAPEUTIC ISSUES IN ADOLESCENT PSYCHIATRY

EDITORS' INTRODUCTION

With our greater understanding of ego development and structural theory, a wide range of dyadic techniques from supportive dynamic psychotherapy to intensive psychoanalytic psychotherapy and psychoanalysis are now being utilized. Gitelson, as early as 1948, proposed that the therapeutic task not only is directed to psychic analysis but rather should result in a synthesis of the adolescent's character. Whatever approach is required to engage the adolescent may be used, but only as a means to the end: eventual dyadic engagement. Chapters by John E. Meeks and Allen J. Cahill and by Henry N. Massie introduce approaches to adolescents with severe behavior problems and adolescents with psychotic defenses. Following this, Allan Z. Schwartzberg introduces a special section on the treatment of substance abuse in adolescents.

Meeks and Cahill explore the historical approach to behavior problems in an aggressive, severely disturbed adolescent. They discuss the extent of the problem, developmental factors, the behavioral control system approach, and milieu therapy. Meeks and Cahill advocate focusing on the "malignant defenses" during inpatient hospitalization of the delinquent adolescent and describe denial, projection, projective identification, and splitting as the chief primitive defenses to be analyzed. The authors describe a hospital approach that begins with a predictable, interpretive milieu and combines concurrent psychotherapy (individual and family). They believe long-term therapy is important but stress the importance of the family in eventual transition to outpatient treatment.

Massie is concerned about the skepticism surrounding treatment of adolescent and young adult psychosis. He believes economic factors have curtailed support for long-term psychoanalytic psychotherapy and reports two cases to illustrate the value of approaches pioneered by Fromm-Reichman and Searles, among others. The author discusses a number of principles regarding treatment and etiology of youth psychosis, including outcome of long-term treatment, onset of psychosis during childhood with impairment of competency, and breakdown of adolescent sexual development as described by the Laufers.

28 THERAPY OF ADOLESCENTS WITH SEVERE BEHAVIOR PROBLEMS

JOHN E. MEEKS AND ALLEN J. CAHILL

We are presently going through another period of doubt regarding the proper management of behaviorally disordered adolescents. This is not a new issue (Eissler 1959; Meeks 1979), but the current climate is worrisome.

After eighty years of child guidance clinics and juvenile court probation consultants, the public is beginning to despair of rehabilitating the aggressive delinquent. Even in the early 1960s, Leonard Bernstein's *West Side Story* signaled society's concern that glib sociological excuses would only worsen the handling of behavior disorders. Public opinion and public institutions are turning back to a punishment model. The pendulum has swung away from the idealization of Rousseau's "noble savage," who would be good if only society did not overcontrol and frustrate him, toward today's bleak cynicism about the essential untreatability of the *Lord of the Flies*.

In the early 1970s, the New York University Institute of Judicial Administration, with solid support from the American Bar Association (ABA), initiated the Juvenile Justice Project, which resulted in the ABA passing resolutions that created sweeping reforms in the juvenile justice system, increasing punishment and limiting rehabilitation. There was clear intent to keep the delinquent away from mental health workers (Benedek and Shetky 1980).

In 1981 Shamsie published an article on juvenile delinquency, asking, "Our treatments do not work—where do we go from here?" The article not only validated the beliefs of many public officials but also rang true to the opinion of many academic psychiatrists.[1]

The current therapeutic nihilism is particularly ironic in that our first good research on the treatment of behavior disorders, our ten-year follow-up studies, initially began to appear in the late 1970s. Tramontana's (1980) classic review of this literature about positive therapy results with behavior disorders appeared a full year before Shamsie's poorly researched article. Suffice it to say that public officials are cynical about treatment of severe behavior disorders. Academic psychiatry has a mind-set that sees behavior disorders as perhaps social rather than medical problems, and only clinicians working daily with families appear aware that an inpatient limit-setting program plus psychotherapy yields a 70–75 percent cure rate for delinquents (Gossett 1983; Tramontana 1980).

The Extent of the Problem

The incidence of serious behavior disorders in the population has been measured by Rutter and Giller (1983) at 4 percent in a rural (the Isle of Wight) and 8 percent in an urban (London) study. Offer (1979) found conduct disorders in the general population (Chicago) at 10 percent (boys 11 percent, girls 8 percent).

The nature of conduct disorders is described in DSM-III as behavior infringing on the rights of others, in violation of society's code—behavior that bothers others. The etiology of behavior disorders extends over the entire range of neuropsychology, including psychosis, brain damage, epilepsy, and attention deficit disorder (Lewis 1979, 1983). The findings concerning the relative frequency of etiology vary from one study to another, but it is probably true that most serious behavior disorders, as McManus (1984) highlights in a recent diagnostic study of serious delinquents in a Michigan juvenile facility, are correlated with a diagnosis either of a serious depressive disorder (40 percent) or of serious characterologic deficits (DSM-III identity disorder or borderline personality—70 percent). We have always had some effective approaches to the major mental illnesses described by Lewis, but it is only in the last two decades that we have refined our techniques for treating depression and borderline personalities. This may account for the better treatment results reported recently with the behaviorally disordered population (see Gossett 1983; Tramontana 1980).

476

Developmental Factors

From a developmental and etiologic standpoint, it must be noted that the behavior disorders do not actually develop in the six-months duration required by DSM-III. They originate in preschool years, with evidence of deficits in social skills, motor control, and cognitive skills often obvious in kindergarten and first grade. Chess and Thomas (1977), in their series of 133 "difficult children," link behavior problems to a temperament showing "intense reactions to stimuli," even in the first year of life. Although organic factors are important, family and psychological issues may be more important. A twenty-year study in Hawaii (Werner 1982) found that the perinatal events (birth difficulties, delayed breathing, and neonatal instability) are associated with delinquency only if the parents later deprive or neglect the child. Intensity of temperament and mismatching of temperaments between parent and child (Chess and Thomas 1966) further complicate the problems of socializing children. Inadequate establishment of behavioral limits by the parents and the resulting inadequately frustrated narcissism in the child set the stage for behavioral explosions at the point of school enrollment, when the child first contends with firm external limits. This is especially likely if the child's needs for affection and support have also been neglected. Lack of socialization about property ("mine" vs. "yours"), which leads to early theft, signals the poorest prognosis (Patterson 1971). The urge to steal is probably also strengthened by neglect and deprivation (Meeks 1979): "I don't need your gifts. I take what I want." There is evidence that genetic factors and sociological factors play a role in causation in addition to the factors already mentioned. However, this chapter will concentrate on psychological factors at the core of the behavioral pattern. The basic issue sounds simple. The vast majority of children and adolescents who cannot appropriately control behavior have never learned to accept "No!" Their problem consists of two deficits, one affective, the other cognitive. They have learned little tolerance for conscious aggression or for anger (theirs or other's), and they have little reality sense of the inevitability of external consequences for their aggressive behavior. Simple, isn't it? They're spoiled kids. Let's punish them!

Is this simply a behavioral problem, or is some mental distortion holding this behavioral pattern in place? Basic tolerance for conscious anger is gained ordinarily between two and five years of age. When the child has to accept a behavioral limit, the child is angry. If the child is faced with the fact that the parent will be angry until the child accepts the limit, he will slowly internalize the rule to avoid the anger of the parent (Cahill 1981). In the borderline adolescent, "malignant" defenses (Meeks 1986), defenses that distort perception of reality and even attempt to change the external human environment, signal the failure of this early process. In healthy or even neurotic development, defenses function primarily to alter and control internal feelings. Malignant defenses, such as projection, projective identification, denial, and splitting, leave the consciousness of the patient generally anger free at the expense of believing he is living in a family and society that is hostile and basically unfair. The world the behaviorally disordered youngster experiences must be placated, misled, or manipulated. When these techniques fail and anger bursts into consciousness, behavior that defies the family's and society's persecutory limits is immediate and is usually felt to be entirely justified. Even if the youngster recognizes that his defiance has gone beyond justification, he still expects to "get away with it."

The family patterns described earlier (inadequate, inconsistent behavioral limits and inadequate anger and external consequences when limits are breached) have allowed the adolescent to be repeatedly rescued from external consequences of misbehavior throughout childhood. Why would the youngster now expect consequences to follow logically on his behavior? Even when adolescents see certain behavior as intrinsically and causally linked to certain results, even after their behavior has repeatedly triggered definite consequences, they expect the laws of cause and effect to be magically suspended *this time*. Often this is not because the children have not been punished—often they have been treated very harshly, in fact (Lewis 1979, 1983). However, they have rarely experienced the consistent, logical consequences of their behavior; they are rather more familiar with their parents' poorly controlled anger, immature impulsiveness, or drunken whim (Patterson and Cogg 1971). The deficits in reality testing about causes and effects of behavior and the difficulties in mastering affect require a treatment plan that combines objective logical application of external consequences and penalties with tolerance (in staff) for intensive affect in themselves and in the adolescent.

478

Traditional psychoanalytic psychotherapy techniques, particularly those developed recently for working with borderline patients, help us to maintain contact with the impulsive teen through veritable fire storms of rage about limits (Masterson 1972, 1980), particularly as omnipotent defenses (which hide work and social incompetence and terror of the real world) are confronted by pragmatic staff. But the major therapeutic contribution of inpatient facilities that initiates change in disturbed teenagers is the milieu: the nurturant, intensely personal social system governed by laws enforced by immediate external consequences. This living environment (Jones 1953; Main 1946; Stanton and Schwartz 1954) provides a "corrective disciplinary experience" that assists the adolescent to assess the external social environment correctly and still modulate affect and avoid being overwhelmed by feelings of helplessness and despair.

A milieu therapy for teens with behavior problems, then, contains two basic elements: (1) a privilege-restriction program based on learning theory research and (2) slowly developing relationships between staff and patient and between the teenager and peers that are carefully analyzed according to psychoanalytic principles until object constancy and object permanence are approached. Then the adolescent is ready for outpatient therapy, capable of making and maintaining a workable therapeutic alliance.

The Behavioral Control System

There is a general conviction among adolescent therapists that complex family factors and sometimes subtle family dynamics may permit or encourage youngsters to ignore or distort social reality (Borzormenyi-Nagy and Spark 1973; Johnson and Szurek 1952; Minuchin, Montalvo, Gueryney, Rosmon, and Schumer 1967; Stierlin 1977). In other cases the explanations for the youngster's arrested development are painfully obvious in the family's disorganization, violent behavior, or even direct abuse of the youngster (Goldston 1971; Isaacs 1972; Jaffe, Wolfe, Wilson, and Zak 1986). The family therapy needed for this range of family dysfunction is beyond the scope of this chapter but does make up a crucial element in successful treatment (Lantz and Thorwald 1985). However, understanding these etiologic factors does not help the staff who deal directly with the devious defenses produced by growing up in such households. Their techniques are better derived from behavior approaches and relatively specific and clear techniques at that. They must know "what to do" to help the adolescent.

A useful exposition of learning theory is contained in Patterson's *Families* (1971). Patterson describes techniques for teaching appropriate behavior to children age two to five and for remedying behavior problems, including aggressive behavior and stealing in older children and adolescents, in a very practical and concrete form. His techniques are supported by research findings, and he offers a clear rationale for beginning with baseline observation and contracting, providing concrete examples of successful and unsuccessful patterns of applying these approaches. Although written with families in mind, the basic techniques provide a theoretical construct for hospital milieu programs.

It is common knowledge that Skinner, Bandura, and their followers have trained animals to do almost anything with rewards for good behavior—positive reinforcement. Patterson notes that in family life there are too many concrete and subtle rewards for bad behavior, especially in view of the fact that sustained attention, intense affect, and lengthy verbalization from parents all serve as positive reinforcers to many children.

The patterns of teaching or at least enabling undesirable behavior vary with the nature of the specific behavior. For example, Patterson distinguishes between parents of ten- to thirteen-year-old children with tantrums and parents of children who steal. The parents of poorly socialized, unpredictable, vaguely angry, impulsive provocative children (the temper-tantrum type) frequently are warm, caring adults with vague, amorphous, "impulsive" (Marohn 1980; Offer and Marohn 1979), "type B" (Singer 1974) responses to a child whom they seem to know fairly well. It is themselves whom they do not know well. They have not decided what they expect of their child and what they will do if the child transgresses. This ambivalent parent needs a systematic, quantifiable technique, a finely honed craft. When the parent says no and the child goes ahead anyway, there needs to be a predictable consequence.

On the other hand, Patterson finds the parents of children who steal (the predatory type) to be cool, distant, inconsistently attentive to the child; they impulsively set harsh, brief penalties (i.e., hitting) but mostly do not see, ignore, and thereby teach that covert misbehavior can succeed undetected (Offer and Marohn 1979; Singer 1974; Szurek 1942). In therapy, these parents are taught to monitor their child continuously to

480

be more mindful of what the child is doing. They are instructed to be more involved, never to let up supervision, to be "always on their case," to be motivated by the full knowledge that the penalty for relaxed vigilance is recidivism.

In the hospital, the temper-tantrum delinquent will have the benefit that expected behavior and penalties for misbehavior will be clearly described. With the predatory patient the program stresses inevitability and consistency. The omnipotent teen will be free to do as he wishes only when he has met fully all the requirements for the privileges he seeks. With both, the clear, concrete, consistent daily routine will make reality immediate and inescapable.

The usefulness of Patterson's ideas for constructing corrective milieu responses for behaviorally disturbed adolescents is that the "why" of the parent-child relationship is never explored. His thesis is simply that certain (ineffective) teaching methods used by parents yield certain defects in children's behavior. He carefully describes corrective and effective teaching methods, systematic, quantifiable techniques that can be taught to child care personnel and applied prescriptively according to the specific defect in socialization that the adolescent reveals.

There are still advantages, however, to the process of trying to understand why and how these interventions succeed within the theoretical framework of dynamic psychiatry. This exercise is particularly important since behavioral management alone cannot eliminate or extensively modify "malignant" defenses. A properly designed and managed milieu can block the effectiveness of the patients' efforts to delude themselves regarding their relationship to the real world, thus freeing both their internal anger and their internal sense of vulnerability so that they can gain a dawning appreciation of the existence and internal origin of these problems. Without concurrent psychotherapy, however, this fledgling insight will quickly disappear beneath the youngsters' chaotic involvement with the environment. The acute hospital treatment—the shock and support of being controlled without being attacked—provides a foothold for the therapist of the adolescent as well as a chance to teach the adolescent's parents to improve their support of reality.[2]

Milieu Therapy: Analysis of Malignant Defenses

It is possible to help delinquent adolescents to begin to develop satisfying object relationships and good reality testing principally by analyzing those defenses against aggressive drives that render the object unstable (Foreman and Marmar 1985). The malignant defenses (denial, projection, projective identification, and splitting) are the chief primitive defenses to be analyzed (or at least "seriously challenged and shaken") during hospital treatment. The most important manifestations of the malignant defenses in the inpatient setting are the following.

1. *Denial* of the importance of the object and the self. "I don't care" ("I'm not involved with you and you're not involved with me") needs to be questioned and interpreted as a distortion—"I don't have to believe that you don't care."

2. *Projection* of internal anger, as well as other ego alien affects and traits, onto the object. "Everybody's unfair, is angry, doesn't like me" needs to be countered by identifying the locus of the anger—"It's OK to be angry as long as you control yourself and get along with others." When the teen is comfortable with his anger during negotiations and perceives that others like him and that he likes others despite the stress of anger and differences, he can give up the distortion of constantly off-loading (projecting) his anger onto others.

3. *Projective identification*, an ability to assume roles that elicit distorted responses from staff. Projective identification precipitates hostile and destructive feelings and fantasies within staff and therapist, who need to process, get comfortable with, and distill out aggressive and assertive feelings to be used in limit setting, so that the teen can reinternalize these aggressive feelings in a manageable form (Ogden 1979).

4. Continual *splitting* whenever frustrated. Splitting is the reflex perception of the self and the other as bad and hateable whenever there is anger; the tendency either to reject the other or to adopt a helpless, "I'm no good" role, ending all energetic negotiations about limits or goals; the stubborn, depressed "I give up" or "I hate you" that keeps the teen intermittently out of therapy each time he perceives anger in the self or in another, with the result that he changes his judgment about whether the other and the self are good and whether the two of them have a relationship at all. Obviously, this splitting defeats the development of an alliance and needs to be gradually replaced by fusion (a balanced blending of good and bad perceptions of the self and others) in therapy. This process must proceed to some success if the teen is ever to set up continuous, predictable relationships with adults and peers.

Once object relationships have become more constant, then the identification process can begin functioning continuously in the therapy sessions and in milieu involvement with supportive adults and integrating peers. This allows development of values, standards, and a personal conscience in tune with constructive peers and the adult world. In training schools or detention centers where malignant defenses are not analyzed and identification and internalization of rules do not take place, patterns and rituals of one or two years of training tend to stay on the surface, are not internalized, and are sloughed off on discharge. Nothing basic has changed, and, not surprisingly, a recidivism rate of 60 percent prevails (Tramontana 1980).

Even with the best inpatient therapy, the transition to essential long-term outpatient treatment is fraught with hazards. These youngsters almost always regress in response to the trauma of discharge, especially if it involves transfer to another therapist. Discharge planning stirs fears of abandonment and reawakens these youngsters' expectations that dependency is dangerous and unrewarding. This often mobilizes acting-out defenses and jeopardizes the fragile identification with inpatient staff. In addition to these symbolically induced problems with leaving the hospital, there are real deprivations involved in the transfer to outpatient care. Instead of constant support and structure, therapy becomes a matter of only two to four hours a week, and much more is required of the youngster. Realistically, the family must be prepared to provide much of the support and structure the inpatient staff has been giving if the transition to outpatient treatment is to succeed.

Conclusions

Hospital treatment of the behavior-disordered teen starts with a milieu that sets predictable limits and consequences and interprets the reality-distorting defenses of the teen who has never set himself the task of accepting and negotiating with "No!" Concurrent psychotherapy utilizes atypical alliances with the therapist to analyze and modify the malignant defenses that defeat the youngster's ability to attach, identify, and grow.

NOTES

1. Shamsie relied on a book by Dennis Romig (1978), in which articles documenting psychotherapy are inaccurately categorized as educational-vocational approaches. One need only read the articles by Persons (1965, 1966, 1967) and by Shore and Massimo (1966, 1969, 1973)

to decide whether traditional ego supportive object relationship therapy was the treatment modality. Romig and Shamsie concluded that therapy did not work but that educational-vocational approaches might.

2. For purposes of simple focus on the inpatient process, we omit entirely any reference to the weekly family therapy that must accompany hospital treatment of the teen.

REFERENCES

Benedek, E., and Shetky, D. 1980. *Child Psychiatry and the Law.* New York: Brunner/Mazel.

Borzormenyi-Nagy, I., and Spark, G. 1973. *Invisible Loyalties.* New York: Harper & Row.

Cahill, A. J. 1981. Aggression revisited: the value of anger in therapy and other close relationships. *Adolescent Psychiatry* 9:539–549.

Chess, S., and Thomas, A. 1966. *Temperament and Behavior Disorders in Children.* New York: Brunner/Mazel.

Chess, S., and Thomas, A. 1977. *Temperament and Development.* New York: New York University Press.

Eissler, K. R., ed. 1959. *Search Lights on Delinquency.* New York: International Universities Press.

Foreman, S. A., and Marmar, C. R. 1985. Therapist actions that address initially poor therapeutic alliances in psychotherapy. *American Journal of Psychiatry* 142(8): 922–926.

Goldston, R. 1971. Violence begins at home: the Parents' Center project for the study and prevention of child abuse. *Journal of the American Academy of Child Psychiatry* 10:336–350.

Gossett, J. T. 1983. *To Find a Way.* New York: Brunner/Mazel.

Isaacs, S. 1972. Emotional problems in childhood and adolescence: neglect, cruelty, battering. *British Medical Journal* 2:756–757.

Jaffe, P.; Wolfe, D.; Wilson, S.; and Zak, L. 1986. Similarities in behavioral and social maladjustment among child victims and witnesses to family violence. *American Journal of Orthopsychiatry* 56:142–146.

Johnson, A. M., and Szurek, S. A. 1952. The genesis of antisocial acting out in children and adults. *Psychoanalytic Quarterly* 21:323–332.

Jones, M. 1953. *The Therapeutic Community.* New York: Basic.

Lantz, J., and Thorwald, S. R. 1985. Inpatient family therapy approaches. *Psychiatric Hospital* 16:85–89.

Lewis, D. O. 1979. Violent juvenile delinquents: psychiatric, neurological, psychological and obese factors. *Journal of the American Academy of Child Psychiatry* 18:307–319.

Lewis, D. O. 1983. Homicidally aggressive young children: neuropsychiatric and experimental correlates. *American Journal of Psychiatry* 140(2): 148–153.

McManus, M. 1984. Psychiatric disturbance in serious delinquents. *Journal of the American Academy of Child Psychiatry* 23(5): 602–615.

Main, T. F. 1946. The hospital as a therapeutic institution. *Bulletin of the Menninger Clinic* 10:66–70.

Marohn, R. 1980. *Juvenile Delinquency: Psychodynamic Assessment and Hospital Treatment.* New York: Brunner/Mazel.

Masterson, J. 1972. *Treatment of the Borderline Adolescent: A Developmental Approach.* New York: Wiley.

Masterson, J. 1980. *From Borderline Adolescent to Functioning Adult: The Test of Time.* New York: Brunner/Mazel.

Meeks, J. E. 1979. Behavioral and antisocial disorders. In J. D. Noshpitz, ed. *Handbook of Child Psychiatry.* New York: Basic.

Meeks, J. E. 1986. *The Fragile Alliance.* 3d ed. Melbourne, Fla.: Krieger.

Minuchin, S.; Montalvo, B.; Gueryney, B. G.; Rosmon, B. L.; and Schumer, R. 1967. *Families of the Slums.* New York: Basic.

Offer, D., and Marohn, R. 1979. *The Psychological World of the Juvenile Delinquent.* New York: Basic.

Ogden, T. H. 1979. On projective identification. *International Journal of Psycho-Analysis* 60:357–373.

Patterson, G. R. 1971. *Families: Applications of Social Learning to Family Life.* Champaign, Ill.: Research Press.

Patterson, G. R., and Cogg, J. A. 1971. A dyadic analysis of "aggressive" behaviors: an additional step toward a theory of aggression. In J. P. Hill, ed. *Minnesota Symposia on Child Psychology,* vol. 5. Minneapolis: University of Minnesota Press.

Persons, R. W. 1965. Degree of affect expression in psychotherapy and degree of psychopathy. *Psychological Reports* 16:1157–1162.

Persons, R. W. 1966. Psychological and behavioral change in delinquents following psychotherapy. *Journal of Clinical Psychology* 22:337–340.

Persons, R. W. 1967. Relationship between psychotherapy with institutionalized delinquent boys and subsequent community adjustment. *Journal of Consulting Psychology* 31:137–141.

Romig, D. A. 1978. *Justice for Our Children*. Lexington, Mass.: Heath.

Rutter, M., and Giller, H. 1983. *Juvenile Delinquency: Trends and Perspectives*. Harmondsworth: Penguin.

Shamsie, S. J. 1981. Anti-social adolescents: our treatments do not work—where do we go from here? *Canadian Journal of Psychiatry* 26:357–364.

Shore, M., and Massimo, J. 1966. Comprehensive emotionally oriented psychotherapy for adolescent delinquent boys: a follow-up study. *American Journal of Orthopsychiatry* 36:609–615.

Shore, M., and Massimo, J. 1969. Five years later: a follow-up study of comprehensive vocationally oriented psychotherapy. *American Journal of Orthopsychiatry* 39:769–773.

Shore, M., and Massimo, J. 1973. After ten years: a follow-up study of comprehensive vocationally oriented psychotherapy. *American Journal of Orthopsychiatry* 43:128–132.

Singer, M. 1974. Family structure, disciplinary configurations, and adolescent psychopathology. *Adolescent Psychiatry* 3:372–386.

Stanton, A. E., and Schwartz, M. S. 1954. *Mental Hospital: A Study of Institutional Participation in Psychiatric Illness and Treatment*. New York: Basic.

Stierlin, H. 1977. *Psychoanalysis and Family Therapy*. New York: Aronson.

Szurek, S. A. 1942. Notes on the genesis of psychopathic personality trends. *Psychiatry* 5:1–6.

Tramontana, M. G. 1980. Critical review of research on psychotherapy outcome with adolescents: 1967–1977. *Psychological Bulletin* 88(2): 429–450.

Werner, E. E. 1982. *Vulnerable but Invincible*. New York: McGraw-Hill.

INTENSIVE PSYCHODYNAMICALLY ORIENTED TREATMENT OF TWO CASES OF ADOLESCENT PSYCHOSIS

HENRY N. MASSIE

In recent years, it has been my experience that trainees, and perhaps therapists in general, are increasingly skeptical about the usefulness—let alone the potential for cure—of intensive long-term psychoanalytically oriented psychotherapy of psychosis in adolescents and young adults. Probably, the main reason for this skepticism is that relatively few trainees now have the opportunity to treat such severely disturbed patients in an extended in-depth manner because third party insurers and community mental health programs have curtailed support for such treatment. Thus, a new generation of therapists is coming to believe that the treatment must be medically excessive or unwarranted when a fiscal reviewer denies permission to treat on the ground that the therapy exceeds the "customary standard of treatment." The trainee may not realize that the insurer has created the limitation to save money and has at the same time cleverly reified the economic customary standard into a medical standard.

To redress some of the ignorance or cynicism about the efficacy of treatment, I have prepared two cases from my own experience that illustrate certain principles and benefits of intensive psychotherapy with psychotic youths—in which I continue the techniques pioneered by Fromm-Reichmann (1950) and Searles (1965), among others. Reported are a girl and a boy who came into treatment in gravely disorganized conditions when they were fourteen and twenty-four years old, respectively, and have been in treatment for ten and two years.

Their treatment descriptions demonstrate two longitudinal courses of psychoses that were etiologically connected with disturbances of body image and sexual identity beginning in childhood; loss of close attachment in early life, which was repeated during the teen years; and the effect of both extensive treatment and adolescent developmental milestones on the illness.

Case Examples

CASE 1: NANCY

In the fall of her fourteenth year, Nancy's behavior changed over a period of several weeks with the onset of increasingly severe, anxious obsessional preoccupations over decisions. Up until this time, Nancy had been an outstandingly successful child. Her grades were always at or near straight A's, and she had the reputation of being her rural community's best girl athlete. She competed on boys' teams since they were the only ones available at her level. Her demeanor with peers and students alike appeared thoughtful and self-assured. She was well liked and had gone about the business of early adolescence without fuss or complaint. She had also had her first menstrual period during the summer, to which she responded matter-of-factly, without show of feeling. Her menses achieved a regular cycle twelve months later. Her idyllic childhood ended during the summer some two months before her psychiatric symptoms began when her pediatrician detected a deteriorating congenital malformation of the hip and fitted Nancy with a leg brace to be worn extensively day and night. He told her that a regimen of brace and exercises for the next three years had a good likelihood for arresting the deterioration so that a fully active life without surgery was likely.

In the fall of the year, Nancy received two more blows. Her brother—two years her senior and her lifelong close buddy—obtained his driver's license. With this key to independence, he also hitched up with his first steady girlfriend and from then on was rarely home. Thus, in effect, he abandoned his sister, who had doted on him. Finally, there was a remote possibility that her stepfather's work would require the family to relocate to a different part of the country. The stepfather had been the child's father since the age of six years; her real father had left the family when she was two years old, although she continued to have weekly contact with him. Nancy had reacted far more intensely than anyone else in the family to the potential move by adamantly saying that she would never go. Likewise, when Nancy developed a minor flu, she overreacted with a fear that she might not recover. At school, she became increasingly paralyzed in her work so that she was unable to complete assignments but rather perseveratively and clingingly asked her teachers and parents about details of assignments and vague questions about the meaning of the behavior of different adults in her life (e.g., "Why was Miss X absent today?" "Why did mother pick this movie to go to?"). The latter question also reflected Nancy's ideas of reference that movies, for example, were delivering special messages to her. Along with failing grades, the girl's dress became disheveled, and she frequently was lost in her own thoughts and unresponsive at school. When I first saw Nancy after a few weeks of these symptoms, she was unmedicated, haphazardly dressed, but attractive. She was not fully in contact but sat with her eyes closed or avoiding eye contact with me. She was quiet with some catatonic posturing. Her thoughts were fragmented with severe blocking, looseness, and ideas of reference that the room had been decorated to receive her and give her a message. Her mood alternated between a detached muteness and moments of anxious clinging, during which she was lucid, fully oriented, and desperate to be helped and not abandoned.

HOSPITAL COURSE

I hospitalized Nancy immediately and over the next three weeks increased haloperidol medication to a level of sixteen milligrams per day. I saw her for five forty-five-minute psychodynamically oriented verbal sessions weekly. In addition, she participated in the ward's therapeutic milieu program, which included school, sports, housekeeping and cooking, and group therapy. Only the parents were allowed two brief visits weekly for the first several weeks, and, after the second week in the hospital, weekly family therapy meetings began with the unit social worker as therapist. Nancy's improvement was slow but steady from the beginning. After a series of successful off-ward and home visits with her family, she was discharged to day treatment after three months. At this time, I decreased individual sessions to three times a week and reduced haloperidol to ten milligrams daily.

In spite of recommendations to the contrary, Nancy shared her family's sense of urgency that she return to her junior high school class immediately, so as not to be stigmatized as abnormal. She attempted this on a part-time basis the week after discharge. As anticipated, her reconstitution was too fragile and her anxiety over performing well and being accepted by her peers too high, and she once more became obsessionally perseverative and blocking in her thinking and had to withdraw from school again. This time, she finished out the school year in the day treatment program with the quality of her work somewhat eroded from its past level. Next fall, once again, I and the others working with the child and family urged a cautious part-time reentry into school and part-time withdrawing from day treatment. But Nancy very much wanted to be with her brother for one year of high school before he graduated. This urgency derived from her desire to share in the companionship of her brother's social life, and her family hesitated to oppose this. Nancy made a surprisingly smooth return to the mainstream. True to her word, she became part of her popular brother's social group so that his friends, including his girlfriend, became her friends. After the third month of school, she no longer took medication. Individual psychotherapy sessions were slowly cut back to once weekly by the time her freshman year in high school was over. By the end of the school year, her academic performance had returned to an A level, and she was again distinguished in sports, though this time on girls' school teams.

To bring us to the present, after that school year Nancy spent a successful two weeks at a tennis camp (her first sleep-away camp). She saw her brother off to college in another state and successfully began her sophomore year in high school. There are two significant and intriguing footnotes to this most recent phase of treatment. They both deal with issues of physical integrity, which are so central to this teen's psychopathology. In midsummer, Nancy sprained an ankle playing tennis, which threatened her sports participation for a time. At the same time, an aged great-grandfather died, and this close-knit family (including Nancy) was at his bedside for the last few hours of his life. During this difficult week marked by death and her minor injury, Nancy again experienced slight blocking of thoughts, a labile mood that included an impulse to laugh at the funeral service, an obsessional attention to detail, and unusual anger at her mother's slight failures. Further, as part of this complex of events and feelings, Nancy worried that her sprained ankle was a harbinger of more serious disability. On the other side of the coin, Nancy's physical fears were counterbalanced by the fact she had overcome the threat of hip disease. She had gambled and had refused to wear her brace when she had returned to school after hospitalization, and follow-up visits to the orthopedist confirmed that the hip deformity was not progressing.

The second footnote to the treatment is that, with her brother gone, Nancy feared loss of his social support and struggled with loneliness. By now, she had physically matured and was tall and attractive, but she did not take special interest in her clothes and wore no makeup. When a high school football star began to ask Nancy on dates, she discussed with me her wish for companionship but was ambivalent about this particular boy's rough manners. Intriguingly, she was hesitant not to go out with him because she feared he might punch her (a fear that was not based on a real threat, a history of violence on this boy's part, or a history of any childhood experiences with physical violence). So, again, we hear from Nancy that there is a recurring conscious profound anxiety over the fear of being physically damaged. First there was the hip disorder and viral illness at the time of her breakdown, then the sprained ankle at the time of the great-grandfather's death one year later, and now the fear of being punched by the football star. Moreover, all this was occurring during the period when Nancy's body was rapidly changing in height and genital maturation under the effect of the intense adolescent hormonal shift.

PSYCHODYNAMIC FORMULATION AND THERAPEUTIC PROCESS

Beneath the surface paint on the canvas of this teenager's life, what unconscious conflicts, fantasies, and psychological structures are there? The answers to these questions emerged during therapy through a two-way process in which the way the treatment was conducted facilitated the emergence of the hidden elements of Nancy's personality. This, in turn, further made it possible to pursue the verbal therapy increasingly effectively and with further production of new information.

From the beginning, my stance was neutral in the psychoanalytic sense with the readiness to address transference as well as to inquire about the patient's present and past life. Very occasionally, I broke neutrality, offering supportive suggestions and answering her questions about my life. This was all directed toward the initial goal of reducing the profound anxiety the patient was suffering. Her terror was manifest in her vigilance, catatonia, desperate clinging and verbalized fear of abandonment, and rambling attempts to understand what was happening to her. It was uncertain at the time how much the terror triggered her psychotic episode, but it was clear that it was maintaining her in a continuing state of disorganization. To reduce the anxiety, I told Nancy that she could depend on me, and we would work together as long and as frequently as necessary to help her relax and understand what was happening so that she could return home and go to school. Thus, I was only setting a stage here in the first few days since I did not have any specific knowledge with which to say anything more precise. But I felt it would be enough to listen, ask clarifying questions, and become a person in this child's life. The real relationship, cemented to a certain extent by Nancy's dependence on me as her physician, would be an anchor in reality to prevent further regression. Resolving the dependency, if the teenager's normal push for autonomy did not accomplish it, could be dealt with later in treatment. Otto Will (1985) describes this from the vantage point of one of his patient's reminiscing many years after the termination of a lengthy treatment for severe psychosis, "I don't know what Dr. Will did, but he was there."

With the stage set, Nancy raised the curtain and began to tell me about herself, albeit mostly in primary process with loose, tangential, and half-finished thoughts. Further, she began a rambling diary with pictures of her family and classmates to help me better understand her. Thus, I repeatedly learned about her concerns that her stepfather's business was not doing as well as hoped and that her mother was the strongest one and so pretty that Nancy could never hope to be her equal. Conversely, at other times, I learned that her mother was weak because she talked to the grandmother daily and that her real father never talked about feelings or shared anything with her. All these observations were corroborated by the family therapists. They gradually helped the stepfather clarify that there was no danger of poverty, helped the mother emotionally separate from the grandmother with less guilt, and helped Nancy urge her real father to be less aloof and ominous.

But none of these issues adequately account for the patient's collapse. They may have been necessary factors but not sufficient explanations. Insight into the underlying causes comes from the two venues of Nancy's unconscious and her overt behavior. Several times, Nancy confused her gender and referred to herself as a boy while talking about things she and her brother and friends did. Nancy did not catch these slips of the tongue, nor did I draw her attention to them, preferring instead to support the healing process of repression of her most disorganizing conflicts. Behaviorally, most striking was Nancy's refusal to wear her leg brace. Her hundred excuses for not wearing the brace (it did not fit, it looked bad, it hurt, she could not play sports with it) obscured for a time the terror it posed for her. Furthermore, during these early weeks, it was not possible for Nancy to talk coherently about her questions concerning the brace or her conscious attitudes about girls and boys. Gradually, however, the strategy of making the patient feel secure paid off, and Nancy was increasingly lucid and in contact and began gathering her courage to leave the hospital, which also carried with it an element of counterphobic denial. It is also likely that the major tranquilizer that Nancy was receiving further diminished the fearsome aspect of her preoccupations and allowed her to organize her thoughts. By this time, at about one month of treatment, I had enough information to formulate the major psychodynamic and etiologic factors in the girl's illness. I felt that Nancy's separation from her father, in her third year of life when her parents divorced, had been especially traumatic for her and had left a fixation point in her development that subsequently would make her vulnerable to intense separation anxiety at times of loss.

At the time of the divorce, Nancy's young mother had herself gone through a period of depression and agitation. Nancy's first attempt at going to nursery school at three years was unsuccessful because she could not leave her mother. A year later it was successful, but then in kindergarten Nancy again regressed when she lost the support of her brother when he was absent from school for a few days. At that time, Nancy also insisted on remaining home.

In fact, the older brother emerged as perhaps the key figure in the girl's history. She apparently had turned to him as the male in her life when her father left. Nancy became the veritable kid sister, always tagging along and making her brother's social life and friends her own. This pattern was likely well established by the time her mother remarried when the patient was six. The regressive, symbiotic, and pseudomature elements of Nancy's attachment to her brother were obscured by her athletic and intellectual talent, which enabled her in many ways to perform as a peer of her brother's group. This attachment to her brother and the absence of her father during the early oedipal phase, I postulated, had also led to faulty development in the areas of gender identity, gender role, and object choice (Tyson 1982). There was some sexual identification with her brother, as revealed in Nancy's referring to herself as "he"; and her comments that her mother was so much prettier than she revealed Nancy's despair at ever being able to compete with her mother on a feminine level. Further, although her ultimate choice of love object seems likely to be heterosexual, as indicated by long evening talks she has with male classmates, the component of bisexuality seems unusually strong in this teenager who now obtains some of her greatest enjoyment from participation in women's athletics.

Thus, Nancy's psychotic episode under the three-pronged assault of loss of her brother to his first girlfriend, the onset of hip illness and the ignominious leg brace that went with it, and the onset of menstruation was more comprehensible. The brace and menses made her feel that she could no longer enjoy her distinctiveness in sports. Also, they further confused her sexual identity, at a time when it should be consolidating, in the sense that she was not "man enough for sports." Nor was she attractive enough, she felt, to compete as a woman for the attention of boys, especially since her brother had thrown her over for another girl.

This formulation now guided the psychotherapy from the time the patient left the hospital at three months in the sense that it helped me to be sensitive to the underlying affective issues of separation and loss and narcissistic issues of gender and attractiveness that were obscured by Nancy's obsessional tendency to isolate herself from affect. For example, there would be long sessions in which the patient complained of nothing to talk about or boredom, of her real father's reticence during their occasional visits, and of loneliness. She talked without emotion about her brother's social life, and she conspicuously avoided talking about her orthopedic problem. Therefore, I slowly chipped away at her defenses of denial, isolation, and intellectualization by calling her attention to what she did not express. For example, I inquired why she had so little feeling about things that were seemingly important and asked for more thoughts in detail about things that she brought up in almost telegraphic fashion and then dropped ("I'm going to summer camp") as if there was nothing more to say or feel about them.

From this approach, Nancy and I slowly were rewarded by insight, memories, dreams; a softening of her defenses and more emotional expression; and a fuller sense of who she was. For example, Nancy's long-held childhood fantasy became conscious—that she needed to be good at sports like a boy to be accepted by her brother. This explained the panic she felt over the brace and occasional minor physical injuries, for they meant she would lose the ability to keep up with her brother. Further, she became conscious of years of repressed anxiety that, whenever there was trouble in the family business, it meant she might lose her stepfather as she had lost her real father.

CONCLUDING REMARKS AND SOME UNANSWERED QUESTIONS

In this manner treatment progressed toward a conclusion in which the patient had in a sense reclaimed her childhood history through experiencing emotions that she had denied because they were too frustrating. In the process, she also softened considerably as she allowed herself to feel more. In the final stages of treatment, she had occasional dreams of being threatened by an out-of-control car (while she was taking her driver's education course), and she understood these dreams as indicating her own wish to keep things under control. She related this to her fear of people trying to dominate her, which she had felt initially in the therapy with me as well. Ultimately, we understood this as connected with her equally troubling impulse to submit to people— thus losing her will and becoming physically vulnerable—out of the hunger for human closeness that apparently began when her real father left home. Finally, it was also related to her recollections of the terror of losing control of her feelings during her psychosis.

There remains the nagging thought that there may be deeper roots to her recurring anxiety about minor injuries. They precipitate fears of physical disintegration for which the fantasy of not being able to keep up with her brother may not be a sufficient explanation. It is possible that the mysterious quality to this panic derives from its origin in developmental interferences with body image consolidation that Nancy experienced during the preverbal period of her life (Greenacre 1958; Roiphe and Galenson 1981; Stoddard 1982). This ties in with data we have of the patient's confusion of her gender identity. Thus, we would postulate that her mother's own anxiety at a failing marriage interfered with an adequate mother-infant symbiosis prior to the psychic separation process (Mahler, Pine, and Bergman 1978), thus derailing preoedipal identity formation. Also, the father's leave-taking prevented a normal oedipal feminine turn to the father that usually facilitates consolidation of genital body schema with accompanying genital sensations. Therefore, when she suffers a risk of physical illness or injury,

495

this patient's fragile sense of body integrity is deeply threatened. Nancy is aware of fear only when she is physically ill, but she more likely actually experiences the threat to her body as an unconscious anxiety that she will be, or has been, castrated since her sense of herself as a woman is so relatively unformed.

CASE 2: JAMES

James's case illustrates the treatment of a youth whose illness was far more chronic than Nancy's. He suffered from paranoid schizophrenia that became evident in his freshman year of college, when he was first hospitalized, although he had been troubled from early childhood. After his first breakdown, he required ten years of treatment before he was sufficiently recovered in terms of having more mature defenses to manage his impulses and adequate insight into his fears so that he could stop regular treatment.

From the beginning life was never very good to James. His mother was an angry, nongiving woman who also had problems with alcohol. Further, when James's sister was born when he was two, his mother apparently dropped him entirely and turned to care for the girl. This was the boy's first loss. Whether it occurred because the mother could not split her attention between two children and had little capacity for nurturance or because there was an additional underlying hostility in the mother toward the male child has never been fully clarified. Nonetheless, with the advent of his sister, James felt increasingly lonely, rejected, helpless to redress this, angry without knowing what to do about the anger, and not even sure that he was angry or what his feelings were throughout childhood. A special unpleasantness was the envy he felt for the attention and favoritism his sister received from his mother. Once, when he was seven, his already compromised sense of male assertiveness was further shamed when, at night, his father away on a trip, his mother left for a brief trip to the store. After she did not return for some time, James became anxious about her safety and walked to the police station. They found the mother at a bar. Instead of being praised for his initiative and concern, a bewildered James was attacked by his mother later when they were alone.

Sadly, James's father was little able to counterbalance the mother's coldness to her son since he was compulsively and ambitiously involved in his highly successful business and often absent from home or preoc-

496

cupied with his work. When the marriage foundered when James was eleven, he went to live with his father.

Looking back on his son's early years, the father recalled that his son seemed paranoid in the sense of never allowing his sister to have one bit more of anything than he had received, whether it was a few cents or a few sips of soda. Further, in latency and early childhood, James began stealing from his parents. By this time he was also suffering from chronic enuresis that persisted until his mid-twenties. In addition, he was awkwardly gregarious with peers in an attempt to hold on to a rare friend. In spite of his good intentions, James's father was not able to make a home for his son, and, in high school, James was sent to boarding school, which he experienced as a further loss and separation from his father. This too failed because of James's petty rule breaking, and he returned to a community high school. By this time, he had begun his habit of episodic drinking when he felt threatened under pressure to conform to what he perceived was the standard for masculine behavior. One day near the end of high school, perhaps under the influence of alcohol and feeling desperate, angry, and unsupported in his attempt to meet family standards of achievement, he had his first break with reality. In a dissociated state, he attempted to assault his best friend's mother sexually. James now recalls how, in that episode, he was taking out both his longing for his mother and his rage at her on his victim.

In the next year, his freshman year in college, he became increasingly disorganized. He began to socialize with his fraternity group and date compulsively in an effort to feel he was "one of the guys." This disorganization only escalated when he was socially rebuffed. He was hospitalized—disheveled, confused, with blocking of thoughts, loose associations, a flat affect, and paranoid ideation and ideas of reference. After this followed seven years of attempts at completing college that were interrupted by profound decompensations and long hospitalizations that ranged from three to eighteen months.

James became my patient during one of these episodes at the age of twenty-four years. The precipitant was typical. He was under pressure to complete a college semester and was living alone. However, he could not talk about anxiety about his studies or about loneliness but only about how he felt everybody intentionally rejected him and slighted him. As the pressure (both inner pressure and pressure from his teachers) built, he became increasingly isolated from affect and flat. He

497

acknowledged both murderous thoughts against peers and professors and suicidal thoughts. He became increasingly unable to care for himself, stopped going to school, wandered, and compulsively telephoned acquaintances until ultimately he was admitted to the hospital. When I met him in the hospital, he was catatonic, incontinent of feces and urine, would not eat for fear the food was poisoned, and refused to bathe because he feared he would be gassed in the shower.

COURSE OF TREATMENT

Four months passed in the hospital—which ultimately proved to be his last hospitalization—without progress. As with Nancy, my initial therapeutic approach was threefold: to understand the nature of the patient's panic, which was driving him from sanity; to forge a dyadic relationship with the patient to draw him back to reality through my frequent daily presence in his life; and to create an ambience of safety and patience so that the patient's own wish for mastery and affiliation with peers might gain some ascendency over his terror-stricken withdrawal from everyday life. However, in James's case, nothing was happening as the weeks passed. During some sessions, he would cringe in his room, mute and partially dressed. In other sessions, he would posture angrily, telling everyone to leave him alone. In still other moods, he would talk compliantly about unrealistic and grandiose discharge plans. However, there was no consistency from session to session or from week to week, and it did no good to interpret one mood as an undoing of a prior mood. Further, a variety of major tranquilizers and antidepressants, including an equivalent of 3,000 milligrams of chlorpromazine daily, was futile.

The breakthrough in James's treatment occurred early in the fifth month of hospitalization in the form of a dream of my own rather than one of the patient's. I dreamed that James was calling to me over and over again and reaching toward me with out-stretched arms but that, at the same time, he was sinking further and further away as if into oblivion. It was a nightmarish dream for me, and, after I thought about it, I understood that James's cry was the desperate cry of a little child for his mother in the middle of the night. He needed his therapist to understand that his psychotic panic was that he felt abandoned and helpless. It is strange because I had already understood this to some extent in an intellectual fashion, but I had never truly appreciated it

498

until James's nightmare became my own. From that day on, what changed with James was not what we talked about for several weeks but that I was more relaxed and more tender than I had been, not in a calculating fashion but just because I felt that way. I had a sense of conviction that I understood James for the first time. In sessions, he steadily improved, and, toward the end of his sixth month, he was in good contact, had improved self-care, and was no longer hallucinating or delusional. His illness was still manifested in some affective flatness, perseverative preoccupations with meeting girls, and not fully realistic plans for out-of-hospital living arrangements. His improvement also must have gathered steam with the threat of not being able to stay at the hospital beyond six months because of the end of his insurance. The hospital to which he was to be transferred had informed him that he would have to consent to electric shock treatment and that I could visit him but would not manage his case. These threats, of course, dovetailed with his fears of punishment and abandonment.

Thus, at six months, he was sufficiently recovered to move into a halfway house. Over the next two years, he finished college, and his phenothiazines were gradually discontinued. Psychotherapy gradually tapered to twice weekly. In sessions, I actively interpreted a variety of warded-off affects such as his wish to be cared for and have things done for him, which was often obscured by the more obvious anger he expressed (and occasionally obscured by a short-lived paranoid delusional rage). I also interpreted his lack of confidence, his anger at women, and his intermittent distrust of his therapist.

However, his progress seemed to plateau and stagnate. The next breakthrough in treatment occurred in almost as dramatic a fashion as the earlier one. A male fellow resident in the partial-care apartment had been bringing in male prostitutes for his own use for months. Observing this threatened James by making him doubt his own ever fragile sense of maleness and by bringing home to him the lonely inadequacy of his awkward attempts at dating. Nonetheless, James masochistically did not call the other man's flagrant rule breaking to the administrator's attention. Nor did he confront the other man until one day James could not stand the humiliation any longer and punched the other man in the chin. The program had a firm rule against physical violence, so James was told to make other arrangements and leave. He came to my office that day with his head low, feeling helpless, and apologetic for, as he said, his "loss of impulse control." My response was, "It's about time. I've been waiting for you to do something like that for weeks." Much to his surprise, we spent the rest of the session talking about why it had taken him so long to stand up for himself and put a stop to the insensitive, rule-breaking behavior that had tormented him so much. Preserving relative neutrality, I made no offer to assist James in finding a place to stay. That night he moved into an apartment with an acquaintance and has had no further contact with the mental health system aside from his sessions with me. It is now six years since James was evicted from his cooperative living apartment. He is now fully self-supporting, pursuing a career in data processing, happily married for three years to a secretary, and contemplating buying a house and having children.

DISCUSSION OF JAMES'S CASE

In one major respect, James's illness was similar to Nancy's in that both broke down under the impact of severe sexual identity confusion (Kubie 1974), Nancy in the sense that the loss of her brother to another girl and her leg brace challenged her sense of attractiveness, and James in that he never had a boy's feeling of masculine competence or attractiveness in his mother's eyes. When James physically, though ambivalently, stood up to another man, the psychotherapeutic intervention, which was critical, was to support his action rather than question it. The event became a touchstone to which we could repeatedly refer as time went by. The episode contained his fears of being feminized through victimization by the other man and, conversely, of asserting himself. It also demonstrated his ability to be a man. It stood out in sharp contrast to his childhood experience of trying to aid his mother by going out at night for help only to be subsequently attacked by her.

Given the severity of James's early childhood developmental trauma, it is not surprising that his conflicts have never been fully resolved. For the first five years of my contact with him, the intensity of his rage and confusion about his mother was so great that he could only idealize her or simply say that she was not a part of his life and had nothing to do with his troubles. In recent years, with increasing self-confidence, he has dared to spend time with her on holidays and can jokingly, yet trenchantly, observe that, since her refrigerator is always almost empty, he and his wife have to bring food with them when they visit to be sure to have enough to eat. I now see James once every three weeks, and, though his life is going well, we still have the familiar themes to talk about. These are his feelings that he is sometimes slighted by his supervisors in favor of other workers and that he is envious of the greater wealth other people have. I have to draw him back to the deeper realization that most of what he wants in the way of attention and money he could get for himself if he did not lack confidence in his ability to develop a certain skill or to study. Rather, James may still panic at the idea that there is no trustworthy authority—that is, no parent surrogate—who will assist him.

Conclusions

Nancy's and James's cases convey several important principles regarding treatment and etiology of youth psychosis. First, the condition can be successfully treated so that patients can recover and become productive and independent. Nonetheless, even under the best of circumstances, when the patient has access to the full range of psychotherapeutic modalities, including intensive long-term treatment, not all patients do as well as these two. In my own experience, if optimum treatment does not resolve the psychosis, it is because the patient's own inner will to master his illness and rejoin his normal peers has been broken. There is a despair and resignation that has set in that makes the person accept that he is a victim of his illness. Thus, he may accept the help of his therapist, but uses it only for a limited good.

This resignation seems to stamp patients if they have been traumatized over and over in their childhood by losses, disappointments, hatred, lack of understanding, and experiences of helplessness so that they have no capacity for confidence or optimism when their breakdown occurs in adolescence. James came close to being one of these irretrievable patients.

As an extension of this, some vulnerable traumatized children develop their psychosis during childhood even though it may not be clinically apparent until failures of maturational steps of adolescence reveal it. If treatment has not occurred prior to adolescence in these children, it is likely that development of basic emotional competencies in the range of effective defenses, socialization, and perception of reality has been so interfered with that there is little hope (in the patient and therapist alike) that a cure of psychosis is possible.

In addition to showing the usefulness of intensive treatment, James and Nancy also epitomize how adolescent sexual development is centrally involved in teen psychotic breakdown. Laufer and Laufer (1984)

501

have drawn our attention to this in a way that is congruent with the two cases reported here. Genital maturation carries with it both the biologic pressure of sexual impulses and the psychological pressure to choose a male or female sexual role and sexual object in keeping with the biologic pressure. For specific developmental reasons described in their histories, neither Nancy nor James was emotionally able either to comply with the heterosexual biologic mandate or adequately to renounce the biologic mandate, as occurs in stable homosexual adaptations.

James frenetically, through action, attempted to assure himself that he was the man his body was telling him he was. But his self-certainty was so impaired by earlier parental deprivation that he was never able to assure himself of the truth of his masculinity. In panic, he repeatedly lost contact with reality. In contrast to James, who very much wanted to follow the lead of his changing body, Nancy did not want to accept her emerging femininity. It implied too many losses, such as the loss of her closeness with her brother and the loss of her psychosexual role as an athlete. Further, the necessity of wearing a brace at this juncture made it impossible for Nancy to feel that she could move forward in the direction of competing with her mother and girlfriends in terms of feminine attractiveness. It also made it impossible for her to move in the other direction of attainment in sports. She also panicked.

From these two cases, we can cull psychotherapeutic principles to apply to adolescents suffering psychosis. A list of suggestions for the initial phases of treatment includes the following. (1) Make the patient feel safe so as to mitigate the underlying terror. (2) Use major tranquilizers initially to assist in controlling the sense of desperation. (3) Initially isolate the patient from family conflicts while simultaneously working to understand the main family conflicts and dynamics, which may involve allowing family and friends very limited visiting with the patient during early weeks of hospitalization. (4) After a time, when the patient is less anxious, begin family sessions with a focus on facilitating communication in the family in order to distinguish those fears that are based on realistic perceptions about the family and its members from the fears that are based on distortions. (5) Insist on maintaining the patient's socialization (whether on the hospital ward or outside) to promote the patient's outward direction rather than an inward, narcissistically focused self-preoccupation. (6) Convey a sense of optimism to the patient to counter primitive fears. (7) As therapist, forge a relationship with the patient (often through encouraging dependency) by utilizing four to seven psychotherapy sessions per week to draw the patient away from further regression; the patient's normative adolescent push for autonomy can be relied on to undo the dependency later. (8) As therapist, build on whatever vestiges remain of the patient's drive toward mastery, including the wish to grow up and be part of a peer group. (9) As therapist, remain largely neutral. However, this does not preclude offering supportive suggestions or responding to personal questions. Likewise, neutrality allows for systematic elucidation and corrections of transference and projections that reveal the patient's core conflicts. The overall goal of the therapist's stance is to identify and reduce the fears that maintain the psychosis and the need for psychotic defenses. (10) There is no value in maintaining a state of regression, or "access to the unconscious," that occurs during acute psychosis. Therefore, foster repression. Interpretations of impulses should not occur until very much later, when normal defenses are again functional and the ego has regained control. (11) Convey the importance to the teenager and family of a gradual course to recovery in order to prevent a denial of a need for therapy and precipitous attempts to prove normalcy by leaving treatment.

REFERENCES

Fromm-Reichmann, F. 1950. *Principles of Intensive Psychotherapy.* Chicago: University of Chicago Press.

Greenacre, P. 1958. Early physical determinants in the development of the sense of identity. *Journal of the American Psychoanalytic Association* 6:612–627.

Kubie, L. 1974. The drive to become both sexes. *Psychoanalytic Quarterly* 43:349–426.

Laufer, M., and Laufer, M. E. 1984. *Adolescence and Developmental Breakdown.* New Haven, Conn.: Yale University Press.

Mahler, M.; Pine, R.; and Bergman, A. 1975. *The Psychological Birth of the Human Infant.* New York: Basic.

Roiphe, H., and Galenson, E. 1981. *Infantile Origins of Sexual Identity.* New York: International Universities Press.

Searles, H. 1965. *Collected Papers on Schizophrenia and Related Subjects.* New York: International Universities Press.

Stoddard, F. 1982. Body image development in the burned child. *Journal of the American Academy of Child Psychiatry* 21:502–507.

Tyson, P. 1982. A developmental line of gender identity, gender role and choice of love object. *Journal of the American Psychoanalytic Association* 30:61–86.

Will, Otto Allen. 1985. Aspects of psychosis in young adults. Paper presented at the McAuley Neuropsychiatric Institute, St. Mary's Hospital, San Francisco.

ADOLESCENT SUBSTANCE ABUSE: INTRODUCTION

ALLAN Z. SCHWARTZBERG

During the past two decades, illicit drug use has reached epidemic proportions in America. Marijuana, the most widely used illegal drug, came of age in the 1960s as a prime symbol of youth protest against the Vietnam War. Abuse of drugs and alcohol have not only contributed to alternative lifestyles but have also triggered a dramatic rise in abuse of other drugs, including cocaine, PCP, LSD, and amphetamine. While originally drug abuse was a preoccupation of adolescents, it has spread rapidly to all ages, occupations, social classes, and regions. Drug abuse has been so pervasive in our culture that it is virtually impossible to avoid some reference daily to drugs in our newspapers and the media. Drug use abounds in schools, colleges, sports, and industry. One recent survey of 3,600 high school seniors revealed that 20 percent used marijuana for at least one month.

The causes of drug dependency are multiple and include genetic, psychological, and social factors. Research increasingly demonstrates a high incidence of chemical dependency in families. Psychological factors in drug use include not only curiosity and the desire for peer group acceptance but for many an attempt to antidote anxiety, depression, and intrapsychic pain. The teenager who abuses alcohol additionally often comes from a family in which there is inconsistent discipline and a high rate of alcoholism. The peer group tends to be friends who are on the "fringe," who lack academic interest and motivation and are underachievers. Often adolescents prone to drug dependency present with low self-esteem, depression, and antisocial behavior and lack strong bonds to family, school, and church.

While there is some confusion about what actually constitutes alcoholism, the National Council on Alcoholism definition is useful: "Alcoholism is a chronic, progressive, and potentially fatal disease characterized by tolerance and physical dependency, pathological organ changes, or both, all of which are the direct or indirect consequences of the alcohol ingested." This definition applies to drug addicts and to many adolescents.

Adolescents who progress to frequent and daily drug use are often motivated by the need to relieve anxiety and depression, bolster low self-esteem, and relieve feelings of emptiness and intrapsychic pain. Drugs are used to avoid dealing with problems of separation and loss as well as the process of individuation. Chronic drug users often have problems of both ego and sexual identity. Psychoactive drugs, by producing altered states of consciousness, contribute to feelings of euphoria and omnipotence, which temporarily reduce feelings of inadequacy, anger, hurt, and guilt.

A major consequence of the development of drug dependency during adolescence is the profound interference with the developmental process. In heavy users, drug abuse produces a developmental arrest, a freezing of the developmental process fostering a postponement of dealing with adolescent developmental tasks. There is often low frustration tolerance. Defense mechanisms of denial, projection, rationalization, and minimization are prominent. The nature of drug use varies from initial experimentation to occasional use, moderate use (two to three times weekly), and heavy, daily use leading to drug dependency and, sometimes, physical addiction.

Adolescents who progress to true drug dependency become increasingly alienated from their families and their predrug peer groups. There is a loss of communication with family, dysphoric mood changes, social isolation, withdrawal, apathy, frequent truancy, and often evidence of drug use and signs of intoxication. The effect on the family is profound. Increasingly, it is apparent that not only is drug abuse a family illness, regardless of genetic factors, but the family must be fully involved in the treatment and recovery process.

The following chapters delineate different aspects of the diagnosis and treatment of adolescent alcohol and chemical dependency.

John E. Meeks focuses on the clinical assessment, etiology, stages, and patterns of adolescent drug abuse. He views drug dependency as a progressive illness in adolescents who present special vulnerability to this illness owing to both genetic and psychodynamic factors. Finally, he describes issues in the treatment of the drug-dependent youngster,

506

stressing the need for inpatient treatment and family therapy for seriously impaired teenagers. As the adolescent gives up drug use, Meeks notes that the basic underlying psychopathology emerges, which can be more amenable to traditional psychotherapy with subsequent development of a transference relationship.

Hospital programs for adolescents presenting both with drug abuse and psychiatric illness (dual diagnosis) are described by Joe W. King and John E. Meeks. They note inherent conflicts in the approach to the dual diagnosis patient between the medical psychiatric treatment approach and the recovering community approach (Alcoholics Anonymous). Differences are discussed involving treatment techniques, training, philosophies, milieu, and effects on the staff. They conclude that there is merit in merging the expertise of the recovering community with the psychiatric approaches in spite of administrative difficulties.

George DeLeon, drawing on extensive experience with the therapeutic community approach to teenage drug abuse, describes the value of a highly structured program with emphasis on a peer model. He reviews the literature, philosophy, milieu, and treatment techniques used at Phoenix House, the nation's largest residential therapeutic community. He observes that the sobriety rate is directly correlated with the length of treatment within the therapeutic community, providing for a good enough "holding" environment long enough to help maintain impulse control and self-regulation.

JOHN E. MEEKS

In numerous studies (DuPont 1984; Goodwin 1985), it has been shown that the rate of alcoholism varies greatly across cultures in direct relation to the social acceptability of drinking and particularly the acceptance of intoxication as a socially condoned state of consciousness. The general acceptance within American society, both adult and adolescent, of drug use and intoxication is obvious to the most casual observer. It is also clear that this has been an increasing fact of cultural life over the past twenty-five years (Johnston, O'Malley, and Bachman 1984). In popular films and television dramas, abstinent individuals are frequently shown as villains or at least uninteresting characters, while meaningful emotional expression, romance, and heart-warming comedy occur when the leading characters are drunk or high on marijuana. A very recent encouraging change is the appearance of recovering alcoholics as heros in some popular media fiction.

The question of what constitutes alcoholism or serious substance abuse in the individual adolescent patient is sometimes difficult for the clinician to determine. The accepted definition of addiction in the past has been the occurrence of withdrawal symptoms on cessation of drug intake or development of clear physical or social damage from drug use. This is a very limiting and clinically inadequate guide, especially in the adolescent population. Because of their youth, physical resilience, and developmental and psychological factors that incline adolescents to disguise situations and feelings through action, adolescents often show no clear-cut physical symptoms of withdrawal even when they have been very heavy users of drugs known to be addictive in adults.

Other definitions of substance abuse or chemical dependency focus on performance factors such as school grades and school attendance, clear changes in dress patterns, and choice of friends, which indicate membership in the "drug culture." These signals are often present in youngsters who are getting into serious problems with drugs, but they are not invariably seen. There are some adolescents who maintain good grades and superficial accommodation to social and family expectations at the same time that they are sliding into serious secret dependence on chemical agents. Schwartz, Cohen, and Bair (1985) have summarized some suggestive findings that suggest serious drug abuse in the adolescent.

A high index of concern and suspicion is definitely justified by the realities of adolescent life today. Psychiatrists and other psychotherapists need particularly to consider the possibility that excess drug use is contributing to the pathological clinical picture in each of their adolescent patients. Self-medication is extremely common in any youngster who is depressed, anxious, lonely, or suffering from significant problems of self-esteem (Marohn 1983; Meissner 1980).

A clinically useful rule of thumb in deciding if a given youngster is chemically dependent is based on deciding the question of whether drugs or people seem most important. It requires careful clinical attention to apply this approach. Almost all chemically dependent youngsters report that they have many friends and that they are deeply attached to them. In fact, they often complain that their parents try to interfere with their friendships and speak of strong devotion and caring relationships with their peers. However, close evaluation of these friendships often reveal that they are shallow, often exploitive, and, most important, focused to a major extent on a shared involvement with active drug use. That is, these "friends" spend a good deal of their time discussing their highs, planning their acquisition of drugs, and distributing their supply within the group often at considerable financial profit. The relationship also often includes mutual support of the denial of the deleterious effects that drugs may be having in each adolescent's life, continued pressure to use drugs regularly, and often support and sharing of an antisocial and alienated position with regard to adults and conventional social values (Kellam, Simon, and Ensinger 1983; Wurmser and Zients 1982). Many drug-involved adolescents have learned a bitter lesson about their "friends" when they have made a decision to stop using drugs only to find that they are dropped by the peer group to whom they felt so close as soon as they refuse to give in to the group's subtle and sometimes blatant efforts to keep them actively involved in drug usage.

The chemically dependent adolescent's gradual move away from people and toward drugs is initially subtle and difficult to detect. It may first appear as a slight loss of sensitivity and empathy in relationships with family and straight friends. Later, it becomes more obvious as the adolescent steals from the family to obtain money to purchase drugs and treats family members as enemies if they oppose drug use in even a mild form. Eventually, the adolescent may reach that desperate and chilling situation in which he will use anyone in order to ensure an uninterrupted supply of his favorite drug. This progression almost always includes a pattern of growing alienation from parents and other family members often accompanied by intense hostility, intimidation, and rejection. These attitudes are not adolescent postures or pretension. They represent the psychological truth that the adolescent no longer needs the parent since he views drugs and drug companions as the important source of comfort, solace, and pleasure. The parents become enemies with the potential power to interfere with the adolescent's crucial sources of emotional supplies. Later, when we discuss the process of chemical dependency, it will become more clear why this pattern of withdrawal and disassociation from people becomes gradually more strident and frenzied as the illness progresses (Newton 1981).

From a clinical perspective, these changes in life-style and attitudes toward important others are more important diagnostically than are signs of acute toxicity or the occurrence of longer-term effect on brain functioning. However, it is obviously true that an adolescent who is observed by the family to be extremely intoxicated on repeated occasions, in the face of family disapproval and efforts at limit setting, should be assumed to have a potentially serious substance-abuse problem. In addition, youngsters who report sleep difficulties, loss of a capacity for concentration, defects in memory, or other cognitive difficulties should have chemical dependency listed as a factor in the differential diagnosis (Schwartz et al. 1985).

Etiology of Chemical Dependency

There is convincing evidence that there is a major hereditary element in vulnerability to severe chemical dependency (Bohman 1978; Cadoret, Cain, and Grove 1980; Goodwin 1985). Most of the solid research data has come in the specific area of alcoholism, but clinical experience suggests that very similar findings will hold for all abused substances. Clinical practitioners who work with chemically dependent patients have long been aware of the high frequency of chemical dependency in the close relatives and the entire family tree of these patients. Studies of children of alcoholics raised since infancy in nondrinking adoptive families and twin studies suggest that the relevant factor is genetic vulnerability rather than learned behavior.

There are other important aspects of family dynamics and developmental experience that seem important, particularly in adolescents who develop severe chemical dependency. The frequency of a history of physical and/or sexual abuse in childhood often accompanied by other experiences of neglect and traumatization is very high (Wurmser and Zients 1982). In our hospital treatment program, about one-third of the patients report this history. Obviously, this finding is not totally independent of the history of chemical dependency in these families since the addictive life-style and the experience of intoxication may have a severely negative effect on the capacity to parent.

Adolescents with severe chemical dependency also have an unusually frequent history of learning disabilities, attention deficit disorder, and other evidences of subtle brain dysfunction (Hartocollis 1982; Kandel 1982; Yendall, Fromm-Auch, and Davies 1982). The role of fetal alcoholism syndrome or other unrecognized or less serious neonatal conditions related to parental drug use is not clear. It is also possible that, whatever the genetic vulnerability toward the development of chemical dependency may be, it may include some other manifestations of ego vulnerability such as these problems in cognitive functioning and control of motor impulses.

It seems clear that there are many different patterns of drug dependency in the adolescent population. Some drug-abusing adolescents seem primarily depressed, lonely, and inhibited. Drugs for them become a vehicle for acceptance, lessening of inhibition, and amelioration of painful social anxiety. Another large group of substance-abusing adolescents seem more sociopathic, grandiose, and arrogant. For them, drugs seem important to maintain their sense of excitement, euphoria, and power over themselves and others. A final group of adolescents seems merely dedicated to self-destruction. They use drugs in such a massive, random, and nondiscriminating manner as regularly to threaten their very existence without showing any concern for their survival, much less their well-being.

Even these three large groups do not fully circumscribe all adolescents who become seriously involved with drugs. We are dealing with a complex interaction of genetic vulnerability, life experience, social expectations, and individual biological responses to specific doses and frequencies of the chemical agents involved. The outline of a general concept or "final common path" to be described has to be viewed as the faintest outline of a possible pattern, which will be influenced in its expression by all the complexities mentioned.

AN ORGANIZING PRINCIPLE FOR THE VULNERABILITY TO SUBSTANCE ABUSE

The developing child needs the combination of gradual mastery of increasingly difficult cognitive and affective tasks along with the support of a "good enough" nurturing environment in order to develop a sense of personal competence. The process requires relinquishing the infantile sense of omnipotence and grandiosity in return for a safe relationship with an idealized parenting figure and satisfying experiences of personal success in a gradually widening world. The emotional investment in the idealized parent becomes richer and deeper and takes on more elements of mature object love with partial resolutions of issues of power and bodily control. As these cognitive and affective issues are worked out with a loving but realistically limit-setting parent figure, internalization and learning occur.

Through the process, the child develops a capacity to self-sooth, provide self-approval, and accept realistic personal limitations without a loss of self-esteem. This combination of self-respect tempered by a readiness to recognize areas of inadequacy permits the child to welcome the learning process and, indeed, to value and love those who know more and are in a position to teach. Ego growth, both in the area of skills of adaptation and richness of emotional and interpersonal experience, continues.

Unfortunately, youngsters who seem vulnerable to the severe forms of chemical dependency show evidence that this progression has been severely disrupted. In all three groups of serious drug abusers described, there is an impaired self-esteem and damaged narcissism. If one is afflicted with attention deficit disorder, a primary learning disability, or hyperkinetic syndrome (indeed, any problem that disrupts the basic ego organization), one will find it difficult to have successes and to internalize the memory of successful mastery of the environment. In addition, the youngster is less likely to experience his parents and other adults as adequately helpful people.

Even if a youngster has the basic adaptive equipment, he also requires a supportive environment. If he encounters experiences of neglect and abuse instead of support and help, it becomes extremely difficult for him to be comfortably dependent and to internalize the parenting figures. He does not develop internalized comforting, supporting images that would permit him to feel safe in an unfamiliar, lonely, or challenging situation.

If the youngster has to struggle with both ego deficiencies and parental traumatization, as is often the reality in the drug-dependent population, the effort to gain a sense of personal competence faces almost insurmountable obstacles. The result is the development of narcissistic character defenses with an unwarranted dependence on maintaining a grandiose image in one's self-expectation and in the eyes of others. This "false self" is difficult to maintain since it is constantly assaulted by the realities of life's complexity, individual limitations, and the growing genuine ego deficits, which the condition itself produces. In other words, if one is pretending an omnipotent superiority to life and its problems and avoiding dependency relationships, the normal learning of ego mastery skills does not occur with the result that the youngster continuously falls further behind peers in important areas of life management. Even though these deficiencies are disguised to some extent by hypertrophied skills in manipulation and an impressive superficial self-presentation, the defects still lead to vulnerabilities that are always a potential source of embarrassment to the narcissistically oriented adolescent.

Of course, there are many adolescents with problems of this kind who do not become seriously drug involved. However, drug use is certainly a tempting support to this defensive structure. The drugs themselves provide a spurious sense of well-being, and some even induce a euphoric confirmation of the desired fantasied omnipotence. The capacity voluntarily and consciously to regulate mental processes by ingesting drugs also lends an illusion of self-control (Wieder and Kaplan 1969). The youngster on drugs feels impervious to events in the surrounding world that normally would have an effect on his or her sense of well-being (Meissner 1980). The narcissistic youngster's difficulty in accepting dependency on people makes depending on a self-administered chemical agent appear attractive (Marohn 1983; Sugarman and Kurash 1982).

In addition, the limited and well-defined pattern of interpersonal interactions on the drug scene provides the youngster with a pseudo–peer group and a sense of belonging that is not threatened by requirements for genuine intimacy or honest emotional interaction. Finally, the drug culture provides an opportunity for living out a "street image" as a tough, fearless, rebellious, and totally independent person who has neither need nor fear in interactions with adults. All these elements of the drug experience act in concert to support the adolescent's desperately needed self-perception as self-sufficient, all knowing, and all conquering. The only problem with this solution to the need for unrealistic self-perception is that the process of serious drug dependency has some unforeseen side effects that will not allow the solution to remain satisfactory.

CHARACTERISTICS OF THE PROGRESSION OF CHEMICAL DEPENDENCY

Chemical agents (except for Soma, the mythical substance in Huxley's *Brave New World*) have two inherent characteristics that play a major role in their unsuitability as final answers to mankind's problems. First, all drugs have a number of simultaneous effects on the body. Those that are desired are seen as the drug's actions; all those that are undesired are seen as side effects. Some of the side effects may be, in fact, definitely damaging to the human body. The second characteristic of all psychoactive drugs is that the body gradually develops tolerance to the desired effects. Ever larger doses are required to produce the same effect if the drug is taken with any frequency. Consequently, the higher dosage produces more and more of the unwanted effects, many of which are unaffected by tolerance, including those that are damaging. Sooner or later, people who use drugs heavily have to recognize, even if only briefly and episodically, that the drug use is producing effects that are a source of considerable concern to them. If an adolescent uses marijuana and alcohol regularly, it is eventually noticed that there is a growing memory deficit. The adolescent who uses cocaine eventually experiences a severe withdrawal depression, damage of the nasal mucosa, or simply severe personal and practical problems occasioned by the escalating cost of their habit.

In addition to these direct physical side effects, there is a concurrent effect on the development of ego skills as mentioned. This affects not only serious skills but also the capacity to have fun and find pleasure in everyday activities. The drug-dependent adolescent maintains few interests or hobbies and, indeed, is unaccustomed to engaging in any leisure activity except in the intoxicated state. Opportunities for gratifying success disappear as both motivation and capacity to work are adversely affected by the drug use. Chronic boredom, only imperfectly relieved by periodic intoxication, becomes a way of life.

Finally, relationships with others (particularly those in positions of authority who would be potential sources of appropriate dependency supply and learning) are severely damaged by the drug use. Partly because of the adolescents' guilt over their behavior and partly because of the actual opposition of caring adults, adolescents come to view many people as enemies who may interfere with access to the desired chemical agents. The adolescents' relationships with others become increasingly dishonest, manipulative, and hostile so that the need for the drug is actually increased since there is diminished opportunity for meeting needs in interpersonal relationships (Schwartz et al. 1985).

The factors just outlined explain why drug dependency is almost always a progressive illness characterized by an increasingly blind and desperate dependency and a narrowing preoccupation with drug use. In a curious way, the adolescent has recreated an infantile dependency relationship. Rather than becoming independent and self-sufficient, he finds himself increasingly helplessly dependent on the availability of the needed drugs and also on the people who will supply the agents to him.

At this point in the illness, there is an astonishing degree of denial. Although the most casual objective observer would see the addict's life as massively affected by a blind dependency on the drug, the patient maintains that this is totally untrue. Often patients will stop using drugs for a period of time to demonstrate that they can "take them or leave them," but, of course, they always return to the same pattern of heavy drug usage in a relatively brief time. The denial probably represents an emergency measure to defend the person against the recognition of the true state of affairs. The recognition of their true situation would be simply too devastating. The adolescent would have to recognize that, rather than being independent, he has become helplessly dependent on someone else to help him out of his situation. Of course, he would also have to recognize the need to give up what at this point he regards as his only reliable source of support, pleasure, and self-esteem, namely, the chemical agents.

ISSUES IN THE TREATMENT OF THE ALCOHOLIC AND SUBSTANCE-ABUSING ADOLESCENT

The outpatient treatment of drug-involved youngsters is complicated by their resistance to forming a strong attachment to the therapist. They are more attached to their drugs of choice than to human beings when chemical dependency reaches an advanced state. This phobic avoidance of dependent attachments will certainly extend to the therapist. In the emotional life of the severe chemically dependent adolescent, a therapist is merely a means to an end, and manipulation and exploitation of the therapist is the common event:

An intelligent seventeen-year-old boy hospitalized after a near fatal accidental drug overdose had been in psychotherapy for over a year on an outpatient basis. Early in his hospital treatment he bragged of convincing his outpatient therapist to prevail on his parents to allow access to the area of the city where he obtained his drugs. He felt no remorse for this and held an attitude of amused contempt toward the therapist, whom he had outsmarted.

The therapist who treats a youngster with a serious drug problem needs to recall that these youngsters have found human dependency uncomfortable and unrewarding. They avoid anxiety about dependent relationships by constantly trying to prove that they are smarter than adults and that they have no need for their help. As a rule, abstinence must be a requirement for successful treatment of these youngsters. If abstinence can be obtained, underlying feelings of depression, yearnings for support, and feelings of anxiety may come to the fore for psychotherapeutic management. However, it is usually not possible for the therapist to compete with the instant solutions to these problems that drugs provide, at least in the early phases of usage. Even as therapy succeeds, temptations develop. As physical and emotional vigor return, the adolescent forgets the negative effects of drug use and begins to idealize the pleasant and gratifying aspects of intoxication.

517

Patients in treatment for severe chemical dependency will periodically be tempted to use drugs. These temptations come both from yearnings for remembered gratifications and from urges to self-medicate in the face of some of the emotional discomfort created by life or indeed by the psychotherapeutic process itself. Progress is occasion for celebration; frustration calls for comfort. To deal with these facts in outpatient therapy, it is usually necessary to provide external support to maintain abstinence. Regular random monitoring of drug urines and membership in such support groups as Alcoholics Anonymous and Narcotics Anonymous that encourage continuing abstinence and remind of the dangers of drug use are important. Family cooperation and supervision is an essential adjunct to outpatient psychotherapy. Obviously, the family can be genuinely helpful only after resolution of enabling behaviors in the family system.

Many seriously drug-involved youngsters cannot maintain abstinence on an outpatient basis even with the support of family and self-help groups. For these youngsters, treatment must be started in a drug-free residential environment in which a period of abstinence can be insured while the youngster gains at least beginning control over compulsive drug use.

In both outpatient and inpatient treatment, trained drug counselors, particularly those who have previously been addicted themselves, are an invaluable aid to the treatment process. They provide both an empathic understanding of the joys and horrors of chemical dependency and a seismographic awareness of the manipulations and self-delusions that characterize the illness. They do not usually need to see gross evidence of a return to drug use in addicted adolescents because they recognize the very subtle evidences of the mind-set that usually precedes or accompanies a relapse. Their comfort in confronting the adolescent drug addict is usually higher than therapists who have not been drug addicted not only because they have the sense of having "been there" but also because they usually have a conviction of the correctness of their assessment, which "straight" therapists find very difficult to maintain in the face of blatant denial by the patient.

The role of family therapy has already been mentioned. Obviously, intensive family therapy focusing on enabling patterns is very important if the adolescent is to be strongly encouraged to find and persist in new life-style patterns (Wegscheider 1981). If the family continues to encourage and support chemical dependency, the adolescent's own temptations to return to drug use will find ready support and likely expression. Adequate therapy for parents includes both major educational efforts to be sure that they understand the nature of chemical dependency, peer support, especially from other families who have successfully dealt with the problem, and appropriate therapy for family-system psychopathology, which might lead to a need for a scapegoated child (Haley 1980).

If these special parameters of therapy are carefully attended to, chemically dependent youngsters will gradually turn away from compulsive drug use. As a rule, as they give up drug use and abandon the fantasy that drug use in the future will solve their problems, the basic underlying psychopathology will tend to become more obvious and more available to traditional psychotherapy. This change is accompanied by the development of a genuine transference relationship and a strong human attachment to the therapist. At this point in treatment, the patient's motivation to maintain this relationship and explore it becomes a very important element in avoiding drug use. Since the therapist is now more important than the chemical substance, the balance has shifted, and traditional psychotherapy becomes possible. (Of course, some youngsters who use drugs can reach that point with traditional psychotherapy alone. These youngsters are usually characterized by better ego functioning, reasonably good family relationships, peer groups that are not deeply drug involved, and a recent onset of drug involvement. Those youngsters are not our topic here.)

At this point, therapy can address the basic problems leading to vulnerability. This will include appropriate remediation, correction of self- and body-image problems, and modification of personality deficits—in short, the kind of individualized, prescribed specific therapy we offer all disturbed adolescents. It should be remembered, however, that a youngster who has been chemically dependent may continue to find the prospect of chemical solutions attractive in the face of unusual stresses, especially those that relate directly to therapy. The time of termination, for example, may be fraught with risk for these youngsters as they deal with the major loss of giving up the therapist. Vacation times and periods of disillusionment with the therapist also raise the specter of relapse as a treatment complication. This reality should be recognized by the therapist and also conveyed to the parents so that these episodes of return to drug use can be seen as neurotic regressions rather than being misdiagnosed as a simple continuation of the drug pattern.

Conclusions

Chemical dependency usually begins as an effort to resolve some of the painful problems of adolescence. The heavy use of drugs is particularly attractive to adolescents who have serious defects in self-regulation, mastery skills, and the capacity for appropriate dependency relationships. These defects result from complex interruptions between heredity, construction, and environment. In many youngsters, the drug use progresses to a disease state that requires recognition and specific treatment. After treatment of the chemical dependency, basic psychotherapy is still often required to ameliorate basic personality deficiencies.

REFERENCES

Bohman, M. 1978. Some genetic aspects of alcoholism and criminality: a population of adoptees. *Archives of General Psychiatry* 35:269–276.

Cadoret, L. J.; Cain, C. A.; and Grove, W. M. 1980. Development of alcoholism in adoptees raised apart from alcoholic biologic relatives. *Archives of General Psychiatry* 37:561–563.

DuPont, R. 1984. *Getting Tough on Gateway Drugs: A Guide for the Family.* Washington, D.C.: American Psychiatric Press.

Goodwin, D. W. 1985. Alcoholism and genetics. *Archives of General Psychiatry* 42:171–174.

Haley, J. 1980. *Leaving Home.* New York: McGraw-Hill.

Hartocollis, P. 1982. Personality characteristics in adolescent problem drinkers: a comparative study. *Journal of the American Academy of Child Psychiatry* 21:348–352.

Johnston, L. D.; O'Malley, P. M.; and Bachman, J. G. 1984. *Drugs and American High School Students, 1975–1983.* Rockville, Md.: National Institute on Drug Abuse.

Kandel, D. B. 1982. Epidemiological and psychological perspectives on adolescent drug use. *Journal of the American Academy of Child Psychiatry* 21:328–347.

Kellam, S. G.; Simon, M.; and Ensinger, M. E. 1983. Antecedents in first grade and teenage drug use and psychological well-being: a ten-year community-wide prospective study. In D. Ricks and B. Dohrenwend, eds. *Origins of Psychopathology: Research and Public Policy.* New York: Cambridge University Press.

Marohn, R. C. 1983. Adolescent substance abuse: a problem of self-soothing. *Clinical Update in Adolescent Psychiatry* 1(10).

Meissner, W. W. 1980. Addiction and paranoid process: psychoanalytic perspectives. *International Journal of Psychoanalytic Psychotherapy* 8:273–279.

Newton, M. 1981. *Gone Way Down: Teenage Drug Use Is a Disease.* Tampa, Fla.: American Studies Press.

Schwartz, R. H.; Cohen, P. R.; and Bair, G. O. 1985. Identifying and coping with a drug-using adolescent: some guidelines for pediatricians and parents. *Pediatrics in Review* 7:133–139.

Sugarman, A., and Kurash, C. 1982. Marijuana abuse, transitional experience and the borderline adolescent. In J. Lichtenberg and S. Smith, eds. *Adolescent Addiction: Varieties and Vicissitudes, Psychoanalytic Inquiry.* Hillsdale, N.J.: Analytic.

Wegscheider, S. 1981. *Another Chance.* Palo Alto, Calif.: Science & Behavior.

Wieder, H., and Kaplan, E. H. 1969. Drug use in adolescents: psychodynamic meaning and pharmacogenic effect. *Psychoanalytic Study of the Child* 24:399–431.

Wurmser, L., and Zients, A. 1982. The return of the denied superego. In J. Lichtenberg and S. Smith, eds. *Adolescent Addiction: Varieties and Vicissitudes, Psychoanalytic Inquiry.* Hillsdale, N.J.: Analytic.

Yendall, L. T.; Fromm-Auch, D.; and Davies, P. 1982. Neurological impairment of persistent delinquency. *Journal of Nervous and Mental Disease* 170:257–260.

521

31 HOSPITAL PROGRAMS FOR PSYCHIATRICALLY DISTURBED, DRUG-ABUSING ADOLESCENTS

JOE W. KING AND JOHN E. MEEKS

A large number of adolescent patients who present with sufficient psychopathology to require hospitalization include among their symptoms the frequent use of alcohol and/or other drugs (Stone 1973; Treffert 1978). For many, the working through of underlying conflict will reduce the behavioral expression of their symptomatology (Rado 1933; Wieder and Kaplan 1969). In a significant number of drug-using patients, however, chemical "highs" have become the primary reason to live. Almost everything they do relates to their preoccupation with and dependency on the direct use of drugs and adjunctive drug interests, including music, dress, behavioral style, choice of peer relationships, career choices, and so forth. Many also demonstrate moderate to severe regression in cognitive and ego functioning. These patients are rarely responsive to traditional inpatient psychiatric care (Meeks 1982; Milman 1982).

Both of us have served as unit directors for the development of coeducational substance abuse programs. The programs were developed to bring young patients the best of a medical model for adolescent psychiatric inpatient care along with a self-help program. The patients participated in an intense, group-process-oriented, unit-centered treatment approach utilizing a team concept. Daily formal group psychotherapy, prescribed individual psychotherapy, family therapy, participation in ancillary services including special education, and a variety of activity therapies were provided. In addition, these youngsters simultaneously participated in a recovering-community treatment approach. They participated in the "Twelve Step" Alcoholics Anonymous (AA) program and had didactic and process-oriented meetings with substance abuse counselors. They attended program meetings regularly, and most parents participated either in a "Next Step" program, consisting of an all-day Saturday meeting and six evening meetings, or in an intensive family therapy program on the unit.

As these substance abuse programs were introduced into traditionally oriented psychiatric settings, a number of areas of fundamental conflict appeared. Some of our experiences were anticipated and some were not. To our surprise, in 1981 we could find no confirmation of this combination therapy approach either in the literature or by personal inquiry to professional colleagues. In this chapter the following areas concerning this approach will be discussed: philosophical differences; training and experiential differences; differences in community attitudes; administrative need differences; and clinical differences.

Philosophical Considerations

We noted two major areas of philosophical differences in the early months of our experience. There was the obvious conflict between the medical psychiatric treatment approach and the recovering-community treatment model (*Alcoholics Anonymous* 1976; Wegscheider 1981). While both treatment approaches are designed to assist the patient in removing defenses in order to face underlying conflicts and problems, the recovering-community model is drastically different from traditional psychiatric and psychological techniques.

The medical model and the recovering-community model have very different techniques for the removal of surface defenses. The primary defense in substance abusers and alcoholics is denial. The more traditional treatment approach deals with the anxiety that is created as a person gradually works through his or her denial. The recovering-community model uses a more direct approach in which the patient is confronted warmly but firmly about his or her denial. Sarcasm, wit, and self-disclosure are routine treatment tools. The traditional substance abuse counselor believes that the substance abuser has, as a cardinal fear, a dread of being alone and different. Such a counselor believes that the technique of self-disclosure offers a beacon of hope to follow during early efforts to tackle Step One of the AA program.

523

Step One requires acknowledgment that patients have been powerless in their efforts to deal with substance abuse (Johnson 1973).

Mary, age fifteen, had been admitted to the substance abuse unit after two previous psychiatric hospitalizations. Both hospitalizations were followed by the patient returning to serious substance abuse. She was frequently truant from school and had fallen two years behind in her studies. She had also participated in many runaways, engaged in sexual promiscuity, and stolen from her parents to support her drug habit. One morning in group therapy Mary was talking about the role drugs had played in her life: "Oh, I've used quite a few drugs—and often too. But I only use them when I want to, and I could certainly quit if I wanted to. I just don't see any reason to quit." One of the substance abuse counselors replied, "Oh sure, Mary! You use drugs but you can quit any time you want to. I know all about that. I've been there! You know damn well you have no control whatsoever over your use of drugs. You think about drugs when you wake up in the morning and that's the last thing you think about before you go to sleep at night. I used to talk just like you do; I was desperate to play like I had some control over something that I was absolutely powerless to control. I can see myself in almost everything you say, and I don't buy your crap about being able to control it."

During this confrontation Mary made direct eye contact with the drug counselor and maintained it throughout the interchange. She initially looked as though she was going to become angry, and then her expression calmed as she said almost inaudibly, "You've got it." Later, in a team meeting, one of us (J.W.K.) commented that, although he understood the substance abuse counselor's wish to work through Mary's resistance, he was sure that it was not the counselor's intent to strip Mary of her defenses as she had in the group. The counselor replied, "Oh yes it was! She can put out that crap about control over her drug use forever if we don't jump in and stop it. I fully intended to strip her naked and hope I did." It should be noted that an important characteristic of a substance abuse counselor is directness and dedication. We have been very impressed with the high degree of genuineness among dedicated substance abuse counselors and members of the recovering community. It is our impression that this degree of genuineness and self-commitment, including self-disclosure, allows a broader spectrum of technique within the recovering-community approach.

There is clinical evidence, however, that direct interpretation cannot be tolerated by some patients with borderline ego integration or other forms of severe psychopathology. We have seen several examples of further ego disintegration, even to the point of transient psychosis, in patients who could not tolerate this degree of direct confrontation. Caution in this area continues as counselors have become more sensitive to the needs of the borderline adolescent. In addition to limits imposed by psychopathology, there are required variations of technique that result from the unique developmental characteristics of adolescents.

The programs have recognized needs of adolescents and preadolescents that differ from those of adult substance abusers. There are usually ego strength differences between substance-abusing adults and substance-abusing adolescents. Most adults have found some psychological baseline that has served them, at least partially, as young adults or adults to provide successful experiences. Most adolescents are searching for that psychological baseline whether they are substance abusers or not. This has implications for the way denial is approached. It also influences some traditional recovery techniques. For example, relaxation techniques including back rubs and other forms of touching are commonplace among adult substance abuse units. It is our observation that most adolescents cannot tolerate this degree of physical contact and almost always misinterpret its intended and sometimes very concretely stated meaning. We do not allow back rubs on the substance abuse units, although we still permit "group hugs" in structured and clearly defined situations.

Adolescent substance abusers and adult substance abusers also have different ego positions regarding dependency and helplessness. Usually, the adult finds dependency and expressed helplessness rather ego syntonic, while the adolescent finds the dependent position ego dystonic and will usually reject it, especially from adults. Also, adolescents frequently eroticize dependency, and in a substance abuse program this process would tend only to confuse and defeat the purpose of forms of physical relaxation if they are not clearly defined and prescribed. Finally, adolescents do not usually have the capacity to reciprocate the dependency position—even with peers—as much as do adults. The patients are encouraged to support and help new patients. They are told, "You can only keep it [sobriety and good mental health] by giving it away." They do make a genuine and successful effort to follow these directions. However, treatment or no treatment, they remain adolescents with a legitimate developmental right to be partially dependent on available adults.

The AA model clearly feels that the "devil is in the drug" and that one is born vulnerable to alcoholism or substance abuse (Jellinek 1960). The traditional psychiatric position is that drug use is a conscious effort to deal with stress or psychological pain (Hartocollis 1982; Kandel 1982; Marohn 1983; West and Allen 1968). The adolescent would be viewed by traditional psychological philosophy as attempting to integrate his life through the maladaptive coping efforts of self-medication. The common thread woven into the two philosophies is biological vulnerability from genetic or experiential sources. Both groups would concur that there is much that we do not yet know about vulnerability and predisposition to substance abuse.

Perhaps the most serious handicap experienced in attempting to set up a high-quality and effective treatment program utilizing both medical model benefits and recovering-community benefits is that there are few existing substance abuse treatment programs for adolescents that incorporate the expertise of both these fields. In fact, very little data are available from which to draw in learning about substance abuse programs for adolescents that are based on the recovering-community model.

Training and/or Experiential Differences

As described, some substance counselors are part of the recovering community. They have been helped personally by being "stripped naked." They believe, then, that this is the correct approach. On the other hand, the mental health professional has been taught to work through the resistances and has had success with that approach (and often personal experience of being helped by a psychoanalytically oriented therapeutic approach). Patients can be caught between the two belief systems.

CLINICAL EXAMPLE 2

Richard, a seventeen-year-old youngster, was transferred to the substance abuse program after being hospitalized for six months. Intensively involved in individual, group, and family therapy, and in spite of significant improvement, Richard continued to be obsessed by drugs, drug use, drug paraphernalia, and the music of drug-oriented groups. When allowed, he chose to wear T-shirts that referred to drugs. Richard entered into the substance abuse program with some degree of fearfulness and doubt. After several days in the program, however, he became staunchly oppositional and demanded to see his individual therapist, who had been working with him for some months. He expressed a great deal of resentment, rage, and righteous indignation that he had been "tricked" into going into the substance abuse program. Richard stated that he had been betrayed because he had learned during hospitalization that his feelings were important and that they would be treated with respect no matter how ridiculous, silly, or bizarre they seemed to be. He stated, "That Betty [a substance abuse counselor on the unit] doesn't respect nothing about nobody. She rips into me and scares me to death and makes me real nervous." Richard went on to state that he would not work with people who "would make me nervous on purpose" and especially with people who would "zap me like that." Richard thus seemed to be experiencing a further sense of betrayal because two of his precious childhood myths were being challenged—the myth that those who loved him would not frustrate him and the myth that those who really cared for him would anticipate his needs and not expect him to assume some responsibility for his destiny.

Richard was shortly thereafter transferred back to the traditional psychiatric treatment program in spite of his serious substance abuse problem. He seemed to be clearly overwhelmed, and his borderline level of ego integration was inadequate to sustain him through the very difficult early phases of the AA program. Our experience with Richard and other youngsters has caused us to use special caution in transferring adolescents into a substance abuse program after several months of hospitalization in a traditional program and also, as mentioned earlier, to examine closely whether a borderline patient can tolerate the ego assault that occurs with such an aggressive approach.

CLINICAL EXAMPLE 3

Several days after the opening of the substance abuse program, Joan was unusually restless during the early morning group therapy session. Other peer group members commented that she thought it might have something to do with "all that tea I am drinking." She commented that she had had a cup of tea "every thirty minutes or so" the day before "just because it was there, and I wanted to try it, and I guess I drank it because I was getting so nervous anyway." Faced with a substance abuser who was on an iatrogenic caffeine high, we were forced to rethink the appropriateness of having coffee, tea, multiple high proteins, and so forth on the unit. The good reasons for the practice on adult substance abuse units simply did not apply to our programs, so we discontinued the practice.

Community Concerns

Although from their beginning both programs utilized counselors, didactic material, and programmatic suggestions from the recovering community, resistance from that group at large was significant. It was felt that we were "creating patients" through the excessive application of psychiatric diagnosis to those who only abused drugs. There was also a fear that we would not return patients to the recovering community but would encourage them to participate only in professional treatment. In addition, we were frequently told that since we were not from the recovering community we were not in a position to understand fully the problems of recovery from substance abuse.

Administrative Differences

Establishing a substance abuse program for children and adolescents in an existing hospital for children and adolescent psychiatric patients is similar to the task of adding adolescent units to an existing general psychiatric hospital. These two programs produced internal concern and some tension in their respective hospitals. Concern was expressed by staff from other units regarding the omnipresence of treats, the initial nonuse of psychotropic medication, allowing patients to go off the grounds to AA or Narcotics Anonymous (NA) meetings early in their treatment, and group hugs. When these concerns were expressed openly and candidly in team meetings, tension was reduced to a level no greater than that on other units after only a few months.

Perhaps the most pressing administrative concern was the twenty-eight-day coverage limit imposed by some third-party systems on substance abuse care. Twenty-eight days is not usually enough time to treat adolescents engaged in substance abuse to an extent that requires hospital treatment. Almost all the youngsters admitted to the programs thus far have carried a psychiatric diagnosis in addition to substance abuse and, therefore, have not been subject to the third-party limitations.

We have also struggled with the difficulties the legal system has in differentiating between adolescents we can treat and those we cannot. This is not limited just to substance abuse problems: the opening of a substance abuse unit has rekindled that concern. Once again we have also had to be careful not to participate in the substitution of hospital care for a correctional placement when the latter is appropriate and indicated. Some of the school systems have become adamant in their position that they do not have to pay for the treatment of adolescents who are hospitalized for substance abuse, sometimes even those school districts that have been cooperative in providing tuition grants for non–substance abuse psychiatric diagnoses.

Clinical Differences

Perhaps one of the most sensitive areas that we have experienced has been the feeling on the part of substance abuse counselors that psychiatric intervention dilutes their treatment approach efforts.

CLINICAL EXAMPLE 4

Chris was hospitalized on one of the new units for his third psychiatric hospital admission. Following his last psychiatric hospital discharge he had done well for approximately one month and then had gradually increased his use of first marijuana, then alcohol, and then more and more drugs, including PCP and LSD. He came into the substance abuse unit as a voluntary patient, frightened of his vulnerability to substance abuse. During the second week of hospitalization, Chris regressed severely. He became loose and disorganized and expressed serious suicidal ruminations. He had blocking and other evidences of ego disintegration. Chris had experienced a similar episode of ego disintegration during his previous hospitalization and responded to small doses of thiothixene. The medication was reintroduced after discussion by the treatment team. Within a couple of days it was apparent that the substance abuse counselors were viewing Chris as "out of treatment," although he had reintegrated and was once again able to participate in the group sessions and other aspects of the treatment program. No amount of discussion served as enough working through to enable the substance abuse counselors not to view Chris as "damaged goods" and in fact as someone who was contaminating the entire program because he was "on medication." Fortunately, over time both units have matured greatly in their acceptance of all effective treatment modalities.

Another area that requires discussion is the issue of counseling versus psychotherapy. This is especially controversial when considering individual psychotherapy, which may be viewed by substance abuse counselors as intrusive to the recovering-community treatment process.

The role of recovering-community treatment model programs as major agents of change in the treatment of substance abuse is a conceptual problem to some psychiatrists. Many feel that the fostering of the recovering-community approach is in essence an institutionalization of the dependency needs and process for patients with substance abuse problems. Rather than have so much free-floating dependency, the patients are sometimes able to sublimate these needs into loyal, meaningful, and sustaining group functions.

This view may contain an unstated value judgment that favors individual psychological autonomy as the pinnacle of adaptation. It is important to recognize that many people in our society regard successful group functioning as an important indication of healthy mental functioning. In any case, we can all agree that, if our drug abusing adolescent patients are able to develop the capacity to function in a group, albeit dependently, it is at a higher order of functioning than they have achieved before and has clear personal and social value as a treatment goal.

Recovering-community groups profess the view that substance abuse is a family disease that is a spin-off of the addiction process. They do acknowledge that some families have other serious problems and that these problems predate the use of drugs. We have found the family work within the recovering-community model to be very compatible with other family therapy efforts (Wegscheider 1982). The question is clearly one of a difference in style and prioritization of content. Alcoholics Anonymous focuses on the ramifications of substance abuse, sometimes with active disinterest in the evidence of other family conflicts or family psychopathology. This is another area in which the adolescent treatment model and the adult treatment model should be differently designed. In the treatment of the adult substance abuser the family may not be involved in an active way; in our adolescent programs we encourage parents to become very actively involved.

Follow-up Data

Since there was significant overlap in the design of the two units, with an active ongoing consultation occurring between the two of us and a general consensus on the development of most elements in each program, there are many programmatic similarities between programs. However, after the programs actually began to function, the extent of this consultation diminished greatly, and each program developed individually with only occasional discussions between us and exchange visits of unit staffs. Because of this, it was felt that it would be interesting to provide some follow-up on the similarities and differences that have evolved from the original designs. We also wanted to question the effectiveness of each program, recognizing that conclusions must be tentative in view of the brief time span involved.

THE PROGRAM'S EVOLUTION

One attitudinal approach that characterizes both programs and seems to have been beneficial in encouraging the exploration of alternative approaches is the open admission that to a large extent we planned experientially. That is, since there was very little in the way of comparable experience, we were not bound by dogma but were open to taking an honest look at the actual results obtained through various technical approaches with a given patient. As mentioned earlier, this process has continued and expanded in the face of desperate patient needs.

An interesting sidelight is the problem that some counselors have had with the need for limit setting around adolescent rebelliousness when this does not relate directly to drug use. Recovering-community staff are usually extremely comfortable about the need for restriction, alertness, and limit setting related to the patient's temptation to return to drug use. For example, they insist on a rather strict dress code because of the feeling that a substantial amount of hidden drug ideation can be expressed through mode of dress and subtle elements of hairstyle and makeup.

531

On the other hand, the NA group, which comes into the hospital to hold weekly meetings, has only gradually accepted the need for staff members to be present in the meetings and for patients to be restricted because of serious clinical problems, although most psychiatric personnel would regard such a restriction as quite routine. It should be noted, however, that with discussion these problems have all been resolved.

DIFFERENCES IN COMMUNITY ACCEPTANCE

We recognized that within the hospital the program would definitely be seen as different. Since both programs were receiving the special attention of the medical director and involved special staffing patterns (in one hospital there were special treats such as high protein snacks), we were worried that the programs might be scapegoated to a degree that would interfere with their effective utilization and, perhaps, with staff morale.

Again we were correct. There clearly has been some jealousy and envy on the part of those involved with other programs and some competitiveness. On one occasion the nurse on the open adolescent unit sent the medical director a strong note protesting the frequency of requests to back up the drug unit staff during crises on their unit. Some psychiatrists at one hospital still insist on treating drug-involved adolescents on units other than the special drug treatment unit. However, it is probably a mark of their true attitude toward the drug program that severe drug abusers and those with complex or puzzling problems are quickly referred to that program. In addition, there has been an encouraging growth of requests for consultation on patients hospitalized on other units in both hospitals. In some cases these result in transfer to the drug units, but in other cases they provide the attending psychiatrist with information that he can utilize in the existing treatment effort.

FAMILY TREATMENT

The treatment of families of youngsters involved with drugs has been, from the beginning, crucial in both programs. We now define substance abuse as a family disease and provide families with traditional family therapy aimed at altering family systems, malfunctions, or inappropriate parenting patterns. We have found most families quite dysfunctional and in need of substantial treatment above and beyond assistance in diminishing their enabling behavior.

One program contracted with a group called "The Next Step," which specializes in providing intensive treatment for parents of substance-abusing adolescents. The other program has developed a family treatment program utilizing hospital staff. In spite of these two somewhat divergent approaches, the end result is remarkably similar. For example, both programs utilize marathon two- to three-day family treatment sessions that serve to orient families, provide a commonality of understanding about the problems they face in helping their youngsters to overcome drug abuse, provide information, and confront the family with their role in perpetuation of the problem.

Conclusions

Two programs for the inpatient treatment of psychiatrically disturbed adolescents who also abuse drugs have developed along surprisingly similar lines. There does seem to be merit in attempting to merge the expertise of the recovering community with the psychological and developmental insights of adolescent psychiatry in spite of the administrative and psychiatric problems in actualizing this joint effort.

REFERENCES

Alcoholics Anonymous. 1976. New York: Alcoholics Anonymous World Services.

Hartocollis, P. 1982. Personality characteristics in adolescent problem drinkers: a comparative study. *Journal of the American Academy of Child Psychiatry* 21(4): 348–353.

Jellinek, E. M. 1960. *The Disease Concept of Alcoholism.* New Haven, Conn.: Hillhouse.

Johnson, V. E. 1973. *I'll Quit Tomorrow.* New York: Harper & Row.

Kandel, D. B. 1982. Epidemiological and psychosocial perspectives on adolescent drug use. *Journal of the American Academy of Child Psychiatry* 21(4): 328–347.

Marohn, R. C. 1983. Adolescent substance abuse: a problem of self-soothing. In R. Marohn, ed. *Clinical Update in Adolescent Psychiatry,* vol. 1, no. 10. Princeton, N.J.: Nassau.

Meeks, J. E. 1982. Some clinical comments on chronic marijuana use in adolescent psychiatric patients. In *Marijuana and Youth: Clinical Observations on Motivation and Learning*. U.S. Department of Health and Human Services Publication no. (ADM) 82-1186. Washington, D.C.: National Institute of Drug Abuse.

Milman, D. H. 1982. Psychological effects of cannabis in adolescence. In *Marijuana and Youth: Clinical Observations on Motivation and Learning*. U.S. Department of Health and Human Services Publication no. (ADM) 82-1186. Washington, D.C.: National Institute of Drug Abuse.

Rado, S. 1933. The psychoanalysis of pharmacothemia. *Psychoanalytic Quarterly* 2:22–23.

Stone, M. H. 1973. Drug-related schizophrenic syndromes. *International Journal of Psychiatry* 11(4): 391–437.

Treffert, D. A. 1978. Marijuana use in schizophrenia: a clear hazard. *American Journal of Psychiatry* 135(1): 1213–1215.

Wegscheider, S. 1981. *Another Chance*. Palo Alto, Calif.: Science & Behavior Books.

West, L. J., and Allen, J. R. 1968. Flight from violence: hippies and the green rebellion. *American Journal of Psychiatry* 125:364–370.

Wieder, H., and Kaplan, E. H. 1969. Drug use in adolescents: psychodynamic meaning and pharmacogenic effect. *Psychoanalytic Study of the Child* 24:399–431.

32 THE THERAPEUTIC COMMUNITY PERSPECTIVE AND APPROACH FOR ADOLESCENT SUBSTANCE ABUSERS

GEORGE DE LEON

The therapeutic community (TC) for substance abuse emerged in the 1960s as a self-help alternative to existing conventional treatments. Inadequately helped by the medical and correctional establishments, recovering alcoholics and drug addicts were its first participant developers. Though its modern antecedents can be traced to Alcoholics Anonymous and Synanon, the TC prototype is ancient, existing in all forms of communal healing and support. Today, the term "therapeutic community" is generic, describing a variety of drug-free residential programs. About a quarter of these conform to the traditional long-term model. These have had the greatest effect on rehabilitating substance abusers.

The Traditional TC

Traditional TCs are similar in planned duration of stay (fifteen to twenty-four months), structure, staffing pattern, perspective, and rehabilitative regime, although they differ in size and client demographics. Staff are a mixture of TC-trained clinicians and human service professionals. Primary clinical staff are usually former substance abusers who themselves were rehabilitated in TC programs. Ancillary staff consist of professionals in mental health, vocational, educational, family, medical, counseling, fiscal, administration, and legal services.

Therapeutic communities accommodate a broad spectrum of substance abusers. Although they originally attracted narcotic addicts, a majority of their client population are nonopioid abusers. Thus, this modality has responded to the changing trend in drug use patterns, treating clients with drug problems of varying severity, different lifestyles, and various social, economic, and ethnic backgrounds.

Most traditional TCs provide service for adolescent substance abusers. Estimates indicate that 20–30 percent of all clients in residential TCs are under age twenty-one and that 10–20 percent are under eighteen. These estimates are based on residential population figures in the age-integrated TCs. A number of programs have evolved special residential facilities exclusively for adolescents; however, much of what is known about the TC approach for the adolescent client is derived from the experience in the traditional TCs, which have not segregated clients by age.

The material in this chapter is drawn from the research and clinical experience in one therapeutic community, Phoenix House. Generalization to other traditional TCs must be cautious, although Phoenix House is representative of the structure, principles, and practices of traditional TCs in the United States for the substance abuse client.

Phoenix House is one of the nation's largest drug-free rehabilitation systems based on the therapeutic community perspective and approach. Residential and nonresidential programs annually admit over 400 adolescents who vary across race, ethnicity, socioeconomic levels, and drug use patterns. This chapter focuses on the residential treatment of adolescents, although modification of the TC model for the nonresidential settings is described elsewhere (e.g., De Leon 1982).

The TC perspective. Full accounts of the TC perspective are described elsewhere (De Leon 1981, 1984, 1986b; De Leon and Beschner 1977; De Leon and Rosenthal 1979; Kaufman and De Leon 1978). Although expressed in a social-psychological idiom, this perspective evolved directly from the experience of recovering participants in therapeutic communities.

The TC perspective can be described in terms of its view of the disorder, of the client, of recovery, and of right living. Though related, these views can be outlined separately.

View of the disorder. Drug abuse is viewed as a disorder of the whole person, affecting some or all areas of functioning. Cognitive and behavioral problems appear, as do mood disturbances. Thinking may be unrealistic or disorganized; values are confused, nonexistent, or antisocial. Frequently, there are deficits in verbal, reading, writing, and marketable skills. And, whether couched in existential or psychological terms, moral or even spiritual issues are apparent.

Abuse of any substance is viewed as overdetermined behavior. Physiological dependency is secondary to the wide range of influences that control the individual's drug use behavior. Invariably, problems and situations associated with discomfort become regular signals for resorting to drug use. For some abusers, physiological factors may be important, but, for most, these remain minor relative to the functional deficits that accumulated with continued substance abuse. Physical addiction or dependency must be seen in the wider context of the individual's life.

Thus, the problem is the person, not the drug. Addiction is a symptom, not the essence of the disorder. In the TC, chemical detoxification is a condition of entry, not a goal of treatment. Rehabilitation focuses on maintaining a drug-free existence.

View of the client. Rather than drug use patterns, individuals are distinguished along dimensions of psychological dysfunction and social deficits. Many clients have never acquired conventional life-styles. Vocational and educational deficits are marked; middle-class mainstream values are either missing or unachievable. Usually, these clients emerge from a socially disadvantaged sector in which drug abuse is more a social response than a psychological disturbance. Their TC experience is better termed "habilitation," the development of a socially productive, conventional life-style for the first time in their lives.

Among clients from advantaged backgrounds, drug abuse is more directly expressive of psychological disorder or existential malaise. The word "rehabilitation" is more suitable, emphasizing a return to a lifestyle previously lived, known, and perhaps rejected.

Nevertheless, substance abusers in TCs share important similarities. Either as cause or consequence of their drug abuse, all reveal features of personality disturbance and/or impeded social function. Thus, all residents in the TC follow the same regime. Individual differences are recognized in specific treatment plans that modify the emphasis, not the course, of their experience in the therapeutic community.

View of recovery. In the TC's view of recovery, the aim of rehabilitation is global. The primary goal is to change the negative patterns of behavior, thinking, and feeling that predispose drug use; the main social goal is to develop a responsible drug-free life-style. Stable recovery, however, depends on a successful integration of these social and psychological goals. For example, healthy behavioral alternatives to drug use are reinforced by commitment to the values of abstinence; acquiring vocational or educational skills and social productivity is motivated by the values of achievement and self-reliance. Behavioral change is unstable without insight, and insight is insufficient without felt experience. Thus, conduct, emotions, skills, attitudes, and values must be integrated to ensure enduring change.

The rehabilitative regimen is shaped by several broad assumptions about recovery.

Motivation. Recovery depends on pressures to change, positive and negative. Some clients seeking help are driven by stressful external pressures; others are moved by more intrinsic factors. For all, however, remaining in treatment requires continued motivation to change. Thus, elements of the rehabilitation approach are designed to sustain motivation or detect early signs of premature termination.

Self-help. Although the influence of treatment depends on the person's motivation and readiness, change does not occur in a vacuum. The individual must permit the effect of treatment or learning to occur. Thus, rehabilitation unfolds as an interaction between the client and the therapeutic environment.

Social learning. A life-style change occurs in a social context. Negative patterns, attitudes, and roles were not acquired in isolation, and they cannot be altered in isolation. Thus, recovery depends not only on what has been learned but also on how and where learning occurs. This assumption is the basis for the community itself serving as teacher. Learning is active, by doing and participating. A socially responsible role is acquired by acting the role. What is learned is identified with the people involved in the learning process, with peer support and staff, as credible role models. Because newly acquired ways of coping are threatened by isolation and its potential for relapse, a perspective on self, society, and life must be affirmed by a network of others.

Treatment as an episode. Residency is a relatively brief period in an individual's life, and its influence must compete with the influence of the years before and after treatment. For this reason, unhealthy "outside" influences are minimized until the individuals are better prepared to engage these on their own, as the treatment regimen is designed for high impact. Thus, life in the TC is necessarily intense, its daily regime demanding, its therapeutic confrontations unmoderated.

View of right living. Therapeutic communities adhere to certain precepts that constitute a view of healthy, proper, social living. Although somewhat philosophical in its focus, this view relates to the TC perspective of the client and of recovery.

Therapeutic communities are explicit in identifying right and wrong behaviors for which there exist appropriate rewards and punishments. Guilt, a moral experience, is a central issue in the recovery process. Particular values are stressed as essential to social learning and personal growth. These include truth and honesty (in word and deed), the work ethic, accountability, self-reliance, responsible concern ("brother's keeper"), and community involvement. On a broader philosophical level, treatment focuses the individual on the personal present (here and now) as opposed to the historical past (then and when). Past behavior and circumstances are explored only to illustrate the *current* patterns of dysfunctional behavior, negative attitudes, and outlook. Individuals are encouraged and trained to assume personal responsibility for their present reality and destiny.

Adolescent and Adult Substance Abusers: Some Differences and Similarities

A critical assumption in the TC's perspective is that adolescent substance abuse usually precedes adult drug abuse. Hence, much of what is known about the adult drug abuser can be applied to the adolescent. Conversely, what is understood about the adolescent drug abuser can be used in treating adult drug abusers. This assumption is supported by research data obtained in therapeutic communities. Social background histories of adult and adolescent abusers in residential treatment vary little with respect to initiation into drug use, the sequence and pattern of substances abused, and chronic problems concerning school performance, truancy, or juvenile delinquency.

Psychological studies also show few age differences either in overall deviancy or in profiles. Tennessee Self-Concept and MMPI profiles reveal a characteristic picture of low self-esteem and mixed features of psychiatric disorder and sociopathic personality. In fact, TC workers view the low self-esteem and character disorder features of many adult abusers as evolving from conduct disorders in adolescence, for example, immaturity, lack of impulse control, the inability to delay gratification or tolerate discomfort, and problems with authority.

Although substance abusers in TCs share similar social and psychological background features, research and clinical evidence have identified certain consistent age differences (e.g., De Leon 1976, 1980, 1984; Holland and Griffin 1984). Compared with adults, adolescents in TCs use drugs at an earlier age, have less involvement with opiates, have shorter periods of abuse, and have greater involvement in alcohol, marijuana, and multiple drug use patterns. Additionally, younger substance abusers have a higher incidence of family deviance and more involvement with previous psychological treatments. As might be expected, adolescent substance abusers have shorter histories of criminal activity and less involvement in the criminal justice system.

Some of these differences reflect the longer periods of illicit drug involvement for older individuals. The drug use differences also parallel those associated with society's changing pattern of substance abuse. For example, multiple drug use and the declining age of first use have been documented for adolescent samples not in drug treatment.

Other important distinctions between adult and adolescent abusers are drawn mainly from clinical experience. These are primarily developmental and reflect the complexity of substance abuse occurring within the unique stage of adolescent physical, social, and psychological growth. For example, the young substance abuser struggles with the general turbulence that characterizes normal adolescent transition (e.g., psychosexual adjustment, emancipation from parents, changes in social role, and physical self-identification). Although these developmental aspects existed for the adult drug abuser, the latter have been tempered by more frequent encounters with reality demands and age-appropriate role expectations.

Adolescent substance abusers remain fascinated with or absorbed in their drug-related or street life-style and less fatigued with cycles of failure or negative social consequences. They disbelieve or reject the possible dire physical, emotional, and social consequences of their life-style. In part, this reflects a realistic assessment of the relatively higher survival potential of young people. However, it also reveals the adolescent propensity for unrealistic thinking concerning their invulnerability.

For adults, the effect of negative consequences of substance abuse is more severe, for they generally suffer tangible and greater losses in money, family, and interpersonal relationships. Moreover, they usually are emancipated, without organized peer groups, and, therefore, more susceptible to personal alienation through their social deviancy. Adolescents, however, have not made substantial investments in the future and have relatively little to lose. They are more often protected from negative consequences by support of peers and family.

Another distinction is in motivation for change. More extrinsic pressure exerted by family or fear of jail is required to keep the adolescent in treatment. For adults, intrinsic pressures are relatively more important. The anxiety associated with the passage of time itself as well as weariness and fatigue with the drug abuse life-style (also associated with time) more often compel adult decisions to seek and remain in treatment. Conversely, adolescents are less conscious of or anxious about the passage of time, the limits of life, fear of disability, or death.

Finally, other practical differences between the adolescent and the adult substance abuser are the relatively greater importance of educational needs and the role of the family in the problems and treatment of the adolescent.

Some indicators for residential treatment. Clinical indicators assigning adolescents to residential treatment are reflected in the following areas: (1) school difficulties (e.g., truancy, maladjustment, violence or chronic conduct difficulties) and poor performance or educational difficulties (e.g., reading, math, communication); (2) antisocial behavior (e.g., "street values," criminal or juvenile delinquency history); (3) family intactness (e.g., broken homes, single parents) or family deviance (e.g., alcoholism, drug use, criminality); (4) drug use patterns (e.g., inability to maintain abstinence from all chemicals in a nonresidential treatment setting); and (5) runaway patterns and family conflict. In general, these indicators portray youths who are perceived as unmanageable by significant others outside a structured setting.

The TC Model and the Adolescent

The treatment approach. For adults and adolescents in the TC, integrated recovery is mediated through its structure—social organization, staff, and daily regimen—and through the process inherent in the individual's passage through phases within that structure (De Leon 1986b).

The TC is a stratified community consisting of peer groups that hold membership in wider subgroups led by individual staff. The collection of peers or subgroups constitutes the community, or family, in a residential facility. This peer-to-community structure strengthens the individual's identification with a perceived and ordered network of others. More important, it arranges relationships of mutual responsibility to others at various levels in their passage through the program—those behind, parallel to, and ahead of the resident.

The management of the community itself is the complete responsibility of the residents, under staff supervision. Job functions are arranged in a hierarchy, according to seniority, individual progress, and productivity. The new client enters a setting of upward mobility. While job assignments generally begin with the most menial tasks (e.g., mopping the floor), they lead vertically to levels of management or coordination. This social organization reflects the fundamental elements of the rehabilitative approach: self-help, responsible performance, and earned successes. Indeed, clients come in as patients and can leave as staff.

Senior staff, as recovered addicts, are visible role models who illustrate the reality of personal change. Their own rehabilitative experience qualifies them to teach, to sanction, and to serve as guides and rational authorities.

The full and varied regimen is designed primarily to facilitate the daily management of the community. Its scope and schedule, however, reflect an understanding of the conditions of drug abuse. Thus, it provides an orderly environment for many who customarily have lived in chaotic or disruptive settings; it reduces boredom and distracts from negative preoccupations that in the past have been associated with drug use; and it offers the opportunity to achieve satisfaction from a busy schedule and the completion of daily chores.

Within this structure, the TC has explicit phases that are prescribed for all clients: orientation (one to sixty days); primary treatment (two to twelve months); early reentry (thirteen to eighteen months); and late reentry (eighteen to twenty-four months), which is usually live-out status. These are sequenced to achieve incremental degrees of psychological and social learning, which prepare the individual for learning at the next stage.

542

The typical therapeutic community day is highly structured, beginning at 7 A.M. wake-up and ending at 11 P.M. This sixteen-hour day consists of morning and evening house meetings, job functions, classroom attendance, therapeutic groups, special seminars, personal time, recreation, and study time as well as individual counseling on an as-needed basis.

The basic components of the TC are relevant to the psychology of youths and to changing their behavior. Several of these are briefly discussed.

Peer pressure. This is a key element in the TC treatment approach. The TC attempts to utilize the positive aspects of peer group strength and, at the same time, weaken their possible negative consequences.

Peers are the primary mediators of the recovery process. As role models, they demonstrate the expected behavior values and teachings of the community.

The peer encounter is the cornerstone group process in the TC. These groups meet at least three times weekly, usually for two hours. Although its process is intense, its aim is modest—to heighten the adolescents' awareness of the images, attitudes, and conduct that should be modified.

Staff as rational authorities. Therapeutic community staff must be firm and reliable mediators of both values and sanctions. Adolescents often have had difficulties with authorities, who have not been trusted or perceived as guides and teachers. Thus, they need a successful experience with a rational authority who is credible (recovered), supportive, correcting, and protecting in order to gain authority over themselves (personal autonomy). Implicit in their role as rational authorities, staff provide the reasons for their decisions and explain the meaning of consequences. They exercise their powers to train, guide, facilitate, and correct rather than punish, control, or exploit.

The rationale for the autocratic regimen of the therapeutic community is relevant to the substance abuser's difficulty with impulse control, which is particularly serious for adolescents who have unclear values and ambiguous environmental cues. For most of these adolescents, their own social-family environment has been either ambiguous or extreme, sharply negative (abusive), or overly indulgent. These imbalances subvert the young person's capacity to acquire firm boundaries for his or her own behavior. Thus, explicit consequences, positive and negative, must be provided along with clear behavioral expectations.

The social structure. The highly structured TC day is designed to keep adolescents busy, stimulated, and absorbed to counter the boredom and understimulation that have been consistently implicated in youth drug abuse. The graduated vertical system teaches goal setting. Establishing explicit landmarks for individual movement counters youths' difficulties in delaying gratification and strengthens the persistence needed for longer-term goals.

The TC process emphasizes mobility—for example, job performance and school behavior earn promotions to positions of increased responsibility. This is based on the assumption that the psychological effect (i.e., reinforcement) of chemicals is less among those who are satisfied through social rewards achieved in schools, sports, work, and social interactions. For the young, in particular, these rewards enhance self-esteem, which in turn reduces identity confusion, image making, and the excessive need for acceptance or approval from others—all factors that tend to exaggerate the importance of peer groups.

For example, an adolescent is promoted to the role of expediter, which in the TC is described as "the eyes and ears of the community." He or she reports to a departmental head or director of the facility concerning a wide variety of daily activities. Satisfactory performance in this role obtains privileges in the program, further promotion, recognition by senior residents and staff, and admiration (or envy) of age peers. These rewards not only provide an opportunity for learning new specific job skills that heighten self-esteem but also strengthen learning through role modeling and community affiliation. Thus, the adolescent's typical need for being accepted by the peer group shifts to striving for success in the larger community.

Participant self-help learning. A critical assumption underlying the TC approach is that, as active contributors, rather than passive recipients, clients are less prone to use drugs. Youths who see themselves as useful and needed by the family or the community acquire responsibility, self-management, and self-reliance—factors that facilitate personal independence. These lessen the anxiety associated with adolescent emancipation, which predisposes substance abuse as relief from a negative reality.

For example, adolescents in TCs are involved in the housekeeping management of the facility. This offers them a certain sense of ownership that tends to strengthen self-management and self-reliance. Additionally, in incremental ways, the adolescents are required to solve problems and make decisions in their work, school, and social roles. In these, they encounter demands, criticisms, and possible failure, experiences not unlike the hassles of the outside world that characteristically have precipitated escape through drug use. Thus, while most adolescents in TCs do not achieve complete social and economic self-reliance, they acquire a certain psychological growth that prepares them for an emancipated role change in the outside world.

Special Treatment Issues for Adolescents

Though adults and adolescents follow the same regimen, certain elements are emphasized or modified for the unique needs of the adolescent. These elements reflect the normal developmental needs of most adolescents but also some distinctive aspects of the adolescent substance abusers in treatment.[1]

Images. Characteristically, adolescents struggle to develop their identity. This often is reflected in the variety of social-personal images they assume. These have been overtly destructive or self-impeding or, at best, associated with the conduct of the outsider.

Images or masks arise in various ways—for example, through imitation, role fulfillment, or positive assertion toward self-differentiation. A primary origin of images, however, is fear—that is, of physical violence, disapproval, nonacceptance, social and sexual impotency, vulnerability, personal weakness, intimidation, or anonymity. Practically all adolescents acknowledge the need to maintain a particular posture, style of speech, and constellation of attitudes, which are designed to mask or contradict a variety of feelings, fears, and perceived threats.

Several approaches and strategies are used to modify the adolescent's predisposition toward developing a negative social image. The first goal is to make the adolescent aware of the phenomenon of image making as well as the range of familiar or recognizable images maintained. Next, an attempt is made to help the adolescents develop self-monitoring methods to assess their own images as well as the images of others and to suggest changes in behaviors, dress, speech, or even posture, where appropriate.

Guilt. Guilt is often the fundamental feeling associated with self-defeating behavior, using drugs, suicidal attempts, or acting out against others (stealing, injuring, or dropping out of treatment). The phrase "guilt kills," often used in the TC, powerfully expresses a vicious cycle in which negative behavior produces guilt, which results in further negative behavior to escape the guilty feelings. Three varieties of guilt are addressed in treatment: guilt relating to the self, to significant others, and to the community.

Community guilt relates to violations of house rules or expectations concerning attitude and conduct in the TC. Thus, even activities as small as borrowing someone else's cigarettes are viewed as moral actions that can hurt the community.

Community guilt can result from "condoning," that is, tacit acceptance of the negative behavior and attitudes of others by not disclosing these attitudes to peers and staff. Individuals may witness cursing in public places, stealing, or the poor attitudes of other people. If they do not make their observations known to peers and staff, they are viewed as condoning the negative behavior and attitude of others and as having strained a moral imperative of the community.

Self-guilt refers to personal secrets relating to past actions that have hurt other people (strangers), including bodily injuries, through criminal activities and varieties of nonviolent criminal behavior; feelings related to lies, deception, and hidden feelings; conduct concerning jealousies, vengeance, and sexuality or betrayal of friends and peer group, teachers, and employers; and failures to meet one's own standards of achievement and good conduct. Not infrequently, these standards are excessively high or distorted, which predisposes a characteristic cycle of failure.

Significant other guilt refers to conduct, attitudes, and hidden feelings relating to parents, siblings, grandparents, and other relatives. These feelings revolve around the theme of being "good or bad" with respect to the expectations of significant others. For example, family members often have been hurt by the adolescent directly (through stealing, physical or sexual abuse, or drug use) and indirectly (through injury to others or getting into trouble outside the home) or, more covertly, by unexpressed feelings of hatred, disrespect, or contempt for parents.

The TC continually addresses the problem of guilt in therapeutic encounter groups, seminars, individual counseling, and special guilt sessions. The first step taken to counteract the feeling of guilt in the TC is confession. Essential to eliciting confession is the psychological and moral neutrality of peers and staff. Although the act itself must be revealed, it is the concealment of the act that must be confronted.

Disclosure of real and imagined guilt feelings is encouraged in group, community, and individual settings. Strategies center on initiating confession in one member toward facilitating confession in others.

The step following confession depends on the reality, recency, and severity of the guilt issue as well as the feasibility of resolution through action. Fundamental to the resolution process is raising the resident's awareness of the powerful relation between guilt and self-destructive behavior. Recognition and acceptance of the pain of guilt provide the experiential basis for new social learning. Thus, some or all of the TC's techniques for raising awareness may be invoked—for example, groups, encounters, one-to-one conversation, and bans on certain behavior. Where appropriate, the resident may be encouraged to accept a "contract" (a disciplinary learning experience) both to raise awareness and as redemptive behavior. Often, however, the final step with respect to guilt is acknowledgment of the unchangeable past followed by a commitment to a changeable future.

Sexuality. The critical relation between physical sexuality, social behavior, and personal identity in the adolescent client is well documented in social and developmental psychology. The problems associated with this aspect of adolescent growth are intensified in young substance abusers. Some of the more common adolescent sexuality issues encountered in the TCs are related to sexual feelings, sex roles, values, and attitudes. For example, both sexes must learn to manage strong sexual impulses; the physiological arousal that characterizes adolescents and young adults affects their physical and psychological adjustment. Some must learn to cope with feelings associated with aberrant historical sexual incidents or relationships.

Problems of self-perceived physical beauty, competition with peers, and adolescent sexuality are worsened for drug abusers insofar as they struggle with a comparatively lower self-esteem than do non-drug-abusing peers. Additionally, there are gender-specific variations on some of these problems. Females, for example, often see themselves as sex objects or use sex for survival, approval, or acceptance. For males, the pressure to sustain a "macho" image often compels inordinate frequency of sexual activity, abusive or exploitative behavior, and negative attitudes toward females.

The issue of sexual adjustment of adolescent drug abusers is further complicated by other problems. These include inadequate information, poor role models, and the history of drug use itself (the psychophar-

547

macological effects of chronic drug use as well as the distortions in attitude, values, and self-perception arising from the socially negative life-style).

Adolescent sexuality remains a difficult question for the TCs to solve. Three general approaches are used, however, each of which attempts to address this issue in a different way—through management and regulation, education, and therapeutic problem solving.

The management approach attempts to minimize sexual activity through rules and sanctions. Male-female interaction is unrestricted during therapy, work, and recreational periods, although separate sleeping arrangements are maintained. A cardinal rule against sexual contact aims to teach the importance of restraint in the management of impulses. Sexual roles, conduct, and feelings have been confused because of the adolescent's inability to manage his or her impulses or a history of a negative sex role. A long period of restraint permits clarification and development of a new social-sexual perspective. In short, restraint is necessary before a new positive sexual role can be acquired. Nevertheless, dating and relationships evolve. These are managed as specific aspects of the developmental learning process. Dating and (nonsexual) relationships are granted as privileges earned through learning self- and social responsibilities, which enhance individual growth and motivation.

The educational approach employs seminars to provide specific information and general sexual education. Seminars held on a periodic basis discuss anatomy, physiology, contraception, abortion, attitude/values, and other related topics (e.g., AIDS and other sexually transmitted diseases).

The therapeutic approach consists of general encounter groups, individual counseling, and special sessions that center around problem solving. Specifically, these are designed to surface individual feelings, attitudes, and concerns about sexuality, in contrast to intellectual understanding. The primary goals are to disclose traumatic and/or abusive sexual histories, vulnerabilities concerning physical image, sexual performance, beauty, and strength and to encourage expressions of fears, anxieties, and expectancies concerning the client's sexual behavior. Clients are helped to understand how one's sexual behavior and attitudes are used for social survival, personal acceptance, coping, and manipulating and how drug taking masks nondrug feelings (often guilt, anger, self-hatred, boredom, insecurity, etc.) or, conversely, how drugs are used to heighten feeling synthetically in attempts to increase potency or desire.

Increased Supervision, Individual Evaluation, and Recreation

Adolescents require more supervision, evaluation, and recreation than do adult residents in TCs. Adolescents display greater physical tension than adults, relating to physiological and social role factors. Their needs for stimulation and their restlessness are often exacerbated by their curiosity and the demands made on them by the TC. Restraint is imposed by the residential setting, which is unchanging (twenty-four hours) compared with the relatively more varied environment of the home, street, neighborhood, and city. Avoidance of this discomfort is often sought through stimulus change reflected in drug taking, sexual preoccupation, and physical acting out (e.g., vandalism).

Staff must be continuously vigilant concerning their own consistency in rule setting and enforcement. In their histories, adolescents' abusers reveal an absence of consistency and explicit rule setting, which has cued uncontrolled behavior.

The frequency of case review in the TC for the adolescent client is considerably greater than for the adult. Primarily, this reflects the complex mandate of treating the adolescent in residence, which includes both clinical and educational goals. These require continuous monitoring by clinical staff and educational staff and early identification of special problems or deficits. Thus, psychological and neurological assessment (e.g., for learning disabilities) and remediation plans are substantially more involved than for the adult.

Addicts in general, and adolescent drug abusers in particular, have typically never learned to make good use of leisure time without drugs. Thus, programs must be prepared to help youngsters obtain the knowledge and skill for constructive use of leisure time. In the TC, regular staff supervise dances, movies, and games that are scheduled into the week within the residence. Athletic sports are less regularly planned since these often require the use of facilities off premises. Much of the effort to introduce the adolescent to new recreational activity is assumed by volunteer staff. Teachers, consultants, and organized voluntary units in TCs such as Phoenix House schedule sport activities, music and theater events, museum and zoo outings, and other programs.

Education

Educational advancement is stressed for adolescent clients in the therapeutic community. Instilling the value of education is an explicit socialization goal of treatment. Moreover, adolescents under eighteen years of age are mandated to obtain a high school education while in residential treatment. Therefore, all residents may attend up to five hours of daily academic classes in the facility during their stay in residence.

Adolescents may not enter into a full school schedule for several months. A period of time is needed to assess and to stabilize clients in the regimen of the therapeutic community before exposing them to another possible failure in the school situation. Moreover, in the TC perspective, attending classes is an earned privilege, a view that (re)establishes the value of and incentive for education for the young client.

The Family

Family involvement is assumed to be particularly important for adolescents since, by definition, they are not emancipated economically or socially. Therapeutic communities have emphasized the involvement of significant others for clients in residential treatment. For adolescents, this almost universally refers to the parent or guardian. For adults, this may involve spouse, mate, or family members.

In Phoenix House, for example, acceptance of the adolescent into residential treatment is often (but not necessarily) contingent on an agreement by a family member to participate in the treatment. (This condition is not set forth for the adult residential client.) The basic objective of a family participation program is to maximize client retention in treatment addressed through a planned curriculum. The program consists of parent group seminars, open houses in the facilities, and other special events involving family, client, and staff. The specific aims of the family participation program are to teach the TC perspective and approach; to modify attitudes and conduct in the family that are countertherapeutic for the adolescent client, particularly the family's role as enabler; and to prepare the family for the adolescent's return after residency.[2]

Effectiveness of the TC

The effectiveness of TCs has been evaluated in a number of large-scale follow-up studies. Many of these have been conducted by investigative teams engaged in modality comparisons that include TCs (e.g., Simpson and Sells 1982). Others have been conducted on and by individual TCs (e.g., Barr and Antes 1981; De Leon 1984; De Leon, Andrews, Wexler, Jaffe, and Rosenthal 1979; De Leon and Jainchill 1981–1982; Holland 1978).

These investigations have consistently demonstrated positive outcomes in social and psychological areas. For example, in clients treated in Phoenix House, significant improvements occur in psychological well-being, accompanied by reductions in drug use, criminality, and increased employment (De Leon 1984).

Most studies show a direct correlation between time spent in residential treatment and positive outcomes (fig. 1). For example, long-term success rates exceed 75 percent for therapeutic community graduates and 50 percent for dropouts who remain at least twelve months in treatment (De Leon, Wexler, and Jainchill 1982).

These findings are similar for adolescents in TCs (De Leon 1986a; Simpson and Sells 1982). However, clients under nineteen years of age generally require more time in treatment to produce the same success rate as adults (see fig. 1) because of their particular problems, needs, and vulnerabilities (De Leon 1986a; De Leon et al. 1979; De Leon et al. 1982).

The Nonresidential TC

Most adolescents with drug, alcohol, and related problems do not require residential treatment. For these, the TC model has been modified for treatment in outpatient settings. For example, Phoenix House maintains a nine-to-five day program for adolescents who require treatment and schooling (Step One) and a second program for youths whose problems have not impeded their attending regular school (Impact). Although clients differ in the severity of their problems and in the degree of social and educational skills, the structure and basic elements of both programs are guided by the TC perspective, concerning self-help recovery and right living. This is illustrated in a brief outline of the after-school program (Impact) (see De Leon 1982).

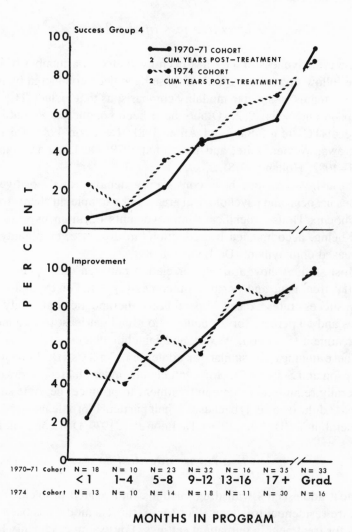

Fig. 1.—Success and improvement rates by time in program through two years of posttreatment follow-up in two cohorts of male opioid users.

The Impact program consists of three main components: youth groups (twenty-four weeks); parent education seminars (eight to twelve weeks); and family effectiveness groups (eight to twelve weeks). The main element of the youth component is the peer encounter group (four days weekly), the goals of which are to raise awareness concerning situation and feelings about drugs; to learn alternative coping behaviors; problem solving and acquisition of values (e.g., self-reliance, work ethic, and honesty); and to take responsibility for conduct and attitudes despite outside influences. Although nonresidential, the youth groups constitute a small community, the strength of which exerts positive influences over all its members to maintain a drug-free life-style.

The parent education component consists of twelve weeks of seminars, the objective of which is to train parents to be rational authorities. Seminars focus on clarification of values (e.g., issues of recreational alcohol and drug use, sexuality, work ethic, materialism, self-reliance, etc.), disciplinary approaches (e.g., eliminating verbal or corporal abuse and substituting positive training methods); position taking (e.g., the child's school performance, social life and curfew, and chore responsibility); forfeiture (how parents lose influence and give their responsibilities to teachers, other professionals, and the peer group); and role modeling (training parents to be role models guided by the precept, "Do as I say *and* do").

The family effectiveness component consists of weekly multiple family sessions involving youths, parents, and significant others. The goals of these sessions are to train communication and listening between youths and nonyouths, problem identification (e.g., parental nonposition taking, lying, and poor conduct), and remediation training (family groups providing alternative solutions as well as serving in a monitorial and supportive function).

Consistent with the TC self-help perspective, a major initiative of the family program is to assist parents in becoming effective community change agents. Since adolescent substance abuse is pervasive, a positive change in the individual family must be accompanied by community change. Toward this purpose, the organizational and informational resources of Phoenix House (as in other TCs) are utilized to catalyze development of parent networks and community action groups to minimize substance abuse and establish values of a drug-free existence in a society that is still ambivalent concerning its own drug and alcohol use.

553

Conclusions

The TC perspective and model is described for treating adolescent substance abusers. Outcome studies indicate that success rates are no different between adults and adolescents treated in residential TCs, documenting the efficacy of this approach for the younger clients. A brief description of the model adapted for adolescents in nonresidential settings highlights the broad applicability of the TC approach.

NOTES

1. A fuller discussion of the special treatment elements for adolescents is contained elsewhere (De Leon and Deitch 1985).
2. Some TCs, such as Phoenix House, also offer family therapy services.

REFERENCES

Barr, H., and Antes, P. 1981. *Factors Related to Recovery and Relapse in Follow-Up*. Final report of project activities under grant no. 1H81 DAO1864. Rockville, Md.: National Institute on Drug Abuse.

De Leon, G. 1976. *Psychologic and Socio-demographic Profiles of Addicts in the Therapeutic Community*. Final report of project activities under National Institute on Drug Abuse Project no. DA-00831.

De Leon, G. 1980. *Therapeutic Communities: Training Self Evaluation*. Final report of project activities under National Institute on Drug Abuse Project no. 1H81-DAO.

De Leon, G. 1981. The role of rehabilitation. In G. Nahas and H. Frick, eds. *Drug Abuse in the Modern World—a Perspective for the Eighties*. New York: Pergamon.

De Leon, G. 1982. Impact: a model for treating the marijuana dependent abuser. In R. De Silva and G. Russell, eds. *Treating the Marijuana Dependent Person*. New York: American Council on Marijuana and Other Psychoactive Drugs.

De Leon, G. 1984. *The Therapeutic Community: Study of Effectiveness*. Treatment Research Monograph Series. Department of Health and Human Services Publication no. (ADM)84–1286. Rockville, Md.: National Institute on Drug Abuse.

De Leon, G. 1986a. Adolescent substance abusers in the therapeutic community: treatment outcomes. In A. Acampora and E. Nebelkopf, eds. *Proceedings of the Ninth World Conference on Therapeutic Communities*. San Francisco: Abacus.

De Leon, G. 1986b. The therapeutic community for substance abuse: perspective and approach. In G. De Leon and J. Ziegenfuss, eds. *Therapeutic Communities for Addictions: Readings in Theory, Research and Practice*. Springfield, Ill.: Charles Thomas.

De Leon, G.; Andrews, M.; Wexler, H.; Jaffe, J.; and Rosenthal, M. 1979. Therapeutic community dropouts: criminal behavior five years after treatment. *American Journal of Drug and Alcohol Abuse* 6(3): 253–271.

De Leon, G., and Beschner, G. 1977. *The Therapeutic Community: Proceedings of Therapeutic Communities of America Planning Conference, January 29–30, 1976*. Services Research Report, Department of Health, Education, and Welfare Publication no. (ADM)77–464. Rockville, Md.: National Institute of Drug Abuse.

De Leon, G., and Deitch, D. 1985. Treatment of the adolescent substance abuser in a therapeutic community. In G. Beschner and A. Friedman, eds. *Treatment Services for Adolescent Substance Abusers*. Department of Health and Human Services Publication no. (ADM)85–1342. Rockville, Md.: National Institute on Drug Abuse.

De Leon, G., and Jainchill, N. 1981–1982. Male and female drug abusers: social and psychological status two years after treatment in a therapeutic community. *American Journal of Drug and Alcohol Abuse* 3(4): 465–497.

De Leon, G., and Rosenthal, M. 1979. Therapeutic communities. In R. Dupont, A. Goldstein, and J. O'Donnell, eds. *Handbook on Drug Abuse*. Rockville, Md.: National Institute on Drug Abuse.

De Leon, G.; Wexler, H.; and Jainchill, N. 1982. The therapeutic community: success and improvement rates 5 years after treatment. *International Journal of the Addictions* 17:703–747.

Holland, S. 1978. Gateway Houses: effectiveness of treatment on criminal behavior. *International Journal of the Addictions* 13:369–381.

Holland, S., and Griffin, A. 1984. Adolescent and adult drug treatment clients: patterns and consequences of use. *Journal of Psychoactive Drugs* 16(1): 79–90.

Kaufman, E., and De Leon, G. 1978. The therapeutic community: a treatment approach of drug abusers. In A. Schecter, ed. *Treatment Aspects of Drug Dependence*. West Palm Beach, Fla.: CRC.

Simpson, D., and Sells, S. 1982. Effectiveness of treatment for drug abuse: an overview of the DARP research program. *Advances in Alcohol and Substance Abuse* 2(1): 7–29.

THE AUTHORS

E. JAMES ANTHONY is Clinical Professor of Psychiatry and Behavior, George Washington University Medical School; and Director of Child and Adolescent Psychotherapy, Chestnut Lodge Hospital, Rockville, Maryland.

ROBERTA J. APFEL is Assistant Professor of Psychiatry, Howard Medical School, Cambridge, Massachusetts.

HOWARD S. BAKER is Clinical Assistant Professor of Psychiatry, University of Pennsylvania; Attending Psychiatrist, the Institute of Pennsylvania Hospital; and Director, Student Mental Health Services, Drexel University, Philadelphia, Pennsylvania.

NORMAN R. BERNSTEIN is Visiting Professor of Psychiatry, Harvard University; and Professor of Psychiatry Emeritus, University of Illinois School of Medicine, Chicago, Illinois.

ALBERT A. BUYTENDORP is Associate Professor of Psychiatry, University of Cincinnati School of Medicine; and Director, Adolescent Psychiatry, Cincinnati Jewish Hospital, Cincinnati.

ALLEN J. CAHILL is Assistant Clinical Professor of Psychiatry, University of Texas Health Science Center; and Adolescent Unit Coordinator, Baylor University Medical Center, Dallas, Texas.

JOHN L. CAUGHEY is Associate Professor, Department of American Studies, the University of Maryland, College Park, Maryland.

557

ADRIAN D. COPELAND is Clinical Professor of Psychiatry and Chief, Adolescent Psychiatry, Jefferson Medical College of Thomas Jefferson University, Philadelphia.

MARIETTA DAMOND is Research Associate, George Washington University, Washington, D.C.

GEORGE DE LEON is Director of Research and Evaluation, Phoenix House, New York.

AARON H. ESMAN is Professor of Clinical Psychiatry, Cornell University Medical College; Director of Adolescent Services, the New York Hospital; Faculty Member, New York Psychoanalytic Institute; and a Senior Editor of this volume.

CARL B. FEINSTEIN is Assistant Professor and Director, Program in Developmental Disabilities, Emma Pendleton Bradley Hospital, Brown University Program in Medicine, Providence, Rhode Island.

SHERMAN C. FEINSTEIN is Clinical Professor of Psychiatry, Pritzker School of Medicine, University of Chicago; Director, Child Psychiatry Research, Michael Reese Hospital and Medical Center; and Editor in Chief of this volume.

SUSAN M. FISHER is Clinical Associate Professor of Psychiatry, Pritzker School of Medicine, University of Chicago.

HEINZ VON FOERSTER is Professor Emeritus, Departments of Biophysics and Physiology, and Electrical Engineering; and Director, Biological Computer Laboratory, University of Illinois, Champaign, Illinois.

ELIO J. FRATTAROLI is Attending Psychiatrist, the Institute of Pennsylvania Hospital, Philadelphia.

RHODA S. FRENKEL is Clinical Professor of Psychiatry, Southwestern Medical School, University of Texas Health Science Center; and Training and Supervising Analyst, Dallas Division of the New Orleans Psychoanalytic Institute, Dallas, Texas.

FRANK GALUSZKA is Chairman, Department of Illustration, Philadelphia College of Art.

HOWARD GARDNER is Professor of Neurology, Boston University School of Medicine; and Codirector, Project Zero, Harvard University, Cambridge, Massachusetts.

JOHN E. GEDO is Clinical Professor of Psychiatry, Abraham Lincoln School of Medicine, University of Illinois; and Training and Supervising Analyst, Chicago Institute of Psychoanalysis.

DAVID A. HALPERIN is Assistant Clinical Professor of Psychiatry, Mount Sinai School of Medicine; and Consulting Psychiatrist, Jewish Board of Family and Children's Services, New York.

ROBERT HORAN is Lecturer in English, University of Wisconsin—Stout, Wisconsin.

HARVEY A. HOROWITZ is Professor of Psychiatry, University of Pennsylvania School of Medicine; and Associate Director, Adolescent Service, the Institute of Pennsylvania Hospital, Philadelphia.

DIANA KELLY-BYRNE is Lecturer, University of Pennsylvania; and Director, Program in Child Culture and Imagination.

JOE W. KING is Associate Clinical Professor of Psychiatry, University of Oklahoma—Tulsa Medical College; Chief Executive Officer and Psychiatrist in Chief, Shadow Mountain Institute; and Vice-President of Medical Affairs, Century Health Care, Tulsa, Oklahoma.

JOHN G. LOONEY is Professor of Psychiatry, Duke University Medical School; Director, Division of Child and Adolescent Psychiatry; Director, Durham Community Guidance Clinic for Children and Youth, Durham, North Carolina; current President of the Society and a Senior Editor of this volume.

HENRY N. MASSIE is Director, Child Psychiatry Training Program, Neuropsychiatric Institute, St. Mary's Hospital, San Francisco, California.

JAY MECHLING is Professor and Director of American Studies, University of California at Davis, California.

JOHN E. MEEKS is Associate Clinical Professor of Psychiatry, George Washington Medical School, Washington, D.C.; and Medical Director, the Psychiatric Institute of Montgomery County, Rockville, Maryland.

CYNTHIA R. PFEFFER is Associate Professor of Clinical Psychiatry, Cornell University Medical College; and Chief, Child Psychiatry Inpatient Unit, New York Hospital—Westchester Division, White Plains, New York.

RUSSELL E. PHILLIPS is Attending Psychiatrist, Institute of Pennsylvania Hospital, Philadelphia.

DAVID REISS is Professor of Psychiatry and Director, Division of Research, Department of Psychiatry and Behavioral Sciences, George Washington University, Washington, D.C.

DONALD B. RINSLEY is Clinical Professor of Psychiatry, University of Kansas School of Medicine, Kansas City; Senior Faculty Member in Adult and Child Psychiatry, Karl Menninger School of Psychiatry and Mental Health Sciences; and Associate Chief for Education, Colmery-O'Neil Veterans Administration Medical Center, Topeka, Kansas.

CARL T. ROTENBERG is Assistant Professor of Psychiatry, Yale University School of Medicine, New Haven, Connecticut.

ROSINA G. SCHNURR is Psychologist, Children's Hospital of Eastern Ontario, Ottawa, Canada.

ALLAN Z. SCHWARTZBERG is Associate Clinical Professor of Psychiatry, Georgetown University School of Medicine, Washington, D.C.; and a Senior Editor of this volume.

ANN D. SIGAFOOS is Research Assistant Professor, George Washington University, Washington, D.C.

MAX SUGAR is Clinical Professor of Psychiatry, Louisiana State University; Director, Children's Unit, Coliseum Medical Center, New Orleans; and a Senior Editor of this volume.

BRIAN SUTTON-SMITH is Professor of Education and Chairman, Interdisciplinary Studies in Human Development, University of Pennsylvania, Philadelphia.

C. K. WILLIAMS is Professor of English Literature, George Mason University, Philadelphia, Pennsylvania; and Member, Creative Writing Faculty, School of Arts, Columbia University, New York.

ELLEN WINNER is Associate Professor of Psychology, Boston College; and Research Associate, Project Zero, Harvard University, Cambridge, Massachusetts.

CONSTANCE WOLF is Research Assistant, Project Zero, Graduate School of Education, Harvard University, Cambridge, Massachusetts.

CONTENTS OF VOLUMES 1–14

564

566

570

574

576

577

580

582

NAME INDEX

594

SUBJECT INDEX

606